Basic Medical Sciences

Boyd & Hoerl	Basic Medical Microbiology
Colton	Statistics in Medicine
Hine & Pfeiffer	Behavioral Science
Kent	General Pathology: A Programmed Text
Levine	Pharmacology
Peery & Miller	Pathology
Richardson	Basic Circulatory Physiology
Roland et al.	Atlas of Cell Biology
Selkurt	Physiology
Sidman & Sidman	Neuroanatomy: A Programmed Text
Siegel, Albers, et al.	Basic Neurochemistry
Snell	Clinical Anatomy for Medical Students
Snell	Clinical Embryology for Medical Students
Streilein & Hughes	Immunology: A Programmed Text
Valtin	Renal Function
Watson	Basic Human Neuroanatomy

Clinical Medical Sciences

Clark & MacMahon	Preventive Medicine
Daube et al.	Medical Neurosciences
Eckert	Emergency-Room Care
Grabb & Smith	Plastic Surgery
Green	Gynecology
Gregory & Smeltzer	Psychiatry
Judge & Zuidema	Methods of Clinical Examination
MacAusland & Mayo	Orthopedics
Nardi & Zuidema	Surgery
Niswander	Obstetrics
Thompson	Primer of Clinical Radiology
Wilkins & Levinsky	Medicine
Ziai	Pediatrics

Manuals and Handbooks

Alpert & Francis	Manual of Coronary Care
Arndt	Manual of Dermatologic Therapeutics
Berk et al.	Handbook of Critical Care
Bochner et al.	Handbook of Clinical Pharmacology
Children's Hospital Medical Center, Boston	Manual of Pediatric Therapeutics
Condon & Nyhus	Manual of Surgical Therapeutics
Friedman & Papper	Problem-Oriented Medical Diagnosis
Gardner & Provine	Manual of Acute Bacterial Infections
Iversen & Clawson	Manual of Acute Orthopaedic Therapeutics
Massachusetts General Hospital	Clinical Anesthesia Procedures
Massachusetts General Hospital	Diet Manual
Massachusetts General Hospital	Manual of Nursing Procedures
Neelon & Ellis	A Syllabus of Problem-Oriented Patient Care
Papper	Manual of Medical Care of the Surgical Patient
Shader	Manual of Psychiatric Therapeutics
Snow	Manual of Anesthesia
Spivak & Barnes	Manual of Clinical Problems in Internal Medicine: Annotated with Key References
Wallach	Interpretation of Diagnostic Tests
Washington University Department of Medicine	Manual of Medical Therapeutics
Zimmerman	Techniques of Patient Care

INTERPRETATION
OF DIAGNOSTIC TESTS

INTERPRETATION
OF DIAGNOSTIC TESTS
A HANDBOOK SYNOPSIS OF LABORATORY MEDICINE

Jacques Wallach, M.D.
Clinical Associate Professor of Pathology,
College of Medicine and Dentistry of New Jersey,
Rutgers Medical School, New Brunswick;
Visiting Assistant Professor of Pathology,
Albert Einstein College of Medicine, New York

Third Edition

Boston
Little, Brown and Company

Library of Congress Catalog Card No. 77-81483

ISBN 0-316-92044-4

Printed in the United States of America

INTERPRETATION OF DIAGNOSTIC TESTS: A HANDBOOK SYNOPSIS OF LABORATORY MEDICINE is published in the following translations:

First Edition

INTERPRETACIÓN DE LOS DIAGNÓSTICOS DE LABORATORIO: MANUAL SINÓPTICO DE BIOLOGÍA MÉDICA

Ἑρμηνεία τῶν Διαγνωστικῶν Ἐξετάσεων καὶ Δοκιμασιῶν: Συνοπτικὸν Ἐγχειρίδιον Ἐργαστηριακῆς Ἰατρικῆς

INTERPRETAÇÃO DOŚ DIAGNÓSTICOS DE LABORATÓRIO

Second Edition

INTERPRETAZIONE DEI TESTS DI LABORATORIO IN MEDICINA

TO DORIS

AND

TO KIM, LISA, AND TRACY

Results of laboratory tests may aid in
- Discovering occult disease
- Preventing irreparable damage (e.g., phenylketonuria)
- Early diagnosis after onset of signs or symptoms
- Differential diagnosis of various possible diseases
- Determining the stage of the disease
- Estimating the activity of the disease
- Detecting the recurrence of disease
- Measuring the effect of therapy
- Genetic counseling in familial conditions
- Medicolegal problems, such as paternity suits

This book is written to help the physician achieve these purposes with the least amount of
- Duplication of tests
- Waste of patient's money
- Overtaxing of laboratory facilities and personnel
- Loss of physician's time
- Confusion caused by the increasing number, variety, and complexity of tests currently available. Some of these tests may be unrequested but performed as part of routine surveys or hospital admission multitest screening.

In order to provide quick reference and maximum availability and usefulness, this handy-sized book features
- Tabular and graphic style of concise presentation
- Emphasis on serial time changes in laboratory findings in various stages of disease
- Omission of rarely performed, irrelevant, esoteric, and outmoded laboratory tests
- Exclusion of discussion of physiologic mechanisms, metabolic pathways, clinical features, and nonlaboratory aspects of disease
- Discussion of only the more important diseases that the physician encounters and should be able to diagnose

This book is not
- An encyclopedic compendium of clinical pathology
- A technical manual
- A substitute for good clinical judgment and basic knowledge of medicine

Deliberately omitted are
- Technical procedures and directions
- Photographs and illustrations of anatomic changes (e.g., blood cells, karyotypes, isotope scans)
- Discussions of quality control
- Selection of a referral laboratory
- Performance of laboratory tests in the clinician's own office
- Bibliographic references, except for the most general reference texts in medicine, hematology, and clinical pathology and for some recent references to specific conditions

The usefulness and need for a book of this style, organization, and content have been increased by such current trends as
- The frequent lack of personal assistance, advice, and consul-

tation in large commercial laboratories and hospital departments of clinical pathology, which are often specialized and fragmented as well as impersonal

Greater demand for the physician's time

The development of many new tests

The lack of adequate teaching of laboratory medicine in most medical schools. Faculty and administrators still assume that this essential area of medicine can be learned "intuitively" as it was 20 years ago and that it therefore requires little formal training. This attitude ignores changes in the number and variety of tests now available as well as their increased sophistication and basic value in establishing a diagnosis

The contents of this book are organized to answer the questions most often posed by physicians when they require assistance from the pathologist. There is no other single adequate source of information presented in this fashion. It appears from numerous comments I have received that this book has succeeded in meeting the needs not only of practicing physicians and medical students but also of pathologists, technologists, and other medical personnel. It has been adopted by many schools of nursing and of medical technology, physicians assistant training programs, and medical schools. Such widespread acceptance confirms my original premise in writing this book and is most gratifying.

A perusal of the table of contents and index will quickly show the general organization of the material by type of laboratory test or organ system or certain other categories. In order to maintain a concise format, separate chapters have not been organized for such categories as newborn, pediatric, and geriatric periods or for primary psychiatric or dermatologic diseases. A complete index provides maximum access to this information.

Obviously these data are not original but have been adapted from many sources over the years. Only the selection, organization, manner of presentation, and emphasis are original. I have formulated this point of view during 30 years as a clinician and pathologist, viewing with pride the important and growing role of the laboratory but deeply regretting its inadequate utilization.

This book was written to improve laboratory utilization by making it simpler for the physician to select and interpret the most useful laboratory tests for his clinical problems.

J. W.

ACKNOWLEDGMENTS

I thank those colleagues whose trust and loyalty have made this book possible. They have stimulated me to find answers to their laboratory questions and clinical needs and to provide these in a format that will be most useful. I have been rewarded by learning much more than I could compress into this small volume. In particular, I am grateful to patients, who have always taught me so much when I have listened.

Ah, if my brush could only catch the faint
Scent of the white plum-blossoms that I paint!*
—Shôha

Special thanks are due to the staff of Little, Brown and Company, especially to Lin Richter for her encouragement and assistance since the start of this project, and to Jane Sandiford and Debra Corman for their work on this edition. The index prepared by Betty Herr Hallinger has been a valuable contribution to the usefulness of this book and has simplified access to the material; her excellent work is much appreciated.

J. W.

*Haiku poem reprinted from Harold Stewart, trans., *A Chime of Windbells*. Rutland, Vt.: Tuttle, 1969.

CONTENTS

III. DISEASES OF ORGAN SYSTEMS

IV. EFFECTS OF DRUGS ON TEST VALUES

Alteration of Laboratory Test Values by Drugs (*Continued*)

TABLES

I

NORMAL VALUES

BLOOD

A review of the texts, reference books, and current literature in clinical pathology often reveals surprising and considerable discrepancy between well-known sources. The following pages of normal laboratory values were summarized from what seemed to be the best and most current sources of data available.

I have used my own experience and clinical judgment in selecting the most useful data to be included.

Table 1. Normal Leukocyte Differential Count in Peripheral Blood

Age	Segmented Neutrophils %	No. per cubic milli-meter	Band[a] Neutrophils %	No. per cubic milli-meter	Eosinophils %	No. per cubic milli-meter	Basophils %	No. per cubic milli-meter	Lymphocytes %	No. per cubic milli-meter	Monocytes %	No. per cubic milli-meter
At birth	47 ± 15	8400	14.1 ± 4	2540	2.2	400	0.6	100	31 ± 5	5500	5.8	1050
12 hr	53	12,100	15.2	3460	2.0	450	0.4	100	24	5500	5.3	1200
24 hr	47	8870	14.2	2680	2.4	450	0.5	100	31	5800	5.8	1100
1 wk	34	4100	11.8	1420	4.1	500	0.4	50	41	5000	9.1	1100
2 wk	29	3320	10.5	1200	3.1	350	0.4	50	48	5500	8.8	1000
4 wk	25 ± 10	2750	9.5 ± 3	1150	2.8	300	0.5	50	56 ± 15	6000	6.5	700
2 mo	25	2750	8.4	1100	2.7	300	0.5	50	57	6300	5.9	650
4 mo	24	2730	8.9	1000	2.6	300	0.4	50	59	6800	5.2	600
6 mo	23	2710	8.8	1000	2.5	300	0.4	50	61	7300	4.8	580
8 mo	22	2680	8.3	1000	2.5	300	0.4	50	62	7600	4.7	580
10 mo	22	2600	8.3	1000	2.5	300	0.4	50	63	7500	4.6	550
12 mo	23	2680	8.1	990	2.6	300	0.4	50	61	7000	4.8	550
2 yr	25	2660	8.0	850	2.6	280	0.5	50	59	6300	5.0	530
4 yr	34 ± 11	3040	8.0 ± 3	710	2.8	250	0.6	50	50 ± 15	4500	5.0	450
6 yr	43	3600	8.0	670	2.7	230	0.6	50	42	3500	4.7	400
8 yr	45	3700	8.0	660	2.4	200	0.6	50	39	3300	4.2	350
10 yr	46 ± 15	3700	8.0 ± 3	645	2.4	200	0.5	40	38 ± 10	3100	4.3	350

12 yr	47	3700	8.0	640	2.5	200	0.5	40	38	3000	4.4	350
14 yr	48	3700	8.0	640	2.5	200	0.5	40	37	2900	4.7	380
16 yr	49 ± 15	3800	8.0 ± 3	620	2.6	200	0.5	40	35 ± 10	2800	5.1	400
18 yr	49	3800	8.0	620	2.6	200	0.5	40	35	2700	5.2	400
20 yr	51	3800	8.0	620	2.7	200	0.5	40	33	2500	5.0	380
21 yr	51 ± 15	3800	8.0 ± 3	620	2.7	200	0.5	40	34 ± 10	2500	4.0	300

[a]Note that these values are higher than those found in other references. They have been obtained by using strict criteria in differentiating segmented from band forms. I do not classify a neutrophil as a segmented form unless a typical threadlike filament is visible.

Source: J. B. Miale, *Laboratory Medicine—Hematology* (4th ed.). St. Louis: Mosby, 1972.

Table 2. Normal Values for Red Corpuscles at Various Ages

Age	Red Cell Count (millions/cu mm)	Hemoglobin (gm/100 ml)	Vol. Packed RBC (ml/100 ml)	Corpuscular Values			
				MCV (cu μ)	MCH (γγ)	MCHC (%)	MCD (μ)
First day	5.1 ± 1.0	19.5 ± 5.0	54.0 ± 10.0	106	38	36	8.6
2–3 days	5.1	19.0	53.5	105	37	35	
4–8 days	5.1	18.3 ± 4.0	52.5	103	36	35	
9–13 days	5.0	16.5	49.0	98	33	34	
14–60 days	4.7 ± 0.9	14.0 ± 3.3	42.0 ± 7.0	90	30	33	8.1
3–5 mo	4.5 ± 0.7	12.2 ± 2.3	36.0	80	27	34	7.7
6–11 mo	4.6	11.8	35.5 ± 5.0	77	26	33	7.4
1 yr	4.5	11.2	35.0	78	25	32	7.3
2 yr	4.6	11.5	35.5	77	25	32	
3 yr	4.5	12.5	36.0	80	27	35	7.4
4 yr	4.6 ± 0.6	12.6	37.0	80	27	34	
5 yr	4.6	12.6	37.0	80	27	34	
6–10 yr	4.7	12.9	37.5	80	27	34	7.4
11–15 yr	4.8	13.4	39.0	82	28	34	
Adults							
Females	4.8 ± 0.6	14.0 ± 2.0	42.0 ± 5.0	87 ± 5	29 ± 2	34 ± 2	7.5 ± 0.3
Males	5.4 ± 0.8	16.0 ± 2.0	47.0 ± 5.0	87 ± 5	29 ± 2	34 ± 2	7.5 ± 0.3

MCV = mean corpuscular volume; MCH = mean corpuscular hemoglobin; MCHC = mean corpuscular hemoglobin concentration; MCD = mean corpuscular diameter.

Source: M. M. Wintrobe, *Clinical Hematology* (7th ed.). Philadelphia: Lea & Febiger, 1974.

NORMAL HEMATOLOGIC VALUES

Fetal hemoglobin	<2% of total
Methemoglobin	<3% of total
Carboxyhemoglobin	<5% of total
Haptoglobins	Adults: 100–300 mg/100 ml
	Age 1–6 months: gradual increase to 30 mg/100 ml
	Newborn: absent in 90%; 10 mg/100 ml in 10%
	Genetic absence in 1% of population
Osmotic fragility of RBC	Begins in 0.45–0.39% NaCl
	Complete in 0.33–0.30% NaCl
Erythrocyte sedimentation rate	
Wintrobe	Males: 0–10 mm in 1 hour
	Females: 0–15 mm in 1 hour
Westergren	Males: 0–13 mm in 1 hour
	Females: 0–20 mm in 1 hour
Blood volume	Males: 75 ml/kg of body weight
	Females: 67 ml/kg of body weight (8.5–9.5% of body weight in kg)
Plasma volume	Males: 44 ml/kg of body weight
	Females: 43 ml/kg of body weight
Red blood cell volume	Males: 30 ml/kg of body weight
	Females: 24 ml/kg of body weight
RBC survival time (^{51}Cr)	Half-life: 25–35 days
Reticulocyte count	0.5–1.5% of erythrocytes
Plasma iron turnover rate	38 mg/24 hours (0.47 mg/kg)

BLOOD COAGULATION TESTS

Platelet count	140,000–340,000/cu mm (Rees-Ecker); 200,000–350,000/cu mm (Coulter Counter Model B)
Bleeding time	
Ivy	<4 minutes
Duke	1–4 minutes
Clot retraction qualitative	Begins in 30–60 minutes
	Complete within 24 hours; usually within 6 hours
Coagulation time (Lee-White)	6–17 minutes (glass tubes)
	19–60 minutes (siliconized tubes)
Fibrinogen split products	Positive at >1:8 dilution (staphylococcal clumping)
Fibrinolysins	0
Partial thromboplastin time (activated)	22–37 seconds
Prothrombin time (one stage)	Same as control (control should be 11–16 seconds)

Prothrombin content	100% (calculated from pro-thrombin time)
Prothrombin consumption	>80% consumed in 1 hour
Thromboplastin generation test	Compared to normal control
Thrombin time	Within 5 seconds of control

BLOOD CHEMISTRIES

The lists of normal blood chemistries are arranged both alpha-betically and by type of chemical component (e.g., enzymes, electrolytes, blood gases, pH) for greatest convenience.

The normal values will vary, depending on the individual labora-tory as well as the methods used.

Acetone	0.3–2.0 mg/100 ml
Aldolase (ALD)	3–8 (Sibley-Lehninger) units/ml
Ammonia	80–110 μg/100 ml
Amylase	60–180 Somogyi units/100 ml
Barbiturates	0
Coma level	
Phenobarbital	$\cong 11$ mg/100 ml
Most other barbitu-rates	2–4 mg/100 ml
Base, total	145–160 mEq/L
Bilirubin	
Direct	0.1–0.4 mg/100 ml
Indirect (= total minus di-rect)	0.1–0.5 mg/100 ml
Total	0.2–0.9 mg/100 ml
Bromides	0
Toxic levels	>17 mEq/L (150 mg/100 ml)
Calcium	8.5–10.5 mg/100 ml (higher in children)
Carbon dioxide	
Content	24–30 mEq/L (20–26 mEq/L in infants)
Tension, pCO_2 arterial	35–45 mm Hg
Carbon monoxide	Symptoms with >20% satura-tion
Ceruloplasmin	27–37 mg/100 ml
Chloride	100–106 mEq/L

Cholesterol, total	*Age (years)*	*Cholesterol (mg/100 ml)*
	1–19	120–230
	20–29	120–240
	30–39	140–270
	40–49	150–310
	50–59	160–330

Esters	60–75% of total
Cholinesterase (Michel method)	
Plasma	0.44–1.63 in men; 0.24–1.54 in females (Δ pH/hour)

RBC	0.39–1.02 for males; 0.34–1.10 for females (Δ pH/hour)
Copper	100–200 μg/100 ml
Creatine phosphokinase (CPK)	0–12 Sigma units/ml
Creatinine	0.7–1.5 mg/100 ml ($\leqq$0.6 mg/100 ml in newborns)
Cryoglobulins	0
Dilantin (phenytoin sodium)	
Therapeutic levels	1–11 μg/ml
Toxic levels	20 μg/ml
Ethanol	
Marked intoxication	0.3–0.4%
Alcoholic stupor	0.4–0.5%
Coma	>0.5%
Fibrinogen	200–400 mg/100 ml
Gamma-glutamyl transpeptidase	Females: 4–18 mU/ml at 25°C, 5.3–24 mU/ml at 30°C
	Males: 6–28 mU/ml at 25°C, 8–37 mU/ml at 30°C
Glucose (fasting)	
O-toluidine	60–100 mg/100 ml
True	70–110 mg/100 ml
Folin	80–120 mg/100 ml
Iron	80–160 μg/100 ml in males; 50–150 μg/100 ml in females
Iron-binding capacity	250–410 μg/100 ml
% saturation	20–55%
Isocitric dehydrogenase (ICD)	50–180 Sigma units/ml
Lactic acid	6–16 mg/100 ml
Lactic dehydrogenase (LDH)	200–680 units/ml
Lead	0–40 μg/100 ml
Leucine aminopeptidase (LAP)	75–230 (Goldbarg-Rutenburg) units/ml
Lipase	<1.5 units (ml of N/20 NaOH)
Lipids, total	450–1000 mg/100 ml
Lipid fractionation	

Cholesterol

Age (years)	Cholesterol (mg/100 ml)
1–19	120–230
20–29	120–240
30–39	140–270
40–49	150–310
50–59	160–330

Phospholipids	60–350 mg/100 ml

Triglycerides

Age (years)	Triglyceride (mg/100 ml)
1–19	10–140
20–29	10–140
30–39	10–150
40–49	10–160
50–59	10–190

Magnesium	1.5–2.5 mEq/L (1.8–3.0 mg/100 ml)

Osmolality	280–295 mOsm/L
Oxygen	
Capacity	16–24 vol% (varies with Hb)
Content	
Arterial	15–23 vol%
Venous	10–16 vol%
Saturation	
Arterial	96–100% of capacity
Venous	60–85% of capacity
Tension, pO_2 arterial	75–100 mm Hg while breathing room air (depends on age)
pH, arterial	7.35–7.45
Phenylalanine	0–2 mg/100 ml
Phosphatase	
Acid	1.0–5.0 King-Armstrong units
	0.5–2.0 Bodansky units
	0.5–2.0 Gutman units
	0–1.1 Shinowara units
	0.1–0.73 Bessey-Lowry units
Alkaline	5.0–13.0 King-Armstrong units (10–20*)
	2.0–4.5 Bodansky units ($\leqq$14 BU in infants: $\leqq$5 BU in adolescents)
	3.0–10.0 Gutman units
	2.2–8.6 Shinowara units
	0.8–2.3 Bessey-Lowry units (3.4–9.0*)
Phosphorus	3.0–4.5 mg/100 ml (<6.0 mg/100 ml up to age 1 year)
Potassium	3.5–5.0 mEq/L
Protein-bound iodine (PBI)	3.6–8.8 μg/100 ml
Proteins, serum	
Total	6.0–8.0 gm/100 ml
Albumin	3.5–5.5 gm/100 ml
Globulin	1.5–3.0 gm/100 ml
Electrophoresis	
Albumin	45–55% of total
Globulin	
Alpha$_1$	5–8% of total
Alpha$_2$	8–13% of total
Beta	11–17% of total
Gamma	15–25% of total
Alpha$_1$ antitrypsin	47–153% normal
Haptoglobin	30–160 mg/100 ml
Transferrin	205–374 mg/100 ml
C3	100–200 mg/100 ml

*Values in children.

Immunoglobulins

	IgG (mg/100 ml)	IgA (mg/100 ml)	IgM (mg/100 ml)
Newborn	900–1500	0–5	5–20
1–3 months	250–550	5–50	20–40
4–6 months	300–600	10–55	30–60
7–12 months	400–900	20–60	35–75
2 years	550–1000	35–75	40–80
3 years	550–1100	50–110	40–85
4–5 years	550–1100	60–150	40–95
6–8 years	550–1200	60–170	40–95
12 years	550–1400	60–200	40–110
Adult	550–1900	60–330	45–145

	IgE (mean units/ml)	IgE (range units/ml)
Cord serum	1.6	0.7–3.4
6 weeks–3 months	4.4	1.1–17
3 months–9 months	16	4.2–60
9 months–2 years	18	6.4–53
2 years–5 years	65	21–198
5 years–10 years	89	18–451
10 years–20 years	86	12–618
20 years–70 years	71	10–506

The level of IgE in normal sera is extremely low. For the Phadebas IgE test the above normal values have been recorded.

Salicylate	0
Therapeutic range	20–25 mg/100 ml
Toxic range	>30 mg/100 ml
Sodium	136–145 mEq/L
Transaminase	
SGOT (glutamic-oxaloacetic)	5–40 units/ml (Sigma-Frankel units)
SGPT (glutamic-pyruvic)	5–35 units/ml (Sigma-Frankel units)
Urea nitrogen (BUN)	10–20 mg/100 ml
Uric acid	3.0–7.5 mg/100 ml in females: ≦8.5 mg/100 ml in males

BLOOD CHEMISTRIES BY TYPE OF COMPONENT

The normal values will vary, depending on the individual laboratory as well as the methods used.

General

Glucose (fasting)	
O-toluidine	60–100 mg/100 ml
True	70–110 mg/100 ml
Folin	80–120 mg/100 ml
Uric acid	3.0–7.5 mg/100 ml in females; ≦8.5 mg/100 ml in males
Urea nitrogen (BUN)	10–20 mg/100 ml

Creatinine	0.7–1.5 mg/100 ml: $\leqq$ 0.6 mg/100 ml in newborns

Bilirubin
Direct	0.1–0.4 mg/100 ml
Indirect	0.1–0.5 mg/100 ml
Total	0.2–0.9 mg/100 ml
Protein-bound iodine (PBI)	3.6–8.8 μg/100 ml
Ammonia	80–110 μg/100 ml

Cholesterol, total

Age (years)	Cholesterol (mg/100 ml)
1–19	120–230
20–29	120–240
30–39	140–270
40–49	150–310
50–59	160–330

Esters	60–75% of total
Lipids, total	450–1000 mg/100 ml

Lipid fractionation
Cholesterol

Age (years)	Cholesterol (mg/100 ml)
1–19	120–230
20–29	120–240
30–39	140–270
40–49	150–310
50–59	160–330

Phospholipids	60–350 mg/100 ml

Triglycerides

Age (years)	Triglyceride (mg/100 ml)
1–19	10–140
20–29	10–140
30–39	10–150
40–49	10–160
50–59	10–190

Enzymes

Amylase	60–180 Somogyi units/100 ml
Lipase	< 1.5 units (ml of N/20 NaOH)

Transaminase
SGOT (glutamic-oxaloacetic)	5–40 units/ml (Sigma-Frankel units)
SGPT (glutamic-pyruvic)	5–35 units/ml (Sigma-Frankel units)

Phosphatase
Acid	1.0–5.0 King-Armstrong units
	0.5–2.0 Bodansky units
	0.5–2.0 Gutman units
	0–1.1 Shinowara units
	0.1–0.73 Bessey-Lowry units
Alkaline	5.0–13.0 King-Armstrong units (10–20*)

*Values in children.

	2.0–4.5 Bodansky units ($\leqq 14$ BU in infants; $\leqq 5$ BU in adolescents)
	3.0–10.0 Gutman units
	2.2–8.6 Shinowara units
	0.8–2.3 Bessey-Lowry units (3.4–9*)
Gamma-glutamyl transpeptidase	Females: 4–18 mU/ml at 25°C, 5.3–24 mU/ml at 30°C
	Males: 6–28 mU/ml at 25°C, 8–37 mU/ml at 30°C
Leucine aminopeptidase (LAP)	75–230 (Goldbarg-Rutenburg) units/ml
Lactic dehydrogenase (LDH)	200–680 units/ml
Hydroxybutyric dehydrogenase (α-HBD)	120–260 Rosalki units/ml
Isocitric dehydrogenase (ICD)	50–180 Sigma units/ml
Creatine phosphokinase (CPK)	0–12 Sigma units/ml
Cholinesterase (Michel method)	
Plasma	0.44–1.63 in males; 0.24–1.54 in females (Δ pH/hr)
RBC	0.39–1.02 in males; 0.34–1.10 in females (Δ pH/hr)
Aldolase (ALD)	3–8 (Sibley-Lehninger) units/ml
Malic dehydrogenase (MDH)	25–100 units/ml
Ornithine carbamyl transferase (OCT)	0–500 Sigma units/ml
5′-Nucleotidase	0.3–3.2 Bodansky units

Erythrocyte Enzymes

Glucose-6-phosphate dehydrogenase	5–15 units
6-Phosphogluconate dehydrogenase	2–5 units
Glutathione reductase	9–13 units
Pyruvate kinase	2–3 units

Electrolytes

Sodium	136–145 mEq/L
Potassium	3.5–5.0 mEq/L
Chloride	100–106 mEq/L
Calcium	8.5–10.5 mg/100 ml (higher in children)
Phosphorus	3.0–4.5 mg/100 ml (<6.0 mg/100 ml up to age 1)
Magnesium	1.5–2.5 mEq/L (1.8–3.0 mg/100 ml)

Blood Gases and pH

Base, total	145–160 mEq/L
Carbon dioxide	
Content	24–30 mEq/L (20–26 mEq/L in infants)
Tension, pCO_2 arterial	35–45 mm Hg

*Values in children.

Oxygen
    Capacity   16–24 vol% (varies with Hb)
    Content
        Arterial   15–23 vol%
        Venous   10–16 vol%
    Saturation
        Arterial   96–100% of capacity
        Venous   60–85% of capacity
    Tension, pO_2 arterial   75–100 mm Hg while breathing
                                       room air (depends on age)
Carbon monoxide   Symptoms with >20% satura-
                                       tion
Osmolality   280–295 mOsm/L
Arterial pH   7.35–7.45
Lactic acid   6–16 mg/100 ml

Blood Proteins
Proteins, serum
    Total   6.0–8.0 gm/100 ml
        Albumin   3.5–5.5 gm/100 ml
        Globulin   1.5–3.0 gm/100 ml
    Electrophoresis
        Albumin   45–55% of total
        Globulin
             $Alpha_1$ 5–8% of total
            $Alpha_2$ 8–13% of total
            Beta   11–17% of total
            Gamma   15–25% of total
Fibrinogen   200–400 mg/100 ml
Cryoglobulins   0
$Alpha_1$ antitrypsin   47–153% normal
Haptoglobin   30–160 mg/100 ml
Transferrin   205–374 mg/100 ml
C3   100–200 mg/100 ml
Immunoglobulins

	IgG (mg/100 ml)	*IgA* (mg/100 ml)	*IgM* (mg/100 ml)
Newborn	900–1500	0–5	5–20
1–3 months	250–550	5–50	20–40
4–6 months	300–600	10–55	30–60
7–12 months	400–900	20–60	35–75
2 years	550–1000	35–75	40–80
3 years	550–1100	50–110	40–85
4–5 years	550–1100	60–150	40–95
6–8 years	550–1200	60–170	40–95
12 years	550–1400	60–200	40–110
Adult	550–1900	60–330	45–145

	IgE *(mean units/ml)*	IgE *(range units/ml)*
Cord serum	1.6	0.7–3.4
6 weeks–3 months	4.4	1.1–17
3 months–9 months	16	4.2–60
9 months–2 years	18	6.4–53
2 years–5 years	65	21–198
5 years–10 years	89	18–451
10 years–20 years	86	12–618
20 years–70 years	71	10–506

*The level of IgE in normal sera is extremely low. For the Phadebas
IgE test, the above normal values have been recorded.*

Hematology

Iron	80–160 μg/100 ml in males; 50–150 μg/100 ml in females
Iron-binding capacity	250–410 μg/100 ml
% saturation	20–55%
Transferrin	205–374 mg/100 ml
Ceruloplasmin	27–37 mg/100 ml
Copper	100–200 μg/100 ml

Toxicology

Salicylate	0
Therapeutic range	20–25 mg/100 ml (35–40 mg/100 ml $\leqq$ age 10)
Toxic range	$>$30 mg/100 ml ($>$20 mg/100 ml after age 60)
Fatal range	45–75 mg/100 ml
Dilantin (phenytoin sodium)	
Optimal therapeutic range	10–20 μg/ml
Therapeutically unsatisfac- tory range	$<$2 μg/ml
Toxic range	$>$20 μg/ml
Ethanol	
Marked intoxication	0.3–0.4%
Alcoholic stupor	0.4–0.5%
Coma	$>$0.5%
Lead	$>$40 μg/100 ml
Barbiturates	0
Phenobarbital	

Therapeutic range
      (anticonvulsant
      therapy)
	20–50 μg/ml

Coma level	$\cong$11 mg/100 ml
Most other barbiturates	1.5 mg/100 ml
Bromides	0
Toxic levels	$>$17 mEq/L (150 mg/100 ml)
Lithium	

Therapeutic level (8–12
    hours after
    administration)
	0.8 mEq/L

Toxic level	1.6 mEq/L
Severe intoxication	3–6 mEq/L

Carbon monoxide	% CO Hb	Symptoms
	0–2%	Asymptomatic
	2–5%	Light or moderate smokers: usually asymptomatic
	5–10%	Heavy smokers: slight dyspnea with severe exertion
	10–20%	Dyspnea with moderate exertion, mild headache
	20–30%	Rapid fatigue, headache, irritability, impaired judgment, defective memory
	30–40%	Confusion, hallucination, hyperventilation, ataxia, collapse
	50–60%	Deep coma, possibly convulsions
	60%	Usually fatal

Digitalis
Serum digoxin

Therapeutic range	0.5–2.0 ng/ml
Overlap range	1.6–3.0 ng/ml
Toxic range	>3.3 ng/ml

Toxic effects almost never found at levels <2.0 ng/ml: patients with toxic effects usually have levels >2.0 ng/ml.

Blood should be drawn at least 6 hours after administration of digoxin to allow for equilibrium.

There may be false decrease due to uremia.

There may be false increase due to hemolysis of samples or jaundice.

There may be interference if patient has received radioisotopes.

Increased sensitivity to digitalis in presence of hypokalemia, alkalosis, chronic lung disease, and cardiopulmonary bypass surgery

Decreased sensitivity to digitalis in infancy, hyperkalemia

Thyroid status, renal function, excess circulating catecholamines, and severe heart disease also factors influencing digitalis sensitivity

Serum digitoxin

No toxic symptoms	26–43 ng/ml (mean = 34)
Overlap range	26–39 ng/ml

Toxic symptoms may occur	3–39 ng/ml (mean = 17)
Procainamide (Pronestyl)	
Therapeutic level	4–6 mg/L
Incomplete protection against arrhythmias	<4 mg
Toxic range	>7 mg/L
Quinidine	
Therapeutic range	about 1 mg/100 ml
Toxic range	Variable

The therapeutic ranges listed may not apply to all patients; some people may have a toxic response within these ranges or have maximal therapeutic response outside these ranges. Clinical response is influenced by many factors (especially concurrent drug use), by other clinical conditions (e.g., uremia), by age, and by size.

Beware of different units used for reporting test results from laboratory to laboratory, as well as of different "normal" ranges.

Sufficient time must pass after medication before collection of blood in order to allow therapeutic levels to occur (e.g., lithium >12 hours; diphenytoin sodium or phenobarbital >3 hours; digoxin >6 hours).

2

URINE

Specific gravity	1.003–1.030
pH	4.6–8.0 (average = 6.0): depends on diet
Total solids	30–70 gm/L (average = 50). To estimate, multiply last two figures of specific gravity by 2.66 (Long's coefficient)
Osmolality	500–1200 mOsm/L
Volume	600–2500 ml/24 hours (average = 1200): night volume usually < 700 ml with specific gravity > 1.018 or osmolality > 825 mOsm/kg of body weight in children: ratio of night to day volume 1:2–1:4
Protein	Qualitative = 0 0–0.1 gm/24 hours
Glucose	Qualitative = 0 ≦ 0.3 gm/24 hours
Ketones	Qualitative = 0
Calcium	< 150 mg/24 hours on low-calcium (Bauer-Aub) diet
Phosphorus	1 gm/24 hours (average): depends on diet
Urobilinogen	0–4 mg/24 hours
Porphyrins	50–300 μg/24 hours; 0–75 μg/24 hours in children weighing < 80 pounds
Amylase	260–950 Somogyi units/24 hours
Lead	< 0.08 μg/ml or 120 μg/24 hours
Delta-aminolevulinic acid	1.3–7.0 mg/24 hours
Homogentisic acid	0
Hemoglobin and myoglobin	0
Creatinine	1.0–1.6 gm/24 hours (15–25 mg/kg of body weight/24 hours)
Creatine	< 100 mg/24 hours (<6% of creatinine); higher in children and during pregnancy
Cystine or cysteine	0
Phenylpyruvic acid	0
Microscopic examination	≦ 1–2 RBC, WBC, epithelial cells/hpf; occasional hyaline cast/lpf
Addis count	RBC ≦ 1,000,000/24 hours Casts ≦ 100,000/24 hours WBC + epithelial cells, ≦ 2,000,000/24 hours

Bulk	100–200 gm
Water	Up to 75%
Total osmolality	200–250 mOsm/L
Color	Brown
	Clay color (gray-white) in biliary obstruction
	Tarry if > 100 ml of blood in upper GI tract
	Red—blood in large intestine or undigested beets or tomatoes
	Black—blood or iron or bismuth medication
	Various colors, depending on diet
pH	7.0–7.5 (may be acid with high lactose intake)
Microscopic examination	RBCs absent
	Epithelial cells present (increased with GI tract irritation); absence of epithelial cells in meconium of newborn may aid in diagnosis of intestinal obstruction in the newborn
	Few WBCs present (increased with GI tract inflammation)
	Crystals of calcium oxalate, fatty acid, and triple phosphate commonly present
	Hematoidin crystals sometimes found after GI tract hemorrhage
	Charcot-Leyden crystals sometimes found in parasitic infestation (especially amebiasis)
	Some undigested vegetable fibers and muscle fibers sometimes found normally
	Neutral fat globules (stained with Sudan), normal 0–2+
Nitrogen	< 2.5 gm/day
Urobilinogen	40–280 mg/24 hours (100–400 Ehrlich units/100 gm)
Coproporphyrin	400–1000 mg/24 hours
Fat	< 7 gm/24 hours during 3-day period
	< 30% of dry weight (on diet of > 50 gm of fat/day)

Calcium $\cong 0.6$ gm/24 hours

Sodium and chloride   Variable but considerably lower than simultaneous concentrations in serum

CEREBROSPINAL FLUID

Simultaneous measurement of blood level should always be performed.

Appearance	Clear, colorless: no clot
Total cell count	0–10/cu mm (all mononuclear cells) in adults
	0–20/cu mm in infants
Glucose	45–80 mg/100 ml (20 mg/100 ml less than blood level)
	Ventricular fluid 5–10 mg/100 ml higher than lumbar
Total protein	15–45 mg/100 ml (lumbar)
	15–25/mg/100 ml (cisternal)
	5–15 mg/100 ml (ventricular)
Gamma globulin	5–12% of total protein
Colloidal gold	Not more than 1 in any tube
Chloride	120–130 mEq/L (20 mEq/L higher than serum)
Sodium	142–150 mEq/L
Potassium	2.2–3.3 mEq/L
Carbon dioxide	25 mEq/L
pH	7.35–7.40
Transaminase (GOT)	7–49 units
Lactic dehydrogenase (LDH)	15–71 units
Creatine phosphokinase (CPK)	0–3 IU
Bilirubin	0
Urea nitrogen	5–25 mg/100 ml
Amino acids	30% of blood level

5

SEROUS FLUIDS (PLEURAL, PERICARDIAL, AND ASCITIC)

Specific gravity	1.010–1.026
Total protein	0.3–4.1 gm/100 ml
Albumin	50–70%
Globulin	30–45%
Fibrinogen	0.3–4.5%
pH	6.8–7.6

Volume	1.0–3.5 ml
pH	Parallels serum
Appearance	Clear, pale yellow, or straw-colored
	Viscous, does not clot
Fibrin clot	0
Mucin clot	Good
WBCs (per cu mm)	<200 (even in presence of leukocytosis in blood)
Neutrophils (%)	<25
Crystals	
Free	0
Intracellular	0
Fasting glucose, uric acid, bilirubin	Approximately the same as serum
Total protein	≅25–30% of serum protein
	Mean = 1.8 gm/100 ml
	Abnormal if >2.5 gm/100 ml; inflammation is moderately severe if >4.5 gm/100 ml
Culture	0

7

SEMEN

Volume	>3 ml
Liquefaction	Complete in 15 minutes
pH	7.2–8.0 (average = 7.8)
Sperm count	>50 million/ml; 250 million/ejaculation
Morphology	>60% of sperm motile and >50% of normal morphology
Smear	Usually no RBCs or WBCs present

LIVER FUNCTION TESTS

Bromsulphalein (BSP) test	<5% retained in serum 45 minutes after IV injection of 5 mg/kg body weight
Cephalin-cholesterol flocculation test	0–2+ in 48 hours
Cholinesterase (pseudocholinesterase)	$\geqq 0.5$ pH units/hour
Galactose tolerance test (GTT)	Excretion of $\leqq 3$ gm galactose in urine 5 hours after ingestion of 40 gm galactose
Prothrombin time	Same as control; if increased, IV administration of synthetic vitamin K returns prothrombin time to normal in obstructive liver disease (or other causes of malabsorption of vitamin K) but not in parenchymal liver disease
Thymol turbidity	0–5 units

Serum bilirubin, serum enzymes (e.g., SGOT, SGPT, LDH, alkaline phosphatase), urine bile, and urobilinogen (see data on differential diagnosis of liver disease [Tables 23, 24, 26, pp. 211–213, 218])

Serum proteins, protein electrophoresis, lipoprotein electrophoresis, fractionation of lipids, etc. (see Chap. 27).

9

RENAL FUNCTION TESTS

Concentration and dilution	Specific gravity > 1.025, specific gravity < 1.003
Phenolsulfonphthalein (PSP) excretion	> 25% in urine in 15 minutes; 55–75% in 2 hours

Clearances (corrected to 1.73 sq m body surface area)

To measure glomerular filtration rate (GFR)

Endogenous creatinine (see Table 9, p. 96)	90–130 ml/minute
Inulin	Males: 110–150 ml/minute Females: 105–132 ml/minute
Urea	Maximum: 60–100 ml/minute Standard: 40–65 ml/minute

To measure effective renal plasma flow (RPF) and tubular function

Para-aminohippurate (PAH)	Males: 560–800 ml/minute Females: 500–700 ml/minute
Diodrast	600–800 ml/minute
Filtration fraction (FF) = GFR/RPF	Males: 17–21% Females: 17–23%
Maximal PAH excretory capacity, Tm_{PAH}	80–90 mg/minute
Maximal Diodrast excretory capacity, Tm_D	Males: 43–59 mg/minute Females: 33–51 mg/minute
Maximal glucose reabsorptive capacity, Tm_G	Males: 300–450 mg/minute Females: 250–350 mg/minute
BUN, creatinine, Addis count (see pp. 40–41, 18)	

BLOOD AND URINE HORMONE LEVELS

*Measurement of Thyroid
Function*	*Blood*
T-3 (concentration)	50–210 ng/100 ml serum (radioimmunoassay)
T-4 (concentration)	4.8–13.2 μg/100 ml serum (mean = 8.6) (radioimmunoassay)
T-3/T-4 ratio	Average 1.3%
T-3 (resin sponge uptake)	24–36%
T-4 (resin sponge uptake)	4–11%
Free thyroxine index (T-3 uptake × T-4 uptake)	96–396
T-4 (thyroxine by column chromatography)	2.9–6.4 μg/100 ml
"Free thyroxine"	1.0–2.1 mμg/100 ml
Thyroxine-binding globulin (TBG)	10–26 μg/100 ml thyroxine
Thyroid-stimulating hormone (TSH)	≦ 0.2 μU/ml
Long-acting thyroid stimulator (LATS)	None detectable
Radioactive iodine uptake (RAIU)	9–19% in 1 hour 7–25% in 6 hours 10–50% in 24 hours
Radioactive iodine excretion	40–70% of administered dose in 24 hours
Protein-bound iodine (PBI)	3.6–8.8 μg/100 ml

Hormone	*Blood*	*Urine*
Pregnanediol	
Male		< 1.5 mg/24 hours
Female	
Proliferative phase		0.5–1.5 mg/24 hours
Luteal phase		2–7 mg/24 hours
Postmenopausal		0.2–1.0 mg/24 hours
Pregnanetriol		< 4 mg/24 hours
Estrogens (total)		Male: 4–25 μg/24 hours Female: 4–60 μg/24 hours (marked increase during pregnancy)

Hormone	Blood	Urine
Testosterone		
Male (adult)	0.30–1.0 μg/100 ml (average = 0.7)	47–156 μg/24 hours (average = 70)
Male (adolescent)	>0.10 μg/100 ml	
Female	0–0.1 μg/100 ml (average = 0.04)	0–15 μg/24 hours (average = <6)
Pituitary gonadotropins (FSH)		6–50 mouse uterine units/24 hours
Chorionic gonadotropin		0
Prolactin	<20 ng/ml	
Progesterone	<1.0 ng/ml during follicular phase >2.0 ng/ml during luteal phase	
Luteinizing hormone	<70 mIU/ml during follicular phase >70 mIU/ml during luteal phase	
Growth hormone	≦6 ng/ml in men ≦10 ng/ml in women	
Aldosterone	0.015 μg/100 ml	3–32/24 hours
Catecholamines (adrenaline, noradrenaline)		Epinephrine <10 μg/24 hours Norepinephrine <100 μg/24 hours
Metanephrines, total		24–288 μg/24 hours
Metanephrine		24–96 μg/24 hours
Normetanephrine		72–288 μg/24 hours
Vanillylmandelic acid (VMA)		≦9 mg/24 hours
Homovanillic acid		<15 mg/24 hours
Serotonin (as 5-Hydroxyindoleacetic acid, 5-HIAA)	0.05–0.20 μg/ml	2–10 mg/24 hours (qualitative = 0)
17-Hydroxycorticoids	(cortisol) 5–25 μg/100 ml at 8 A.M. <10 μg/100 ml at 8 P.M. Falls to <10 μg/100 ml by 9 P.M.	3–8 mg/24 hours (lower in women)
Glenn-Nelson		Males: 3–10 mg/24 hours Females: 2–6 mg/24 hours

Hormone	Blood	Urine
17-Ketogenic steroids		Males: 5–23 mg/24 hours Females: 3–15 mg/24 hours

17-Ketosteroids — 25–125 µg/100 ml

Age (years)	Males (mg/24 hours)	Females (mg/24 hours)
10	1–4	1–4
20	6–21	4–16
30	8–26	4–14
50	5–18	3–9
70	2–10	1–7

Hormone	Blood
ACTH	9 A.M.: 5–95 pg/ml Midnight: 0–35 pg/ml
Insulin	6–26 µU/ml (fasting) <20 µU/ml (during hypoglycemia) <150 µU/ml (after glucose load)
Gastrin	0–200 pg/ml
Calcitonin	Absent in normal (>100 pg/ml in medullary carcinoma)

11

BLOOD VITAMIN LEVELS

Vitamin A	65–275 IU/100 ml
	20–60 μg/100 ml
Carotene	100–300 IU/100 ml
	50–300 μg/100 ml
Vitamin C (ascorbic acid)	0.2–2.0 mg/100 ml
Vitamin D	0.7–3.3 IU/100 ml (procedure not generally available) Indirect estimate by measuring serum alkaline phosphatase, calcium, and phosphorus)
Vitamin E (tocopherol)	0.5–2.0 mg/100 ml
Vitamin B_{12}	330–1025 pg/ml
Folic acid	5–21 ng/ml
Thiamine	1.6–4.9 μg/100 ml

URINE VITAMIN LEVELS*

Age	Deficient	Low	Acceptable	High
Urinary Riboflavin Excretion (unit of measurement: μg/gm creatinine)				
Adults	<27	27–79	80–269	>270
1–3 yr	<150	150–499	500–900	>900
4–6	<100	100–299	300–600	>600
7–9	<85	85–269	270–500	>500
10–15	<70	70–199	200–400	>400
Urinary Niacin Excretion (unit of measurement: mg of N-methylnicotinamide/gm of creatinine)				
Adults	<0.5	0.5–1.59	1.6–4.29	>4.3
Urinary Thiamine Excretion (unit of measurement: μg/gm creatinine)				
Adults	<27	27–65	66–129	>130
1–3 yr	<120	120–175	176–600	>600
4–6	<85	85–120	121–400	>400
7–9	<70	70–180	181–350	>350
10–12	<60	60–180	181–300	>300
13–15	<50	50–150	151–250	>250

*Determined by microbiologic assay.

AMNIOTIC FLUID

COMPARISON OF VARIOUS CHEMICAL COMPONENTS IN AMNIOTIC FLUID, MATERNAL SERUM, AND FETAL SERUM DURING NORMAL PREGNANCY

	Amniotic Fluid	Maternal Serum	Fetal Serum
Total protein (gm/100 ml)	0.28 (0.3)	6.5 (0.6)	5.8 (0.7)
Albumin (% by electrophoresis)	65.2 (4.8)	46.4 (3.1)	60.8 (4.8)
A/G ratio	1.9 (0.7)	0.8 (0.1)	1.5 (0.3)
Urea (mg/100 ml)	33.9 (11.7)	17.1 (8.7)	16.5 (8.14)
Uric acid (mg/100 ml)	7.5 (0.3)	3.1 (0.8)	2.6 (0.9)
Creatinine (mg/100 ml)	2.4 (0.3)	1.1 (0.2)	1.3 (0.3)
Glucose (mg/100 ml)	10.7 (5.2)	66.6 (8.7)	49.7 (10.4)
Lactic dehydrogenase (units/ml)	112.3 (64.8)	199.5 (46.4)	328.2 (114.0)
Aldolase (units/ml)	10.1 (7.5)	9.5 (7.0)	23.3 (9.4)
Total cholesterol (mg/100 ml)	42.8 (3.2)	258.6 (47.2)	83.5 (39.7)
Triglycerides (mg/100 ml)	19.3 (9.4)	153.7 (51.4)	16.1 (10.7)

Values are mean values. Numbers in ( ) represent one standard deviation.

Source: L. Castelazo-Ayala, S. Karchmer, and V. Shor-Pinsker, The Biochemistry of Amniotic Fluid During Normal Pregnancy. Correlation with Maternal and Fetal Blood. In A. A. Hodari and F. Mariona (Eds.), *Physiological Biochemistry of the Fetus, Proceedings of the International Symposium.* Springfield, Ill.: Thomas, 1972. Pp. 32–53.

COMPARISON OF VARIOUS CHEMICAL COMPONENTS IN AMNIOTIC FLUID DURING SECOND TRIMESTER OF NORMAL PREGNANCY AND AT TERM

	Second Trimester[b]	*At Term*[b]
Uric acid[a]	3.7 mg	9.9 mg (represents increased urinary output and increased muscle mass of fetus)
Creatinine[a]	0.9 mg	2.0 mg (represents increased muscle mass of fetus)
Total protein	0.6 gm	0.3 gm
Albumin	0.4 gm	0.05 gm
Transaminase (GOT)	17 IU	40 IU
Alkaline phosphatase	25 IU	80 IU (≤ 350 IU in some cases)
Bilirubin[c] Urea nitrogen Calcium Phosphorus Glucose Lactic dehydrogenase Cholesterol	Values do not change significantly during gestation	

[a]Could be useful in determining fetal age in utero.
[b]Values are mean values per 100 ml as determined by SMA-12 Autoanalyser (Technicon).
[c]Useful in following course of hemolytic disease of newborn as an indication for continued observation and retesting, intrauterine transfusion, or immediate delivery (see L. K. Diamond, *Am. J. Clin. Pathol.* 62:311, 1974).

Source: T. Tsudaka, D. Bloch, and P. L. Wolf, An automated profile of amniotic fluid. *Lab. Med.* 32:6, 1971.

AMNIOTIC FLUID TESTS TO MONITOR FETAL STATUS

Fetal Lung Maturity
Determination of lecithin and sphingomyelin in amniotic fluid (by thin-layer chromatography) predicts fetal lung maturity. This is the single most accurate test of fetal maturity.

Immature lungs (up to 30th week of gestation)	Lecithin-sphingomyelin (L/S) ratio < 1
Lungs on threshold of maturity	L/S ratio = 1
Mature lungs (35th week of gestation)	L/S ratio > 2
Postmature lungs	Abundant lecithin with trace or no sphingomyelin

Respiratory distress syndrome (RDS) is unlikely when the L/S ratio is >2. A significant number of infants with L/S ratio <1.5 will develop RDS. L/S ratio of 1.5–1.9 is intermediate pattern and a much smaller percentage of infants delivered with such L/S ratios will develop RDS.

L/S ratio may be affected by
    Accelerated maturation of lungs
        Hypertensive disorders
        Renal disease
        Sickle cell anemia
        Diabetes mellitus
        Heroin addiction
        Glucocorticoid administration
        Abruptio placentae
        Membranes ruptured more than 36 hours
        Intrauterine transfusion
    Delayed maturation
        Hydrops fetalis
        Diabetes mellitus

"Foam" or "shake" test is a bedside qualitative expression of L/S ratio.

If amniotic fluid is not available, L/S ratio or "foam" test can be done on gastric aspirate of infant.

Nile-blue stain of amniotic fluid differentiates fetal squamous cells from anucleated fat cells. More than 20% fat cells indicates mature fetus (>36 weeks) and also correlates with occurrence of RDS. *Maternal diabetes may cause spurious elevation of fat cell count.*

Creatinine content of 1.8–2 mg/100 ml corresponds to pregnancy of 36 weeks or more and represents muscle mass of fetus and the presence of 1 million functioning glomeruli. May be decreased in mature but low birth weight infants. May be spuriously increased by hypertensive disorders of pregnancy (e.g., preeclampsia) and maternal renal disease; therefore serum creatinine of mother should also be determined.

Bilirubin virtually disappears by 36 weeks of gestation, but artifactual increase may be due to maternal hyperbilirubinemia (e.g., hepatitis, hemolytic anemia, cholestasis) or to administration of drugs (e.g., phenothiazines) that make the test useless.

Determination of fetal maturity is indicated to predict development of RDS and determine when it is safe to interrupt gestation because of threat to fetus (e.g., erythroblastosis fetalis, maternal diabetes) or threat to mother (e.g., toxemia, hypertension).

OTHER FUNCTIONAL TESTS

Other tests to determine the functioning status of the various organ systems are outlined in the chapters dealing with specific diseases.

Gastrointestinal Diseases (Chap. 26)

Hepatobiliary Diseases and Disorders of the Pancreas (Chap. 27)

Metabolic and Hereditary Diseases (Chap. 31)

Endocrine Diseases (Chap. 32)

SPECIFIC LABORATORY EXAMINATIONS

BLOOD

CHEMISTRIES

SERUM GLUCOSE

May Be Increased In
Diabetes mellitus, including
    Hemochromatosis
    Cushing's syndrome (with insulin-resistant diabetes)
    Acromegaly and gigantism (with insulin-resistant diabetes in
      early stages: hypopituitarism later)
Increased circulating adrenalin
    Adrenalin injection
    Pheochromocytoma
    Stress (e.g., emotion, burns, shock, anesthesia)
Acute pancreatitis
Chronic pancreatitis (some patients)
Wernicke's encephalopathy (vitamin B_1 deficiency)
Some CNS lesions (subarachnoid hemorrhage, convulsive states)
ACTH administration

May Be Decreased In
Pancreatic disorders
    Islet cell tumor, hyperplasia
    Pancreatitis
    Glucagon deficiency
Extrapancreatic tumors
    Carcinoma of adrenal gland
    Carcinoma of stomach
    Fibrosarcoma
    Other
Hepatic disease
    Diffuse severe disease (e.g., poisoning, hepatitis, cirrhosis,
      primary or metastatic tumor)
Endocrine disorders
    Hypopituitarism and Addison's disease
    Hypothyroidism
    Adrenal medulla unresponsiveness
    Early diabetes mellitus
Functional disturbances
    Postgastrectomy
    Gastroenterostomy
    Autonomic nervous system disorders
Pediatric anomalies
    Prematurity
    Infant of diabetic mother
    Ketotic hypoglycemia
    Zetterstrom's syndrome
    Idiopathic leucine sensitivity
    Spontaneous hypoglycemia in infants

Enzyme diseases
    von Gierke's disease
    Galactosemia
    Maple syrup urine disease
    Fructose intolerance
Other
    Exogenous insulin
    Oral hypoglycemic medications
    Leucine sensitivity
    Malnutrition
    Hypothalamic lesions

SERUM UREA NITROGEN (BUN)

Increased In

Impaired kidney function (see Serum Creatinine, p. 15)
Prerenal azotemia—any cause of reduced renal blood flow
    Congestive heart failure
    Salt and water depletion (vomiting, diarrhea, diuresis, sweating)
    Shock
    Etc.
Postrenal azotemia—any obstruction of urinary tract
    (ratio of BUN creatinine increases above normal of 10:1)
Increased protein catabolism (serum creatinine remains normal)
    Hemorrhage into gastrointestinal tract
    Acute myocardial infarction
    Stress

Decreased In

Severe liver damage (liver failure)
    Drugs
    Poisoning
    Hepatitis
    Other
Increased utilization of protein for synthesis
    Late pregnancy
    Infancy
    Acromegaly
Diet
    Low-protein and high-carbohydrate
    IV feedings only
    Impaired absorption (celiac disease)
Nephrotic syndrome (some patients)

A low BUN of 6–8 mg/100 ml is frequently associated with states of overhydration.
A BUN of 10–20 mg/100 ml almost always indicates normal glomerular function.
A BUN of 50–150 mg/100 ml implies serious impairment of renal function.
Markedly increased BUN (150–250 mg/100 ml) is virtually conclusive evidence of severely impaired glomerular function.

In chronic renal disease, BUN correlates better with symptoms of uremia than does the serum creatinine.

SERUM NONPROTEIN NITROGEN (NPN)

NPN is not as useful as BUN as an index of renal function because it represents a heterogeneous group of substances not all of which are excreted by the kidney. The increase parallels that of BUN.

SERUM CREATININE

Increased In
Diet
    Ingestion of creatinine (roast meat)
Muscle disease
    Gigantism
    Acromegaly
Prerenal azotemia (see Serum Urea Nitrogen, p. 40)
Postrenal azotemia (see Serum Urea Nitrogen, p. 40)
Impaired kidney function
    Ratio of BUN:creatinine > 10:1
        Excess intake of protein
        Blood in small bowel
        Excess tissue breakdown (cachexia, burns, high fever, corticosteroid therapy)
        Urinary tract obstruction (postrenal)
        Inadequate renal blood flow (e.g., prerenal congestive heart failure, dehydration, shock)
        Urine reabsorption (e.g., ureterocolostomy)
    Ratio of BUN:creatinine < 10:1
        Low protein intake
        Repeated dialysis
        Severe diarrhea or vomiting
        Hepatic insufficiency

Serum creatinine is a more specific and sensitive indicator of renal disease than BUN. Use of simultaneous BUN and creatinine determinations provides more information.

Decreased In
Not clinically significant

SERUM CREATINE

Increased In
High dietary intake (meat)
Destruction of muscle
Hyperthyroidism (this diagnosis almost excluded by normal serum creatine)
Active rheumatoid arthritis
Testosterone therapy

Decreased In
Not clinically significant

SERUM URIC ACID

Levels are very labile and show day-to-day and seasonal variation in same person; also increased by emotional stress, total fasting.

Increased In
Gout
25% of relatives of patients with gout
Renal failure (does not correlate with severity of kidney damage; urea and creatinine should be used)
Increased destruction of nucleoproteins
    Leukemia, multiple myeloma
    Polycythemia
    Lymphoma, especially postirradiation
    Other disseminated neoplasms
    Cancer chemotherapy (e.g., nitrogen mustards, vincristine, mercaptopurine)
    Hemolytic anemia
    Sickle cell anemia
    Resolving pneumonia
    Toxemia of pregnancy (serial determinations to follow therapeutic response and estimate prognosis)
    Psoriasis (one-third of patients)
Diet
    High-protein weight reduction diet
    Excess nucleoprotein (e.g., sweetbreads, liver)
Asymptomatic hyperuricemia (e.g., incidental finding with no evidence of gout; clinical significance not known but people so afflicted should be rechecked periodically for gout). The higher the level of serum uric acid, the greater the likelihood of an attack of acute gouty arthritis.
Miscellaneous
    von Gierke's disease
    Lead poisoning
    Lesch-Nyham syndrome
    Maple syrup urine disease
    Down's syndrome
    Polycystic kidneys
    Calcinosis universalis and circumscripta
    Some drugs (e.g., thiazides, furosemide, ethacrynic acid, small doses of salicylates [see Chap. 37])
    Hypoparathyroidism
    Primary hyperparathyroidism
    Hypothyroidism
    Sarcoidosis
    Chronic berylliosis
    Some patients with alcoholism
    Patients with arteriosclerosis and hypertension (*Serum uric acid is increased in 80% of patients with elevated serum triglycerides.*)
    Certain population groups (e.g., Blackfoot and Pima Indians, Filipinos, New Zealand Maoris)

Decreased In
Administration of ACTH

Administration of uricosuric drugs (e.g., high doses of salicylates, probenecid, cortisone, allopurinol, coumarins)
Wilson's disease
Fanconi's syndrome
Acromegaly (some patients)
Celiac disease (slightly)
Pernicious anemia in relapse (some patients)
Xanthinuria
Administration of various other drugs (x-ray contrast agents, glyceryl guaiacolate)
Neoplasms (occasional cases) e.g., carcinomas, Hodgkin's disease
Healthy adults with isolated defect in tubular transport of uric acid (Dalmatian dog mutation)

Unchanged In
Colchicine administration

SERUM CHOLESTEROL
(see also Serum Lipoproteins, p. 70)

Increased In
Idiopathic hypercholesterolemia
Biliary obstruction
    Stone, carcinoma, etc., of duct
    Cholangiolitic cirrhosis
von Gierke's disease
Hypothyroidism
Nephrosis (due to chronic nephritis, renal vein thrombosis, amyloidosis, systemic lupus erythematosus, periarteritis, diabetic glomerulosclerosis)
Pancreatic disease
    Diabetes mellitus
    Total pancreatectomy
    Chronic pancreatitis (some patients)
Pregnancy

Decreased In
Severe liver cell damage (due to chemicals, drugs, hepatitis)
Hyperthyroidism
Malnutrition (e.g., starvation, terminal neoplasm, uremia, malabsorption in steatorrhea)
Chronic anemia
    Pernicious anemia in relapse
    Hemolytic anemias
    Marked hypochromic anemia
Cortisone and ACTH therapy
Hypo-beta- and a-beta-lipoproteinemia
Tangier disease

SERUM SODIUM
(see also Table 4, pp. 48–49)

Increased In
Excess loss of water
    Conditions that cause loss via gastrointestinal tract (e.g., in

vomiting), lung (hyperpnea), or skin (e.g., in excessive sweating)

Conditions that cause diuresis
  Diabetes insipidus
  Nephrogenic diabetes insipidus
  Diabetes mellitus
  Diuretic drugs
  Diuretic phase of acute tubular necrosis
  Diuresis following relief of urinary tract obstruction
  Hypercalcemic nephropathy
  Hypokalemic nephropathy

Excess administration of sodium (iatrogenic), e.g., incorrect replacement following fluid loss

"Essential" hypernatremia due to hypothalamic lesions

Decreased In (serum osmolality is decreased)
  Dilutional (e.g., congestive heart failure, nephrosis, cirrhosis with ascites)
  Sodium depletion
    Loss of body fluids (e.g., vomiting, diarrhea, excessive sweating) with incorrect or no therapeutic replacement, diuretic drugs (e.g., thiazides)
    Adrenocortical insufficiency
    Salt-losing nephropathy
    Inappropriate secretion of antidiuretic hormone
  Spurious (serum osmolality is normal or increased)
    Hyperlipidemia
    Hyperglycemia (serum sodium decreases 3 mEq/L for every increase of serum glucose of 100 mg/100 ml)

SERUM POTASSIUM
(see also Table 4, pp. 48–49)

Increased In
Renal failure
  Acute with oliguria or anuria
  Chronic end-stage with oliguria (glomerular filtration rate <3–5 ml/minute)
  Chronic nonoliguric associated with dehydration, obstruction, trauma, or excess potassium
Decreased mineralocorticoid activity
  Addison's disease
  Hypofunction of renin-angiotensin-aldosterone system (see p. 408)
  Pseudohypoaldosteronism
  Aldosterone antagonist (e.g., spironolactone)
Increased supply of potassium
  Red blood cell hemolysis (transfusion reaction, hemolytic anemia)
  Excess dietary intake or rapid potassium infusion
  Striated muscle (status epilepticus, periodic paralysis)
  Potassium-retaining drugs (e.g., triamterene)
  Fluid-electrolyte imbalance (e.g., dehydration, acidosis)

Laboratory artifacts (e.g., hemolysis during venipuncture, conditions associated with thrombocytosis, incomplete separation of serum and clot)

Decreased In (see Table 49, p. 346)
Renal and adrenal conditions with metabolic alkalosis
    Administration of diuretics
    Primary aldosteronism
    Pseudoaldosteronism
    Salt-losing nephropathy
    Cushing's syndrome
Renal conditions associated with metabolic acidosis
    Renal tubular acidosis
    Diuretic phase of acute tubular necrosis
    Chronic pyelonephritis
    Diuresis following relief of urinary tract obstruction
Gastrointestinal conditions
    Vomiting, gastric suctioning
    Villous adenoma
    Cancer of colon
    Chronic laxative abuse
    Zollinger-Ellison syndrome
    Chronic diarrhea
    Ureterosigmoidostomy

HYPOXEMIA
(arterial blood pO_2 < 100 ± 10 mm Hg at rest at sea level; decreases with age and higher altitude)
Due To
Generalized alveolar hypoventilation
    Skeletal abnormalities (e.g., kyphoscoliosis, flail chest due to trauma)
    Neuromuscular conditions affecting respiration (e.g., phrenic nerve paralysis, tetanus, acute poliomyelitis, status epilepticus, depression of respiratory centers of brain by drugs, head injury, cerebrovascular accident)
    Pickwickian syndrome of massive obesity
    Restricted diaphragmatic breathing (e.g., abdominal distention or pain)
    Environmental (e.g., carbon monoxide exposure, smoke inhalation, anesthesia, near drowning)
Decreased pulmonary diffusing capacity
    Alveolar block syndrome (e.g., lymphangitic carcinomatosis, pulmonary adenomatosis, sarcoidosis, berylliosis, Hamman-Rich syndrome, pulmonary hemosiderosis secondary to mitral stenosis)
    Decreased alveolocapillary membrane surface area by restricted expansion or destruction or loss of lung tissue (e.g., resection), compression of lung (e.g., pneumothorax)
Right-to-left cardiac shunt (e.g., congenital heart disease) or increased venous admixture (e.g., pulmonary hemangioma)

Very often, more than one of these mechanisms is operative simultaneously.

Ventilation-perfusion abnormality or mismatched distribution of inspired air with pulmonary blood flow causing regional hypoventilation
    Diffuse bronchopulmonary disease (chronic and acute) (e.g., bronchitis, asthma, emphysema, bronchiectasis, atelectasis, pneumoconiosis, granulomata, neoplasm, infarction, pneumonia, mucoviscidosis)
    Airway obstruction (e.g., foreign body, croup, neoplasm, retained secretions)

HYPOCAPNIA
(see Tables 3 and 4, pp. 47, 48–49)

Due To Any Mechanism of Hyperventilation
Physiologic (e.g., pregnancy, high altitude)
Psychogenic
Mechanically controlled
Compensatory secondary to metabolic acidosis
Compensatory secondary to anoxemia (e.g., severe anemia, pneumonia, asthma) (see Hypoxemia, p. 45)
Drug (e.g., salicylate poisoning)
Central nervous system lesion
Liver failure
Gram-negative sepsis

Arterial pCO_2 promptly reflects changes in depth and rate of ventilation.

HYPERCAPNIA

Due To
Severe electrolyte disturbances
Acute intermittent porphyria
Severe hypothyroidism

See also causes of hypoxemia, p. 45.

BLOOD pH
(normal arterial pH at sea level is 7.40 ± 0.05) (see Table 3, p. 47)

Decreased In
Metabolic acidosis (see pp. 342–343)
Respiratory acidosis (see p. 347 and Table 3, p. 47)

Increased In
Metabolic alkalosis (see pp. 344, 347)
Respiratory alkalosis (see p. 347 and Table 3, p. 47)

Table 3. Summary of Pure and Mixed Acid-Base Disorders

	Decreased pH	Normal pH	Increased pH
Increased pCO₂	Respiratory acidosis with or without incompletely compensated metabolic alkalosis or coexisting metabolic acidosis	Respiratory acidosis and compensated metabolic alkalosis	Metabolic alkalosis with incompletely compensated respiratory acidosis or coexisting respiratory acidosis
Normal pCO₂	Metabolic acidosis	Normal	Metabolic alkalosis
Decreased pCO₂	Metabolic acidosis with incompletely compensated respiratory alkalosis or coexisting respiratory alkalosis	Respiratory alkalosis and compensated metabolic acidosis	Respiratory alkalosis with or without incompletely compensated metabolic acidosis or coexisting metabolic alkalosis

Source: Adapted from H. H. Friedman and Solomon Papper, *Problem-Oriented Medical Diagnosis*. Boston: Little, Brown, 1975.

Table 4. Urine and Blood Changes in Electrolytes, pH, and Volume in Various Conditions

Measurement	Pulmonary Emphysema	Congestive Heart Failure	Excessive Sweating	Diarrhea	Pyloric Obstruction	Dehydration	Starvation	Malabsorption	Salicylate Intoxication	Primary Aldosteronism
Blood										
Sodium	N	N or D	D	D	D	I	N	D	N	I
Potassium	N	N	N	D	D	N	D	D	N or D	D
Bicarbonate	I	N	N	D	I	N or D	D	N or D	D	I
Chloride	D	D	D	D	D	I	N	N	I	D
Volume	N or I	I	N	D	D	D	N or D	D	N	N
Urine										
Sodium	D	D	D	D	D	I	N or I	D	I	D
Potassium	N	N	N	N or D	N	I	I or N	D	N or I	I
pH	D	N	N	D	I	D	D	N or D	I	N or D
Volume	N	D	N	D	D	D	I	N	N	I

N = normal; D = decreased; I = increased; V = variable.

Measurement	Adrenal Cortical Insufficiency	Diabetes Insipidus	Diabetic Acidosis	Mercurial Diuretic Administration	Thiazide Diuretic Administration	Ammonium Chloride Administration	Diamox Administration	Renal Tubular Acidosis	Chronic Renal Failure	Acute Renal Failure
Blood										
Sodium	D	N or I	D	D	D	D	D	D	D	D
Potassium	I	N	N or I	D	D	D	D	D	N or D	I
Bicarbonate	N or D	N	D	I	D	D	D	D	D	D
Chloride	D	I	D	D	D	I	I	I	D or N	I
Volume	D	D	D	D	D	D	D	D	V	I
Urine										
Sodium	I	N	I	I	I	I	I	I	I	D
Potassium	N or D	N	I	I	I	I	I	I	I	D
pH	N or I	N	D	D	N or I	I	I	I	I	N or I
Volume	N or D	I	I	I	I	I	I	I	V[a]	D

[a] Usually increased.

SERUM OSMOLALITY
(freezing point determination)

Hyperosmolar State

Clinical picture: A middle-aged or older person with diabetes of recent onset or unrecognized diabetes, who shows neurologic symptoms (e.g., convulsions or hemiplegia) and then becomes stuporous or comatose.

Serum glucose is very high but, as expected in diabetic coma, ketosis is minimal and plasma acetone is not found.

Increased serum osmolality (normal = 285–295 mOsm/L). In mildly drowsy patients, mean is 320 mOsm/L: in stuporous or comatose patients, mean is 365 mOsm/L. State of consciousness does not correlate with height of acidemia. *Osmolality should be determined routinely in grossly unbalanced diabetic patients.*

Determinations of blood sodium and potassium levels are not useful in diagnosis or in estimating net ion losses but are performed to monitor changes in sodium and potassium ions during therapy.

Laboratory findings are those due to complications (e.g., pneumonia, pancreatitis, stroke).

Due To

Alcohol ingestion, the commonest cause of hyperosmolar state and of coexisting coma and hyperosmolar state

Increased serum sodium accelerated because of loss of water (e.g., diabetes insipidus, hypercalcemia, diuresis during severe hyperglycemia or during early recovery from renal shutdown)

Hyposmolality

Due To

Low serum sodium often combined with excess water

Treatment with diuretic drugs and low-salt diet in patients with heart failure, cirrhosis, etc.

Adrenal disease (e.g., Addison's disease, adrenogenital syndrome)

"Inappropriate secretion of antidiuretic hormone" (e.g., in bronchogenic carcinoma, severe hypothyroidism, porphyria, cerebral disease [such as tumor, trauma, infection, vascular abnormalities], idiopathic disorders)

Postoperative state—especially with excessive water replacement therapy

SERUM MAGNESIUM

Increased In

Renal failure

Diabetic coma before treatment

Hypothyroidism

Addison's disease and after adrenalectomy

Controlled diabetes mellitus in older patients

Administration of antacids containing magnesium

Decreased In

GI disease showing malabsorption and abnormal loss of GI fluids (e.g., nontropical sprue, small bowel resection, biliary and intes-

tinal fistulas, abdominal irradiation, prolonged aspiration of in-
testinal contents, celiac disease and other causes of steatorrhea)
Acute alcoholism and alcoholic cirrhosis
Insulin treatment of diabetic coma
Hyperthyroidism
Aldosteronism
Hyperparathyroidism
Hypoparathyroidism
Lytic tumors of bone
Diuretic drug therapy (e.g., ethacrynic acid, furosemide)
Some cases of renal disease (e.g., glomerulonephritis, pyelone-
phritis, renal tubular acidosis)
Acute pancreatitis
Excessive lactation
Idiopathic disorders

*Magnesium deficiency may cause apparently unexplained
hypocalcemia and hypokalemia; the patients may have
neurologic and GI symptoms.*

SERUM CALCIUM
(see also p. 82, and Table 56, pp. 386–387)

Increased In
Hyperparathyroidism, primary (due to hyperplasia or adenoma of
parathyroids) or secondary
Hyperparathyroidism due to parathormone-secreting cancer (see
Table 57, p. 390)
Hematologic malignancies (e.g., myeloma, lymphoma, leukemia)
Excess vitamin D intake
Bone tumor
    Metastatic carcinoma (10% of patients)
Acute osteoporosis (e.g., immobilization of young patients or in
Paget's disease)
Milk-alkali (Burnett's) syndrome
Idiopathic hypercalcemia of infants
Infantile hypophosphatasia
Berylliosis
Hyperthyroidism (some patients)
Cushing's syndrome (some patients)
Addison's disease (some patients)
Myxedema (some patients)
Hyperproteinemia
    Sarcoidosis
    Multiple myeloma (some patients)
Thiazide drugs
Artifactual (e.g., venous stasis during blood collection, use of
cork-stoppered test tubes)

Decreased In
Hypoparathyroidism
    Surgical
    Idiopathic
    Pseudohypoparathyroidism

Malabsorption of calcium and vitamin D
  Obstructive jaundice
Hypoalbuminemia
    Cachexia
    Nephrotic syndrome
    Sprue
    Celiac disease
    Cystic fibrosis of pancreas
Chronic renal disease with uremia and phosphate retention
Acute pancreatitis with extensive fat necrosis
Insufficient calcium, phosphorus, and vitamin D ingestion
    Bone disease (osteomalacia, rickets)
    Starvation
    Late pregnancy

Total serum protein should always be known for proper interpretation of serum calcium levels.

SERUM PHOSPHORUS
(see also Table 56, p. 386)

Increased In
Hypoparathyroidism
    Idiopathic
    Surgical
    Pseudohypoparathyroidism
Excess vitamin D intake
Secondary hyperparathyroidism (renal rickets)
Bone disease
    Healing fractures
    Multiple myeloma (some patients)
    Paget's disease (some patients)
    Osteolytic metastatic tumor in bone (some patients)
Addison's disease
Acromegaly
Childhood
Myelogenous leukemia
Acute yellow atrophy
High intestinal obstruction
Sarcoidosis (some patients)
Milk-alkali (Burnett's) syndrome (some patients)

Artifactual increase by hemolysis of blood

Decreased In
Alcoholism*
Diabetes mellitus*
Hyperalimentation*
Nutritional recovery syndrome* (rapid refeeding after prolonged starvation)
Alkalosis, respiratory (e.g., gram-negative bacteremia) or metabolic
Acute gout

*Indicates conditions associated with severe hypophosphatemia.

Salicylate poisoning
Administration of glucose intravenously (e.g., recovery after severe burns, hyperalimentation)
Administration of anabolic steroids, androgens, epinephrine, glucagon, insulin
Acidosis (especially ketoacidosis)
Hyperparathyroidism
Renal tubular defects (e.g., Fanconi syndrome)
Hypokalemia
Hypomagnesemia
Administration of diuretics
Prolonged hypothermia (e.g., open heart surgery)
Malabsorption
Vitamin D deficiency and/or resistance, osteomalacia
Malnutrition, vomiting, diarrhea
Administration of phosphate-binding antacids*
Primary hypophosphatemia

Mechanisms of hypophosphatemia are intracellular shift of phosphate, increased loss (via kidney or intestine), or decreased intestinal absorption; usually associated with prior phosphorus depletion. Often, more than one mechanism is operative.

SERUM ALKALINE PHOSPHATASE
(see also Table 56, pp. 386–387)

Increased In
Increased deposition of calcium in bone
    Osteitis fibrosa cystica (hyperparathyroidism)
    Paget's disease (osteitis deformans)
    Healing fractures (slightly)
    Osteoblastic bone tumors (osteogenic sarcoma, metastatic carcinoma)
    Osteogenesis imperfecta
    Familial osteoectasia
    Osteomalacia
    Rickets
    Polyostotic fibrous dysplasia
    Late pregnancy; reverts to normal level by 20th day postpartum
    Children
    Administration of erogosterol
Liver disease—any obstruction of biliary system (see pp. 222–223)
    Nodules in liver (metastatic tumor, abscess, cyst, parasite, amyloid, tuberculosis, sarcoid, or leukemia)
    Biliary duct obstruction (e.g., stone, carcinoma)
    Cholangiolar obstruction in hepatitis
    Adverse reaction to therapeutic drug (e.g., chlorpropamide) (progressive elevation of serum alkaline phosphatase may be first indication that drug therapy should be halted)
Marked hyperthyroidism
Hyperphosphatasia

*Indicates conditions associated with severe hypophosphatemia.

Primary hypophosphatemia (often increased)
Intravenous injection of albumin; sometimes marked increase (e.g., 10 times normal level) lasting for several days
Some patients with myocardial or pulmonary infarction, usually during phase of organization

Decreased In
Excess vitamin D ingestion
Milk-alkali (Burnett's) syndrome
Scurvy
Hypophosphatasia
Hypothyroidism
Pernicious anemia in one-third of patients
Celiac disease
Malnutrition
Collection of blood in EDTA, fluoride, or oxalate anticoagulant
Alkaline phosphatase isoenzyme determinations are not clinically useful; heat inactivation may be more useful to distinguish bone from liver source of increased alkaline phosphatase.

SERUM LEUCINE AMINOPEPTIDASE (LAP)
Parallels serum alkaline phosphatase except that
LAP is usually normal in the presence of bone disease or malabsorption syndrome.
LAP is a more sensitive indicator of choledocholithiasis and of liver metastases in anicteric patients.
When serum LAP is increased, urine LAP is almost always increased; but when urine LAP is increased, serum LAP may have already returned to normal.

5'-NUCLEOTIDASE (5'-N)

Increased Only In
Obstructive type of hepatobiliary disease

May be an early indication of liver metastases in the cancer patient, especially if jaundice is absent.

Normal In
Pregnancy and postpartum period (in contrast to serum LAP and alkaline phosphatase); therefore may aid in differential diagnosis of hepatobiliary disease occurring during pregnancy.

Whenever the alkaline phosphatase is elevated, a simultaneous elevation of 5'-N establishes biliary disease as the cause of the elevated alkaline phosphatase. If the 5'-N is not increased, the cause of the elevated alkaline phosphatase must be found elsewhere, e.g., bone disease.

SERUM GAMMA-GLUTAMYL TRANSPEPTIDASE

Increased In
Liver disease. Generally parallels changes in serum alkaline phosphatase, LAP, and 5'-nucleotidase but is more sensitive.

Acute hepatitis. Elevation is less marked than that of other liver enzymes, but it is the last to return to normal and therefore is useful to indicate recovery.

Chronic hepatitis. Increased more than in acute hepatitis. More elevated than SGOT and SGPT. In dormant stage, may be the only enzyme elevated.

Cirrhosis. In inactive cases, average values are lower than in chronic hepatitis. Increases greater than 10–20 times in cirrhotic patients suggest superimposed primary carcinoma of the liver.

Primary biliary cirrhosis. Elevation is marked.

Fatty liver. Elevation parallels that of SGOT and SGPT but is greater.

Obstructive jaundice. Increase is faster and greater than that of serum alkaline phosphatase and LAP.

Liver metastases. Parallels alkaline phosphatase; elevation precedes positive liver scans.

Pancreatitis. Always elevated in acute pancreatitis. In chronic pancreatitis is increased when there is involvement of the biliary tract or active inflammation.

Renal disease. Increased in lipoid nephrosis and some cases of renal carcinoma.

Acute myocardial infarction. Increased in 50% of the patients. Elevation begins on fourth to fifth day, reaches maximum at 8–12 days. With shock or acute right heart failure, may have early peak within 48 hours, with rapid decline followed by later rise.

Heavy use of alcohol, barbiturates, or phenytoin sodium (Dilantin). Is the most sensitive indicator of alcoholism, since elevation exceeds that of other commonly assayed liver enzymes.

Normal In

Women during pregnancy (in contrast to serum alkaline phosphatase and LAP) and children over 3 months of age; therefore may aid in differential diagnosis of hepatobiliary disease occurring during pregnancy and childhood.

Bone disease or patients with increased bone growth (children and adolescents); therefore useful in distinguishing bone disease from liver disease as a cause of increased serum alkaline phosphatase.

Renal failure.

SERUM ACID PHOSPHATASE

Increased In

Carcinoma of the prostate (see p. 452)

Infarction of the prostate (sometimes to high levels)

Operative trauma or instrumentation of the prostate (may cause transient increase)

Gaucher's disease (only when certain substrates are used in the laboratory determination)

Excessive destruction of platelets, as in idiopathic thrombocytopenic purpura *with* megakaryocytes in bone marrow

Thromboembolism, hemolytic crises (e.g., sickle cell disease) due to hemolysis (only when certain substrates are used in the laboratory determination)

In the absence of prostatic disease, increased acid phosphatase is seen occasionally in
    Partial translocation trisomy 21
    Diseases of bone
        Advanced Paget's disease
        Metastatic carcinoma of bone
        Multiple myeloma (some patients)
        Hyperparathyroidism
        Other
    Various liver diseases ($\leqq 9$ King-Armstrong units)
        Hepatitis
        Obstructive jaundice
        Laennec's cirrhosis
        Other
    Acute renal impairment (not related to degree of azotemia)
    Other diseases of the reticuloendothelial system with liver or bone involvement
        Niemann-Pick disease
        Other

Decreased In
Not clinically significant

SERUM AMYLASE

Increased In*
Acute pancreatitis. Increase begins in 3–6 hours; reaches maximum in 20–30 hours; may persist for 48–72 hours. May increase up to 40 times normal. Level should be at least 500 Somogyi units/100 ml to be significant evidence of acute pancreatitis. Urine levels reflect serum changes by a time lag of 6–10 hours.

Acute exacerbation of chronic pancreatitis

Perforated or penetrating peptic ulcer, especially with involvement of pancreas

Postoperative upper abdominal surgery, especially partial gastrectomy (up to 2 times normal in one-third of patients)

Obstruction of pancreatic duct by
    Stone or carcinoma
    Drug-induced spasm of sphincter (e.g., opiates, codeine, methyl choline, chlorothiazide) to levels 2–15 times normal
    Partial obstruction + drug stimulation (see Pancreozymin-Secretion Test, p. 144)

Acute alcohol ingestion or poisoning

Salivary gland disease (mumps, suppurative inflammation, duct obstruction due to calculus)

---

*It has been suggested that a level of > 1000 Somogyi units is usually due to surgically correctable lesions (most frequently stones in biliary tree), the pancreas either being negative or showing only edema; but 200–500 units is usually associated with pancreatic lesions that are not surgically correctable (e.g., hemorrhagic pancreatitis, necrosis of pancreas).

Advanced renal insufficiency. Often increased even without pancreatitis

Macroamylasemia

Increased serum amylase with low urine amylase may be seen in renal insufficiency and macroamylasemia.

May also be increased in acute cholecystitis, intestinal obstruction with strangulation, mesenteric thrombosis, ruptured aortic aneurysm, ruptured tubal pregnancy, viral hepatitis, carcinoma of lung

Decreased In
Extensive marked destruction of pancreas (e.g., acute fulminant pancreatitis, advanced chronic pancreatitis, advanced cystic fibrosis)
Severe liver damage (e.g., hepatitis, poisoning, toxemia of pregnancy, severe thyrotoxicosis, severe burns)
Decreased levels are clinically significant only in occasional cases of fulminant pancreatitis.

SERUM LIPASE

Increased In
Acute pancreatitis. May remain elevated for as long as 14 days after amylase returns to normal
Perforated or penetrating peptic ulcer, especially with involvement of pancreas
Obstruction of pancreatic duct by
    Stone
    Drug-induced spasm of sphincter (e.g., by opiates, codeine, methyl choline) to levels 2–15 times normal
    Partial obstruction + drug stimulation

Usually Normal In
Mumps

SERUM BILIRUBIN

Increased In (see Chap. 27, p. 207 and following)
Hepatic cellular damage
Biliary duct obstructions
Hemolytic diseases
Prolonged fasting

A 48-hour fast produces a mean increase of 240% in normal patients and 194% in those with hepatic dysfunction.

SERUM TRANSAMINASE (SGOT)

Increased In
Acute myocardial infarction
Liver diseases, with active necrosis of parenchymal cells
Musculoskeletal diseases, including trauma and intramuscular injections

Acute pancreatitis
Other
    Myoglobinuria
    Intestinal injury (e.g., surgery, infarction)
    Local irradiation injury
    Pulmonary infarction (relatively slight increase)
    Cerebral infarction (increased in following week in 50% of
       patients)
    Cerebral neoplasms (occasionally)
    Renal infarction (occasionally)
"Pseudomyocardial infarction" pattern. Administration of opiates
  to patients with diseased biliary tract or previous cholecystec-
  tomy causes increase in LDH and especially SGOT. SGOT increases by 2–4 hours, peaks in 5–8 hours, and increase may
  persist for 24 hours: elevation may be 2½–65 times normal.

Falsely Increased In (because enzymes are activated during test)
Therapy with Prostaphlin, Polycillin, opiates, erythromycin
Calcium dust in air (e.g., due to construction in laboratory)

Falsely Decreased In (because of increased serum lactate–
consuming enzyme during test)
Diabetic ketoacidosis
Beriberi
Severe liver disease
Chronic hemodialysis (reason unknown)
Uremia (proportional to BUN level) (reason unknown)

Normal In
Angina pectoris
Coronary insufficiency
Pericarditis
Congestive heart failure without liver damage

Varies <10 units/day in the same person.

SGPT generally parallels SGOT, but the increase is less marked in
  myocardial necrosis, chronic hepatitis, cirrhosis, hepatic metastases, and congestive changes in liver, and is more marked in
  liver necrosis and acute hepatitis.

SERUM LACTIC DEHYDROGENASE (LDH)

Increased In
Acute myocardial infarction
Serum LDH is almost always increased, beginning in 10–12 hours
  and reaching a peak (of about 3 times normal) in 48–72 hours.
  The prolonged elevation of 10–14 days is particularly useful for
  late diagnosis when the patient is first seen after sufficient time
  has elapsed for CPK and SGOT to become normal. Levels
  >2000 units suggest a poorer prognosis. Because many other

diseases may increase the LDH, isoenzyme studies should be performed. Increased serum LDH, with a ratio of LDH_1/LDH_2 >1 ("flipped" LDH), occurs in acute renal infarction and hemolysis associated with hemolytic anemia or prosthetic heart valves as well as in acute myocardial infarction. In acute myocardial infarction, flipped LDH usually appears between 12 and 24 hours and is present within 48 hours in 80% of patients; after 1 week it is still present in $<50\%$ of patients, even though total serum LDH may still be elevated; flipped LDH never appears before CPK MB isoenzyme. LDH_1 may remain elevated after total LDH has returned to normal; with small infarcts, LDH_1 may be increased when total LDH remains normal. (See Serum Creatine Phosphokinase [CPK] Isoenzymes, p. 61.)

Acute myocardial infarction with congestive heart failure. May show increase of LDH_1 and LDH_5

Congestive heart failure alone. LDH isoenzymes are normal.

Insertion of intracardiac prosthetic valves consistently causes chronic hemolysis with increase of total LDH and of LDH_1 and LDH_2. This is also often present before surgery in patients with severe hemodynamic abnormalities of cardiac valves.

Cardiovascular surgery. LDH is increased up to 2 times normal without cardiopulmonary bypass and returns to normal in 3–4 days; with extracorporeal circulation, it may increase up to 4–6 times normal; increase is more marked when transfused blood is older.

Hepatitis. Most marked increase is of LDH_5, which occurs during prodromal stage and is greatest at time of onset of jaundice. Total LDH is also increased in 50% of the cases. LDH_5 is also increased with other causes of liver damage (e.g., chlorpromazine hepatitis, carbon tetrachloride poisoning, exacerbation of cirrhosis, biliary obstruction) even when total LDH is normal.

Untreated pernicious anemia. Total LDH (chiefly LDH_1) is markedly increased, especially with hemoglobin <8 gm/100 ml. Only slightly increased in severe hemolytic anemia. Normal in iron-deficiency anemia, even when very severe.

Malignant tumors. Increased in about 50% of patients with carcinoma, especially in advanced stages. Increased in $\cong 60\%$ of patients with lymphomas and lymphocytic leukemias. Increased in $\cong 90\%$ of patients with acute leukemia; degree of increase is not correlated with level of WBCs; relatively low levels in lymphatic type of leukemia. Increased in 95% of patients with myelogenous leukemia. (See also Chap. 30, Hematologic Diseases.)

Diseases of muscle (see pp. 260–265)

Pulmonary embolus and infarction. See next section.

Renal diseases. Occasional increase but to no clinically useful degree.

Other causes of hemolysis
    Artifactual (e.g., poor venipuncture, failure to separate clot from serum, heating of blood)
    Various hemolytic conditions in vivo (e.g., hemolytic anemias)

Decreased In
X-ray irradiation

SERUM LACTIC DEHYDROGENASE (LDH) ISOENZYMES
This test must be correlated with clinical status of the patient. Do serial determinations to obtain maximum information.

Condition	LDH Isoenzyme Increased
Myocardial infarction	I and II (see previous section)
Pernicious anemia	I
Sickle cell crisis	I and II
Mother carrying erythroblastotic child	IV and V
Acute myocardial infarction with acute congestion of liver	I and V
Early hepatitis	V (may become normal even when SGPT is still rising)
Malignant lymphoma	III and IV (may even increase II) (also useful for following effect of chemotherapy)
Disseminated lupus erythematosus	III and IV
Dermatomyositis	V
Carcinoma of prostate	V
Pulmonary embolus and infarction	
Without hemorrhage into lung	III
With hemorrhage into lung	I, II, III
Embolus with acute cor pulmonale causing acute congestion of liver	III and V

Increased total LDH with normal distribution of isoenzymes may be seen in myocardial infarction, arteriosclerotic heart disease with chronic heart failure, various combinations of acute and chronic diseases (this may represent a general stress reaction).
About 50% of patients with carcinoma have altered LDH patterns. This change often is nonspecific and of no diagnostic value.

SERUM ALPHA-HYDROXYBUTYRIC DEHYDROGENASE (ALPHA-HBD)

Increased In
Acute myocardial infarction. Is more specific than SGOT and LDH but less specific than CPK and LDH isoenzymes.
Other conditions that cause elevation of fast-moving LDH in serum (e.g., muscular dystrophy, megaloblastic anemia)

Increase is always accompanied by increased LDH activity.

May Be Slightly Increased In
Heart failure
Nephrosis

Normal In
Angina pectoris

SERUM CREATINE PHOSPHOKINASE (CPK)

Increased In
Necrosis or acute atrophy of striated muscle
  Acute myocardial infarction
  Severe myocarditis
  Progressive muscular dystrophy
  Polymyositis
  Myoglobinuria
  Traumatic injury of muscle. Increase may last for 2 weeks, especially if associated with arterial obstruction.
  Severe or prolonged exercise (transient increase, some patients)
  Status epilepticus
  Postoperative state. Increase may last up to 5 days. Greater increase with use of electrocautery in surgery.
Half of patients with extensive brain infarction. Maximum levels in 3 days; increase may not appear before 2 days; levels usually less than in acute myocardial infarction and remain increased for longer time; return to normal within 14 days; high mortality associated with levels >300 IU. Elevated serum CPK in brain infarction may obscure diagnosis of concomitant acute myocardial infarction.
Parturition and frequently last few weeks of pregnancy

Slight Increase Occasionally In
Hypothyroidism
Intramuscular injections. Variable increase after intramuscular injection to 2–6 times normal level. Returns to normal 48 hours after cessation of injections.
Muscle spasms or convulsions in children
Electrical cardiac defibrillation or countershock in 50% of patients; returns to normal in 48–72 hours.

Normal In
Angina pectoris
Pericarditis
Pulmonary infarction
Renal infarction
Liver disease
Biliary obstruction
Neurogenic muscle atrophy
Pernicious anemia
Malignancies
Following cardiac catheterization and coronary arteriography unless myocardium has been injured by catheter

SERUM CREATINE PHOSPHOKINASE (CPK) ISOENZYMES

MB isoenzyme is increased in acute myocardial infarction, cardiac surgery, and muscular dystrophy; it is not increased by cardiac catheterization or transvenous pacemakers even though total serum CPK may be elevated. In acute myocardial infarction, MB isoenzyme is evident at 4–8 hours, peaks at 24 hours, is present in 100% of patients within the first 48 hours; by 72 hours, two-thirds of patients still show some elevation. CPK isoenzyme studies provide the best laboratory discrimination between the presence or absence of myocardial necrosis. MB isoenzyme is not increased in brain injury or infarction, even though total serum CPK or MM isoenzyme may be elevated (CPK in these patients is probably from skeletal muscle rather than of brain origin).

BB isoenzyme is increased in malignant hyperthermia, uremia, cardiac arrest with brain anoxia, necrosis of large intestine, Reye's syndrome. It is rarely encountered clinically.

SERUM ISOCITRATE DEHYDROGENASE (ICD)

Increased In
Liver disease
  Early viral hepatitis, hepatitis of infectious mononucleosis and of liver poisons—ICD >25 IU, becomes normal in 2–3 weeks
  Metastatic carcinoma—ICD <20 IU
  Cirrhosis—normal or slightly increased
  Extrahepatic biliary obstruction—normal
  Neonatal biliary atresia—may be increased
  With protein malnutrition—may be increased
Active placental degeneration
  Placental infarction
  Preeclampsia

Normal In
Acute myocardial infarction
Pregnancy

SERUM ALDOLASE (ALD)

Increased In
Cell destruction
  Acute myocardial infarction
  Burns
  Acute hepatitis
  Muscular dystrophies (especially Duchenne type), myopathies, polymyositis
  Carcinoma of prostate
  20% of cancer patients—more frequent with liver involvement

Normal In
Neurogenic muscle atrophy
Cirrhosis (or may be slightly increased)
Obstructive jaundice (or may be slightly increased)

SERUM ORNITHINE CARBAMYL TRANSFERASE (OCT)
Increased In
Liver cell damage (e.g., hepatitis, metastatic carcinoma, cirrhosis, acute cholecystitis)

Alcohol consumption
Prolonged exercise (some patients)

SERUM CHOLINESTERASE

Decreased In
Poisoning with organic phosphate insecticides
Liver diseases
> Especially hepatitis. Lowest level corresponds to peak of disease and becomes normal with recovery.
> Cirrhosis with ascites or jaundice. Persistent decrease may indicate a poor prognosis.
> Some patients with metastatic carcinoma, obstructive jaundice, congestive heart failure

Congenital decrease. Such patients are particularly sensitive to administration of succinylcholine during anesthesia.
Some conditions that may have decreased serum albumin (e.g., malnutrition, anemias, infections, dermatomyositis, acute myocardial infarction, liver diseases—see above)

SERUM FRUCTOSE 1-PHOSPHATE ALDOLASE

Decreased In
Heterozygous carrier state for Tay-Sachs disease

SERUM PROTEIN GAMMOPATHIES
(localized or general increase in immunoglobulins demonstrated by serum immunoelectrophoresis)

Monoclonal (hyperproteinemia very frequent)
IgG gammopathy with or without Bence Jones protein (60% of patients)
IgA gammopathy (16% of patients)
IgM gammopathy (15% of patients)
Bence Jones gammopathy (light-chain disease) (9% of patients)
IgE gammopathy (heavy-chain disease), very rare
IgD gammopathy, very rare

Only two-thirds of patients with monoclonal gammopathy are symptomatic (IgG, IgA, IgD, and Bence Jones gammopathies are associated with classic picture of multiple myeloma—see pp. 322–324; IgM gammopathy is associated with classic picture of macroglobulinemia—see p. 324).
Classic (associated with increased serum M-protein >3 gm/100 ml and increased number of plasma cells in marrow >25%)
> Multiple myeloma
> Waldenström's macroglobulinemia
> Certain malignant lymphomas

Idiopathic (not associated with diseases in classical group) (serum M-protein usually <2 gm/100 ml; plasma marrow cells usually 5–25% of total marrow white cells)
> In apparently healthy persons
> Associated with various diseases (e.g., diabetes mellitus, cirrhosis, abnormalities of lipid metabolism, chronic infections,

Table 5. Serum Protein Electrophoretic Patterns in Various Diseases[a]

Condition	Total Protein	Albumin	Alpha$_1$ Globulin	Alpha$_2$ Globulin	Beta Globulin	Gamma Globulin	Comment
Multiple myeloma	I	D	Dyscrasia of beta$_{2A}$ or gamma$_2$ Ig				Total globulin, marked I Variable location of M globulin
Macroglobulinemia	I	D	Dyscrasia of beta$_{2M}$			Marked I	Electrophoresis same as multiple myeloma
Hodgkin's disease	D	D	I	I		V	
Lymphatic leukemia and lymphoma	D	D			D	D	
Myelogenous and monocytic leukemia	D	D			D	I	Gamma globulin to differentiate types of acute leukemias
Hypogammaglobulinemia	D	N	N	N	N	D	
Analbuminemia	Marked D	Marked D	N	I	I	I	
Gastrointestinal diseases Peptic ulcer	D	D	May be I	May be I			

Condition						Comments
Ulcerative colitis	D	May be I	May be I	D		
Protein-losing enteropathy	Marked D	I	I	I	D	
Acute cholecystitis	D			D	N	
Nephrosis	D	I	I	D	D	Typical pattern
Chronic glomerulonephritis	D	N	N	N	N	
Laennec's cirrhosis	D	N	N	N	I	Characteristic pattern of beta-gamma "bridging"
Acute viral hepatitis	D	D (means acute hepatocellular damage)	D	D	V	
Stress	D	I	I	D		"Three-fingered" pattern
Hypersensitivity			I		I	
Sarcoidosis	I	D	Stepwise increase of alpha$_2$, beta, and gamma			"Sarcoid steps" help differentiate from other lung disease

I = increased or elevated; D = decreased or diminished; V = variable; N = normal; blank = no significant change.

[a]Nonspecific changes of decreased albumin and increased globulin occur in many conditions (e.g., infections, neoplasms, metabolic diseases).

Table 5 (Continued)

Condition	Total Protein	Albumin	Alpha₁ Globulin	Alpha₂ Globulin	Beta Globulin	Gamma Globulin	Comment
Collagen diseases Lupus erythematosus (SLE)		D		I		I	Gamma globulin levels of prognostic value
Polyarteritis nodosa		D		I		N	
Rheumatoid arthritis		D		I	I	I	
Scleroderma						V	No significant changes
Acute rheumatic fever		D		I	No significant changes		Albumin D due to hemodilution
Essential hypertension Congestive heart failure	D	D	No significant changes				(Hemodilution, diminished hepatic synthesis, and possible excessive enteric loss)
Metastatic carcinomatosis		D	I	I	D		Nonspecific pattern

Certain infections (meningitis, pneumonia, osteomyelitis)	D				I	
Myxedema						Changes due to hemodilution
Hyperthyroidism	D		N	N	N	
Diabetes mellitus	D	I	N	I	N	

I = increased or elevated; D = decreased or diminished; V = variable; N = normal; blank = no significant change.

[a] Nonspecific changes of decreased albumin and increased globulin occur in many conditions (e.g., infections, neoplasms, metabolic diseases).

Source: Adapted from F. W. Sunderman, Jr., Recent Advances in Clinical Interpretation of Electrophoretic Fractionations of the Serum Proteins. In F. W. Sunderman and J. C. Sunderman (Eds.), *Serum Proteins and the Dysproteinemias*. Philadelphia: Lippincott, 1964.

collagen diseases, myeloproliferative diseases and neoplasms not of lymphocyte or plasma cell origin)

Either type may be familial.

Polyclonal Gammopathy with Hyperproteinemia
Collagen diseases (e.g., systemic lupus erythematosus, rheumatoid arthritis, scleroderma)
Liver disease (e.g., chronic hepatitis, cirrhosis)
Chronic infection (e.g., chronic bronchitis and bronchiectasis, lung abscess, tuberculosis, osteomyelitis, subacute bacterial endocarditis, infectious mononucleosis, malaria)
Miscellaneous (e.g., sarcoidosis, malignant lymphoma, acute myeloid and monocytic leukemia, diabetes mellitus)
Idiopathic (family of patients with lupus erythematosus)

SERUM BETA$_{2M}$ GLOBULIN
(gamma$_{1M}$ globulin; 19S gamma globulin; gamma$_1$ globulin; beta$_2$ macroglobulin)

Increased In
Waldenström's macroglobulinemia (marked increase)
Symptomatic macroglobulinemia
    Cirrhosis
    Nephrosis
    Rheumatoid arthritis
    Eosinophilic granulomatosis
    Hyperglobulinemic purpura
    Other

SERUM BETA$_{2A}$ GLOBULIN
(gamma$_{1A}$ globulin)

Increased In
Multiple myeloma (occasionally)

Decreased In
Multiple myeloma
Lipoid nephrosis
Macroglobulinemia

SERUM ALPHA$_1$-ANTITRYPSIN

Decreased In
Alpha$_1$-antitrypsin deficiency (see p. 325 and Table 7, p. 73)

Increased In
Infections
Neoplasia
Pregnancy and use of birth control pills

IMMUNODIFFUSION OF SERUM PROTEIN

Diagnosis of Specific Diseases
Multiple myeloma
Waldenström's macroglobulinemia

Hypogammaglobulinemia
    Agammaglobulinemia
    Agamma-A-globulinemia
Analbuminemia
Bisalbuminemia
Afibrinogenemia
Atransferrinemia
Wilson's disease

Other Changes
Nonspecific changes in serum proteins
Protein pattern changes in urine, cerebrospinal fluid, peritoneal
fluid, etc.

IMMUNOGLOBULIN A (IgA)

Increased In (in relation to other immunoglobulins)
γA myeloma (M component)
Cirrhosis of liver
Chronic infections
Rheumatoid arthritis with high titers of rheumatoid factor
Systemic lupus erythematosus (some patients)
Sarcoidosis (some patients)
Wiskott-Aldrich syndrome
Other

Decreased In (alone)
Normal persons (1:700)
Hereditary telangiectasia (80% of patients)
Type III dysgammaglobulinemia
Malabsorption (some patients)
Systemic lupus erythematosus (occasionally)
Cirrhosis of liver (occasionally)
Still's disease (occasionally)
Recurrent otitis media (occasionally)

Decreased In (combined with other immunoglobulin decreases)
Agammaglobulinemia
    Acquired
        Primary
        Secondary (e.g., multiple myeloma, leukemia, nephrotic
           syndrome, protein-losing enteropathy)
    Congenital
Hereditary thymic aplasia
Type I dysgammaglobulinemia (decreased IgG and IgA and in-
creased IgM)
Type II dysgammaglobulinemia (absent IgA and IgM and normal
levels of IgG)

IMMUNOGLOBULIN E (IgE)

Increased In
Atopic diseases
    Exogenous asthma in ≅60% of patients
    Hay fever in ≅30% of patients
    Atopic eczema

Influenced by type of allergen, duration of stimulation, presence of symptoms, hyposensitization treatment

Parasitic diseases (e.g., ascariasis, visceral larva migrans, hookworm disease, schistosomiasis, *Echinococcus* infestation)
E-myeloma

IMMUNOGLOBULIN D (IgD)

Increased In
Chronic infection (moderately)
IgD myelomas (greatly)

IMMUNOGLOBULIN M (IgM)

Increased In
Liver disease
Chronic infections
Waldenström's macroglobulinemia

SERUM LIPOPROTEINS
A-beta-lipoproteinemia (Bassen-Kornzweig syndrome). Low-density lipoproteins (beta-lipoproteins) are absent; high-density lipoproteins (alpha-lipoproteins) are normal. Marked decrease in plasma triglycerides (<15 mg/100 ml), decrease in plasma cholesterol (usually <50 mg/100 ml). Patients also have acanthotic RBCs and low serum carotene levels (see p. 255). (The condition is an autosomal recessive trait.)
Hypo-beta-lipoproteinemia. Low-density lipoproteins are 10–20% of normal. Plasma triglycerides are normal; cholesterol is decreased (≅ 50–60 mg/100 ml). May be caused by malabsorption of fats, infection, anemia, hepatic necrosis, hyperthyroidism, acute myocardial infarction, acute trauma; or may be familial, i.e., absence of causative disease and presence of a similar pattern in first-degree relatives. (It is an autosomal dominant trait.)
Hyper-beta-lipoproteinemia. See Table 50, pp. 352–355.
Hyper-alpha-lipoproteinemia. This disorder may be caused by alcoholism, extensive exposure to chlorinated hydrocarbon pesticides, exogenous estrogen supplementation: or it may be familial (it is an autosomal dominant trait). High-density lipoproteins (alpha-lipoproteins) are increased (>70 mg/100 ml). Total serum cholesterol is somewhat increased; triglycerides are normal.
Tangier disease. There is a marked decrease (heterozygous) or absence (homozygous) of high-density lipoprotein (alpha-lipoprotein). Pre-beta lipoprotein is absent. Serum cholesterol and phospholipid are decreased; triglycerides are normal or increased.

See Table 50, pp. 352–355.

TRIGLYCERIDES
(see Serum Lipoproteins, preceding section)

Increased In (see section on lipoprotein electrophoresis in Table 50, pp. 352–355)
Familial hyperlipedemia

Liver diseases
Nephrotic syndrome
Hypothyroidism
Diabetes mellitus (higher values correlate with hyperglycemia and poorer control of diabetes; reduced by insulin therapy)
Alcoholism
Gout
Pancreatitis
von Gierke's disease
Acute myocardial infarction (rise to peak in 3 weeks: increase may persist for 1 year)

Table 6. Serum Immunoglobulin Changes in Various Diseases

Disease	IgG	IgA	IgM
Immunoglobulin disorders (see Table 44, pp. 326–327)			
Lymphoid aplasia	D	D	D
Agammaglobulinemia	D	D	D
Type I dysgammaglobulinemia (selective IgG and IgA deficiency)	D	D	N or I
Type II dysgammaglobulinemia (absent IgA and IgM)	N	D	D
IgA globulinemia	N	D	N
Ataxia-telangiectasia	N	D	N
Multiple myeloma, macroglobulinemia, lymphomas (see pp. 321–324)			
Heavy-chain disease	D	D	D
IgG myeloma	I	D	D
IgA myeloma	D	I	D
Macroglobulinemia	D	D	I
Acute lymphocytic leukemia	N	D	N
Chronic lymphocytic leukemia	D	D	D
Acute myelogenous leukemia	N	N	N
Chronic myelogenous leukemia	N	D	N
Hodgkin's disease	N	N	N
Liver diseases			
Hepatitis	I	I	I
Laennec's cirrhosis	I	I	N
Biliary cirrhosis	N	N	I
Hepatoma	N	N	D
Miscellaneous			
Rheumatoid arthritis	I	I	I
Systemic lupus erythematosus	I	I	I
Nephrotic syndrome	D	D	N
Trypanosomiasis	N	N	I
Pulmonary tuberculosis	I	N	N

N = normal; I = increased; D = decreased.

Decreased In
Congenital a-beta-lipoproteinemia
Malnutrition

THYMOL TURBIDITY

Increased In
Active liver disease (e.g., in acute hepatitis, thymol turbidity becomes positive later than transaminase elevation; may remain positive after cephalin flocculation has become negative. In cirrhosis may be normal.)
Altered serum proteins (e.g., multiple myeloma, sarcoidosis, lupus erythematosus)
Lipemic serum (e.g., postprandial lipemia)

Thymol turbidity and cephalin flocculation should be replaced by more specific tests, e.g., serum alkaline phosphatase, SGOT, SGPT, gamma glutamyl transpeptidase.

CEPHALIN FLOCCULATION TEST
Parallels thymol turbidity test. See preceding section.

SERUM TRIIODOTHYRONINE (T-3) UPTAKE
(see Table 54, pp. 380–382)

This test should be used only with a simultaneous measurement of serum T-4 to exclude the possibility that an increased T-4 is due to an increase in T-4–binding globulin. Measurement of serum T-3 concentration should be done by radioimmunoassay for diagnosis of hyperthyroidism (see pp. 378–379).

Increased In
Hyperthyroidism
Certain drugs (e.g., testosterone, androgens, anabolic steroids, prednisone, heparin, Dicumarol, salicylates, Butazolidin, penicillin, Dilantin)
Threatened abortion
Infants (up to about age 2 months)
Severe nephrosis
Metastatic neoplasms

Decreased In
Hypothyroidism
Pregnancy (from about tenth week of pregnancy until up to 12th week postpartum)
Certain drugs (e.g., estrogens alone or in birth control pills, large amounts of iodine, propylthiouracil in hyperthyroidism)

Normal In
Pregnancy with hyperthyroidism
Nontoxic goiter
Carcinoma of thyroid
Diabetes mellitus

Table 7. Changes in Serum Immunoproteins in Various Conditions

Condition	Albumin	Alpha$_1$ Antitrypsin	Haptoglobin	Transferrin	C3
Acute inflammation	D	I	I	D	Slight I
Chronic inflammation	D	V–I	V–I	D	Slight I
Chronic liver disease	D	V–I	V	D	V–D
Obstructive jaundice	N	N	V–I	N	I
Hemolytic anemia	N	N	D	N	N
Iron deficiency	N	N	N	I	N
Acute glomerulonephritis	N	N	N	N	D
Systemic lupus erythematosus	D	I	D[a]	D	V–D[b]
Alpha$_1$ antitrypsin deficiency	N	D	N	N	N
Analbuminemia	D	N	N	N	N
Agammaglobulinemia	N	N	N	N	N
IgG myeloma	D	N	N	N	N
IgA myeloma	D	N	N	N	N
Waldenström's macro-globulinemia	D	N	N	N	N

N = normal; D = decreased; I = increased; V = variable.
[a] D with associated hemolytic anemia.
[b] N if immunosuppressive treatment is effective.

Addison's disease
Anxiety
Certain drugs (mercurials, iodine)

Variable In
Liver disease

SERUM PROTEIN-BOUND IODINE (PBI)
(see Table 54, pp. 380–382)
This test has been largely replaced by the more specific thyroxine (T-4) assay.

Usually Increased In
Hyperthyroidism
Hereditary increase in thyroxine-binding protein and other causes of increased TBG
Pregnancy (from about fourth week of pregnancy until up to sixth week postpartum)
Infancy
Certain drugs (especially iodine-containing drugs, e.g., radiopaque substances for x-ray studies, expectorants, estrogens, levo-thyroxine, birth control pills; also iodine-containing products, e.g., toothpaste, suntan lotion, antidandruff preparation, food coloring)
About half of very ill euthyroid patients

Occasionally Increased In
Certain tumors (dermoid cyst of ovary, hydatidiform mole, metastatic choriocarcinoma, breast carcinoma, embryonal carcinoma of testicle)
Hashimoto's thyroiditis
Acute intermittent porphyria
Certain drugs (e.g., Bromsulphalein in BSP test, barium sulfate as in x-ray studies of GI tract)

Usually Decreased In
Hypothyroidism
Hereditary decrease in thyroxine-binding protein and other causes of decreased TBG
Nephrosis
Dietary iodine deficiency
Certain drugs (e.g., phenytoin sodium [Dilantin], salicylates, thiouracil, thiocyanates, therapeutic ^{131}I)

Occasionally Decreased In
Starvation
Hypothermia
Certain drugs (e.g., ACTH, corticosteroids, androgens, PAS)

Normal In
Leukemia, polycythemia
Diabetes mellitus, acromegaly, Addison's disease

Certain drugs (e.g., diuretics, digitalis, antibiotics, gonadotropins, desiccated thyroid)

In hypothyroidism, PBI level attained with sufficient therapy to make patient euthyroid depends upon the particular thyroid hormone product.

Levothyroxine (Synthroid)	PBI higher than normal
Liothyronine (Cytomel)	Low PBI
U.S.P. thyroid	PBI normal to low normal
Thyroglobulin (Proloid)	PBI may be low

SERUM BUTANOL-EXTRACTABLE IODINE (BEI)
This test has been largely replaced by the more specific thyroxine (T-4) assay.

Altered in same conditions as listed for PBI, above, except that BEI is not affected by the presence of excess *inorganic* iodine.
BEI measures thyroxine-like compounds.
BEI may be as falsely increased as PBI by organic iodine compounds.
BEI is lower than simultaneous PBI in thyroiditis.

SERUM TOTAL THYROXINE ASSAY (T-4)
(see Table 54, pp. 380–382)

Increased In
Hyperthyroidism
Pregnancy
Certain drugs (estrogens, birth control pills, *d*-thyroxine, thyroid extract, TSH)

Decreased In
Hypothyroidism
Hypoproteinemia
Certain drugs (phenytoin sodium [Dilantin], triiodothyronine, testosterone, ACTH, corticosteroids)

Not Affected By
Radiopaque substances for x-ray studies
Mercurial diuretics
Nonthyroidal iodine

FREE THYROXINE INDEX (T-7)
This is the product of T-3 uptake and T-4 (or T-3 uptake and PBI).
It permits correction of misleading results of T-3 and T-4 (or PBI) determinations caused by pregnancy, estrogens (including especially birth control pills), and other conditions that alter the thyroxine-binding protein concentration.

Condition	T-3	T-4	Free Thyroxine Factor (T-7) (T-3 × T-4)
Normal			
Range	24–36	4–11	96–396
Mean	31	7	217
Hypothyroid	22	3	66
Hyperthyroid	38	12	456
Pregnancy, estrogens (especially birth control pills)	20	12	240[a]

[a]Normal even though T-3 and T-4 alone are abnormal.

FREE THYROXINE ASSAY (NORMALIZED THYROXINE)
(see Table 54, pp. 380–382)

This determination gives corrected values in patients in whom the total thyroxine (T-4) is altered on account of changes in serum proteins or in binding sites.

    Pregnancy

    Drugs (e.g., androgens, estrogens, birth control pills, Dilantin)

    Altered levels of serum proteins (e.g., nephrosis)

This is the best single screening test for thyroid dysfunction.
It is paralleled by the free thyroxine factor.

Increased In
Hyperthyroidism
Hypothyroidism treated with thyroxine
Very ill euthyroid patients (frequently)

Decreased In
Hypothyroidism
Hypothyroidism treated with triiodothyronine

SERUM THYROXINE-BINDING GLOBULIN (TBG)
(see Table 54, pp. 380–382)

Increased In
Pregnancy
Excess TBG, genetic or idiopathic
Hypothyroidism (some patients)
Certain drugs (estrogens, birth control pills)
Gross iodine contamination
Acute intermittent porphyria

Decreased In
Nephrosis and other causes of marked hypoproteinemia
Deficiency of TBG, genetic or idiopathic
Certain drugs (androgenic and anabolic steroids)

An increase of TBG is associated with an increase in PBI, BEI, and T-4 by column and a decrease in T-3; converse association for decrease of TBG.

SERUM TSH (THYROID-STIMULATING HORMONE; THYROTROPIN)
(hormone secreted by anterior pituitary; measured by radioimmunoassay)
Primary usefulness is in diagnosis of hypothyroidism and in differentiation of primary and secondary hypothyroidism.

Increased In
Primary untreated hypothyroidism. Increase is proportionate to the degree of hypofunction, varying from 3 times normal in mild cases to 100 times normal in severe myxedema. A single determination is usually sufficient to establish the diagnosis. Especially useful in early or subclinical hypothyroidism before the patient develops clinical findings, goiter, or abnormalities of routine laboratory thyroid tests. In very early cases with only marginal elevation the thyroid-releasing hormone stimulation test offers a more refined diagnostic procedure. Serum TSH suppressed below normal level is the best monitor of dosage of thyroid hormone for treatment of hypothyroidism, but it does not indicate overtreatment.

Hashimoto's thyroiditis, including those with clinical hypothyroidism and about one-third of those patients who are clinically euthyroid

Other conditions (test is not clinically useful)
Iodide deficiency goiter
Iodide-induced goiter
External neck irradiation
Post-subtotal thyroidectomy

Decreased In
Secondary (pituitary) hypothyroidism
Hypothalamic hypothyroidism
Hyperthyroidism. Some patients have normal levels and it may not be possible to differentiate low range of normal from an abnormally decreased value. A TRH stimulation test may be required to establish the diagnosis (see p. 78).

Normal In
Cushing's syndrome
Acromegaly
Pregnancy at term

TRH (THYROID-RELEASING HORMONE) STIMULATION TEST (TRF [THYROTROPIN-RELEASING FACTOR])
(see Fig. 1)
Serum TSH is measured before and after the intravenous administration of TRH (usually 500 or 200 μg).

The TSH response to TRH is modified by thyroxine, antithyroid drugs, corticosteroids, estrogens, and levodopa. Response is increased during pregnancy.

Normal response—a significant rise from a basal level of about 1 μU/ml by 8 μU/ml at 20 minutes and return to normal by 120 minutes. Response is usually greater in women than in men.

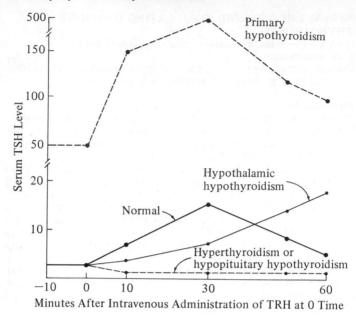

Fig. 1. Sample curves of serum TSH response to administration of TRH in various conditions.

Hyperthyroidism—shows no rise in the depressed TSH level. A normal rise virtually excludes hyperthyroidism. This test may be particularly useful in T-3 toxicosis in which the other tests are normal or in patients clinically suspicious for hyperthyroidism with borderline serum T-3 levels. When serum TSH measurements are available, the TRH stimulation test is superior to the T-3 suppression test of RAIU (see p. 153).

Primary hypothyroidism—an exaggerated rise of an already increased TSH level.

Secondary (pituitary) hypothyroidism—no rise in the decreased TSH level.

Hypothalamic hypothyroidism—low serum T-3 and T-4 and TSH levels, with a TRH response that may be exaggerated or normal or (most characteristically) with a peak delayed 45–60 minutes. Diagnosis must be based on clinical studies that exclude the pituitary gland as the site of the disease.

	Serum TSH	Serum TSH Response to TRH Stimulation
Primary hypothyroidism	I	N or exaggerated
Pituitary hypothyroidism	D	Absent
Hypothalamic hypothyroidism	D	Delayed peak or exaggerated or N

I = Increased; D = Decreased; N = Normal

SERUM LONG-ACTING THYROID STIMULATOR (LATS)
(not used in routine clinical diagnosis)

Normal Condition
None detectable

Increased In (frequently but not invariably)
Graves' disease
Exophthalmos (some euthyroid patients)
Pretibial myxedema

THYROID ANTIBODIES TEST
Precipitin test
    High titers in Hashimoto's disease
    May be positive but with lower titers in other thyroid diseases
      (e.g., primary myxedema)
Tanned red cell titers
    $\geq 1:250,000$—Hashimoto's disease
    May be this high in primary myxedema
    $\leq 1:250$ in hyperthyroidism, carcinoma of thyroid, and simple
      goiter
Fluorescent antibody studies

BLOOD AMMONIA

Increased In
Liver failure (e.g., acute hepatic necrosis, terminal cirrhosis, hepatectomy)

In cirrhosis, blood ammonia may be increased after portacaval anastomosis.
Not all cases of hepatic coma show increased blood ammonia.

Some aminoacidurias (see Table 51, pp. 356–358)

BLOOD LACTIC ACID
(see p. 343)

SERUM CAROTENOIDS

Increased In
Excessive intake (especially carrots)
Postprandial hyperlipemia
Hyperlipemia (e.g., essential hyperlipemia)
Diabetes mellitus
Hypothyroidism

Decreased In
Carotenoid-poor diet—blood level falls within 1 week (*vitamin A level unaffected by dietary change for 6 months because of much larger body stores*)
Malabsorption syndromes (*a very useful screening test for malabsorption*)
Liver disease
High fever

PLASMA RENIN ACTIVITY (PRA)

Blood should be drawn in an ice-cold tube and the plasma immediately separated in a refrigerated centrifuge. Renin level should be indexed against 24-hour level of sodium in urine.

PRA is particularly useful to diagnose curable hypertension (e.g., unilateral renal artery stenosis, primary aldosteronism).

Increased In
15% of patients with essential hypertension
Renal hypertension (see below)
Renin-producing tumors of the kidney
Reduced plasma volume due to low-sodium diet, diuretics, hemorrhage, Addison's disease
Secondary aldosteronism (usually very high levels) (see pp. 406–407)
10% of patients with chronic renal failure
Normal pregnancy
Estrogen-containing birth control pills
Last half of menstrual cycle (twofold increase)
Erect posture for 4 hours (twofold increase)
Ambulatory patients compared to bed patients
Bartter's syndrome

Decreased In
Increased plasma volume due to high-sodium diet, administration of salt-retaining steroids
20% of patients diagnosed at the present time as having "essential hypertension"
Advancing age in both normal and hypertensive patients (decrease of 35% from the third to the eighth decade)
Primary aldosteronism. Usually absent or low and can be increased less or not at all by sodium depletion and ambulation in contrast to secondary aldosteronism. *PRA may not always be suppressed in primary aldosteronism; repeated testing may be necessary to establish the diagnosis.*
Cushing's syndrome (see p. 399)
In diagnosis of renal hypertension, renin is assayed in blood from each renal vein, inferior vena cava, and aorta. The test is considered diagnostic when the level from the ischemic kidney is at least 1½ times greater than the level from the normal kidney (which is equal to or less than the level in the aorta that serves as the standard). This is due to high PRA in peripheral blood, increase in PRA in the renal vein compared to the renal artery of the affected kidney, and suppression of PRA in the other kidney. Maximum renin stimulation accentuates the difference between the two kidneys and should *always* be obtained by pretest conditions (avoid antihypertensive, diuretic, and oral contraceptive drugs for at least 1 month if possible; low-salt diet for 7 days; administer thiazide diuretic for 1–3 days; upright posture for at least 2 hours). This is the most useful diagnostic test in renovascular hypertension as judged by surgical results but is not a sufficiently reliable guide to nephrectomy in patients with hyper-

tension due to parenchymal renal disease. *In renovascular hypertension, if renal plasma flow is impaired in the "normal" kidney, surgery often fails to cure the hypertension.* *

PLASMA INSULIN
Not clinically useful for diagnosis of diabetes mellitus because of the very wide range in both normal and diabetic patients and because results may be influenced by many other factors.

Increased In
Insulinoma. Fasting blood insulin level over 50 μU/ml in presence of low or normal blood glucose level. Intravenous tolbutamide or administration of leucine causes rapid rise of blood insulin to very high levels within a few minutes with rapid return to normal.

Untreated obese diabetics (mild cases). The fasting level is often increased.

Acromegaly (especially with active disease) after ingestion of glucose

Reactive hypoglycemia after glucose ingestion, particularly when diabetic type of glucose tolerance curve is present

Absent In
Severe diabetes mellitus with ketosis and weight loss. In less severe cases, insulin is frequently present but only at lower glucose concentrations.

Normal In
Hypoglycemia associated with nonpancreatic tumors

Idiopathic hypoglycemia of childhood, except after administration of leucine

SERUM C-PEPTIDE
C-peptide is formed during conversion of proinsulin to insulin; C-peptide serum levels correlate with insulin levels in blood, except in islet cell tumors and possibly in obese patients. Therefore test is useful for estimating insulin levels in the presence of circulating insulin antibodies that interfere with insulin assay. Also useful in factitious hypoglycemia due to surreptitious administration of insulin in which high serum insulin levels will occur with low C-peptide levels.

PLASMA TESTOSTERONE
Male hypogonadism—levels lower than in normal male

Klinefelter's syndrome—levels lower than in normal male but higher than in normal female and orchiectomized male

Stein-Leventhal syndrome—variable; increased when virilization is present

*E. F. Fraley and B. H. Feldman, Current concepts: Renal hypertension. *N. Engl. J. Med.* 287:550, 1972.

Adrenogenital syndrome—with virilization (due to tumor or hyperplasia) level is much higher than in normal female; decreases following adrenal suppression
Idiopathic hirsutism—inconclusive
Ovarian stromal hyperthecosis

PLASMA ACTH

Decreased In
Cushing's syndrome due to adrenal tumor
Secondary hypoadrenalism

Increased In
Pituitary Cushing's syndrome
Primary adrenal insufficiency
Ectopic ACTH syndrome (e.g., carcinoma of lung)—levels very high, with no diurnal variation

SERUM PARATHYROID HORMONE

	Parathyroid Hormone Elevated	Parathyroid Hormone Decreased
Serum calcium low	Secondary hyperparathyroidism (chronic renal disease) Pseudohypoparathyroidism (or normal hormone level)	Hypoparathyroidism (surgical or idiopathic)
Serum calcium high	Primary hyperparathyroidism	Hypercalcemia not due to hyperparathyroidism (e.g., various malignancies, milk-alkali syndrome, various osteolytic diseases, others)
Serum calcium normal	Pregnancy Nephrolithiasis Secondary hyperparathyroidism (chronic renal disease)	

There is considerable overlap of serum parathyroid hormone levels in normal patients and those with proven hyperparathyroidism. "Normal" level depends on the serum calcium level, which should always be determined simultaneously. Selective catheterization of veins draining the thyroid-parathyroid region for determination of parathyroid hormone levels may confirm the diagnosis of hyperparathyroidism by showing a significant elevation at one site compared to at least one other site.

SERUM PROLACTIN

Increased in
Syndromes of galactorrhea-amenorrhea (see p. 416)

Other lesions of pituitary-hypothalamus (e.g., primary or metastatic neoplasms, sarcoidosis, histiocytosis X, postoperative pituitary surgery)

Ectopic prolactin production by neoplasms (e.g., bronchogenic carcinoma, hypernephroma)

Irritative lesions of chest wall (e.g., trauma, surgery, herpes zoster)

Hypoglycemia

Stress (e.g., anesthesia, surgery, exercise, anxiety)

Nipple stimulation

Fetal life through first week of infancy, with decrease to adult level by age 3–6 months

Pregnancy (serum level doubles each trimester to peak just before delivery)

Postpartum state (up to 4 weeks in non-nursing mothers; nursing causes marked but transient increases during next 3 months)

SERUM ALPHA-FETOPROTEIN (AFP)

Normal (<40 ng/ml)
Absent after first several weeks of life

Increased In
Primary cancer of liver (hepatoma) in 50% of whites and 75–90% of nonwhites; levels may be markedly elevated (>1000 ng/ml). Elevated in almost 100% of cases in children and young adults.

Some patients with liver metastases from carcinoma of stomach or pancreas

Embryonal carcinoma (in 27% of cases) or malignant teratoma (in 60% of cases) of ovary and testis

Neonatal hepatitis. Most patients with this disorder have levels >40 ng/ml, but in neonatal biliary atresia most patients have levels <40 ng/ml.

Pregnancy; increased above normal level in fetal open spina bifida or anencephaly. (*Increased blood levels of AFP in pregnancy is a valuable screening test but diagnosis should be confirmed by finding of increased levels in amniotic fluid; serum should be drawn after the 15th week of gestation.*)

Ataxia-telangiectasia

Absent In
Various types of cirrhosis and hepatitis in adults

Seminoma of testis

Choriocarcinoma, adenocarcinoma, and dermoid cyst of ovary

SERUM CARCINOEMBRYONIC ANTIGEN (CEA)
(radioimmunoassay detection in plasma)

This is a recently developed test, the usefulness of which is still being evaluated. There is a wide overlap in values between benign and malignant disease.

Because of considerable publicity, the following limitations must be remembered:

CEA test is not a screen for the detection of early cancer.

CEA titers <2.5 ng/ml do not rule out malignant disease (primary, metastatic, or recurrent).

CEA is not an absolute test for malignant disease or for a specific type of malignancy.

CEA level should never be used as the sole criterion for diagnosis.

Summary of current data

97% of healthy nonsmokers have plasma CEA levels <2.5 ng/ml.

19% of heavy smokers and 7% of former smokers have CEA levels >2.5 ng/ml.

75% of patients with carcinoma of entodermal origin (colon, stomach, pancreas, lung) have CEA titers >2.5 ng/ml, and two-thirds of these titers are >5 ng/ml.

Titers >20 ng/ml are usually associated with metastatic disease or with a few types of cancer (e.g., cancer of the colon or pancreas); however, metastases may occur with levels <20 ng/ml.

50% of patients with carcinoma of nonentodermal origin (especially cancer of the breast, head, and neck) have CEA titers >2.5 ng/ml, and 50% of the titers are >5 ng/ml.

40% of patients with noncarcinomatous malignant disease have increased CEA levels, usually 2.5–5.0 ng/ml.

Active cases of nonmalignant inflammatory diseases (especially of the digestive tract, e.g., ulcerative colitis, regional enteritis, diverticulitis, cirrhosis) frequently have elevated levels that decline when the disease is in remission.

In patients with carcinoma of entodermal origin, a CEA level >5 ng/ml before therapy suggests localized disease and a favorable prognosis, but a level > 10 ng/ml suggests extensive disease and a poor prognosis. A fall of CEA to <2.5 ng/ml after the therapy suggests adequate treatment, but persistent elevation may indicate residual tumor. A rising CEA level may indicate recurrent carcinoma of entodermal origin, even if the pretreatment level was normal. However, for an individual patient it is difficult to predict the outcome on the basis of these data. The carcinoma may precede clinical evidence of recurrence.

Do not test heparinized patients or collect plasma in heparinized tubes, since this may interfere with accuracy of CEA assay.

SERUM GASTRIN
(determined by radioimmunoassay of serum)

Normal levels: from absent to ≦200 pg gastrin/ml serum

Elevated levels: >500 pg/ml

Condition	Serum Gastrin	*Serum Gastrin After Intragastric Administration of 0.1N HCl*
Peptic ulcer without Zollinger-Ellison syndrome	Normal range	—
Zollinger-Ellison syndrome	Very high	No change
Pernicious anemia	High level may approach that in Z-E syndrome	Marked decrease

Calcium infusion (IV calcium gluconate, 5 mg/kg body weight/hour for 3 hours) with pre-infusion blood specimen compared to specimens every 30 minutes for up to 4 hours. Normal patients show minimal serum gastrin response to calcium. Patients with Zollinger-Ellison syndrome show excessive increase in serum gastrin.

Secretin infusion (IV of 9 units/kg body weight for 1 hour) with blood specimens drawn before and at 15-minute intervals. Normal patients and patients with duodenal ulcer show no increase in serum gastrin. Patients with Zollinger-Ellison syndrome show increased serum gastrin that usually peaks in 45–60 minutes.

INCREASED SERUM GASTRIN WITHOUT GASTRIC ACID HYPERSECRETION

Atrophic gastritis, especially when associated with circulating parietal cell antibodies

Pernicious anemia in $\cong 75\%$ of patients

Some patients have carcinoma of body of stomach, a reflection of the atrophic gastritis that is present.

Vertigo due to high frequency of associated achlorhydria and pernicious anemia

Chronic renal failure with serum creatinine >3 mg/100 ml; occurs in 50% of patients

INCREASED SERUM GASTRIN WITH GASTRIC ACID HYPERSECRETION

Zollinger-Ellison syndrome (gastrinoma) (see pp. 396–397)

Hyperplasia of antral gastrin cells

Isolated retained antrum—a condition of gastric acid hypersecretion and recurrent ulceration following antrectomy and gastrojejunostomy that occurs when the duodenal stump contains antral mucosa.

Pyloric obstruction with gastric distention

Short-bowel syndrome due to massive resection or extensive regional enteritis

SERUM CALCITONIN
(radioimmunoassay measurement)
Basal level is increased in $\cong 75\%$ of patients with medullary carcinoma of the thyroid even when there is no palpable mass in the thyroid. In some of these patients, the levels may vary from diagnostic to nondiagnostic.

Calcium infusion is used as a provocative test in patients with normal pre-infusion levels, especially those with a family history of medullary thyroid carcinoma or of associated features (e.g., pheochromocytoma, hyperparathyroidism). Infusion will also increase levels in nonthyroid tumors, causing a twofold to fourfold increase over baseline levels.

Also useful for detecting recurrence of medullary carcinoma or metastases after primary tumor has been removed or for confirming complete removal of the tumor.

Increased levels have been reported in some patients with
> Carcinoma of the lung
> Carcinoma of the breast
> Zollinger-Ellison syndrome
> Pernicious anemia
> Chronic renal failure

FUNCTIONAL TESTS

BROMSULPHALEIN (BSP) RETENTION IN SERUM
This test measures the rate of removal of dye from blood by the liver. It is a very sensitive and specific test of hepatic function. *It must be performed while the patient is fasting because postprandial increased hepatic blood flow produces increased excretion and falsely normal result.*

Increased In
Fever (without liver disease)

Liver disease of any type (e.g., chronic hepatitis, cirrhosis, chronic congestion)

Acute cholecystitis

Ingestion (without liver damage) of certain drugs and dyes (e.g., morphine, methadone, monoamine oxidase inhibitors, barbiturates, probenecid, Telepaque, phenolphthalein, phenolsulfonphthalein (PSP), Pyridium), estrogens, and birth control pills.

Upper GI tract hemorrhage. *BSP retention of >20% suggests presumptive diagnosis of cirrhosis. BSP retention $\leqq 20\%$ suggests absence of cirrhosis.*

False Values In
Albuminuria. *BSP dye may be lost in urine.* Results may falsely appear normal.

Ascites. *BSP dye may be lost into abdomen.* Results may falsely appear normal.

Any appreciable jaundice

ORAL GLUCOSE TOLERANCE TEST (GTT)

An appropriate prior diet of ≧ 250 gm of carbohydrate daily and no alcohol for 3 days before the test should be prescribed. Patient should be fasting for 10–12 hours before test, with no smoking or drinking of coffee. Do not test in presence of fever or infection.

For older persons without elevated fasting levels, without glycosuria (alone or during oral GTT), without positive family history of diabetes, limits of normal at 1 and 2 hours should be increased 10 mg/100 ml at age 50 and an additional 10 mg for each subsequent decade (e.g., 30 mg/100 ml at age 70).

To detect early diabetes in pregnancy, upper limits of normal are 165 at 1 hour, 145 at 2 hours, 125 at 3 hours. If results are equivocal test should be repeated in 3 months or IV GTT should be done. If suggestive diagnosis of diabetes is not definite during pregnancy, additional workup should be done after delivery.

U.S. Public Health Service criteria for diagnosis of diabetes: Assign 1 point each to elevated fasting and 3-hour levels, and ½ point each to the 1- and 2-hour levels. Total of two points or more is considered diagnostic.

Decreased Tolerance In
Excessive peak
    Increased absorption (normal IV GTT curve) with normal return to fasting level
        Mechanical (e.g., gastrectomy, gastroenterostomy)
        Hyperthyroidism
        Excess intake of glucose

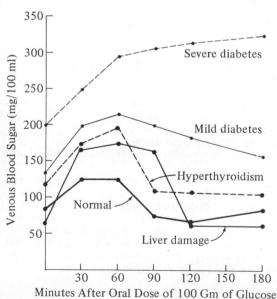

Fig. 2. Sample oral glucose tolerance curves in various conditions.

Decreased utilization with slow fall to fasting level
  Diabetes mellitus
  Hyperlipidemia, types III, IV, V
  Hemochromatosis
  Steroid effect (Cushing's disease, administration of ACTH
    or steroids)
  CNS lesions
Decreased formation of glycogen with low fasting levels and
  subsequent hypoglycemia
    von Gierke's disease
    Severe liver damage
    Hyperthyroidism (normal return to fasting level)
    Increased adrenalin (stress, pheochromocytoma) (normal
      return to fasting level)
    Pregnancy (normal return to fasting level)

Increased Tolerance In
Flat peak
  Pancreatic islet cell hyperplasia or tumor
  Poor absorption from GI tract (normal IV GTT curve)
    Intestinal diseases (e.g., steatorrhea, sprue, celiac dis-
      ease, Whipple's disease)
    Hypothyroidism
    Addison's disease
    Hypoparathyroidism
Late hypoglycemia
  Pancreatic islet cell hyperplasia or tumor
  Hypopituitarism
  Liver disease
See Table 79, pp. 550–555, for effect of drugs.

INTRAVENOUS GLUCOSE TOLERANCE TEST
Administer 20% glucose (0.5 gm/kg body weight) intravenously
  over 30 minutes.
Normal
  Peak 200–250 mg/100 ml immediately
  Return to fasting level by 90 minutes
  Below fasting level by 2 hours
  Return to fasting level by 3 hours
Intestinal disease and hypothyroidism—normal (in contrast to oral
  GTT)
Liver disease—delayed fall after peak; return to fasting level in 3–5
  hours (variable in oral GTT)
Addison's disease and hypopituitarism—normal peak (flat peak in
  oral GTT); severe hypoglycemia later
Acromegaly—IV GTT abnormal more frequently than oral GTT
Oral GTT is more useful for diagnosis of diabetes mellitus and
  pancreatic cell hyperactivity. IV GTT is useful to clarify or rule
  out the influence of absorption factors in the curve.

SOSKIN'S INTRAVENOUS GLUCOSE TOLERANCE TEST
Administer 50% glucose (0.3 gm/kg body weight) intravenously
  within 3–5 minutes.

Normal. Blood sugar returns to fasting level in <60 minutes.
Diabetes. Blood sugar returns to fasting level in >120 minutes.
Liver disease. Blood sugar returns to fasting level in <120 minutes. In 25% of patients with liver disease blood sugar returns to fasting level in <60 minutes.

TOLBUTAMIDE TOLERANCE TEST
Administer 1 gm sodium tolbutamide intravenously within 2 minutes. *Always keep IV glucose available to prevent severe reaction.*
Adrenal insufficiency—normal or low curve
Severe liver disease—low curve
Test is most useful for diagnosis of secreting islet cell tumor and to rule out functional hyperinsulinism.
In islet cell tumor the fall in blood sugar is usually more marked than in functional hypoglycemia; more important, the blood sugar fails to recover even after 2–3 hours.
In functional hypoglycemia, return of blood sugar to normal is usually complete by 90 minutes.

Table 8. Serum Glucose Change Induced by Tolbutamide in Various Conditions

Disease	% of Fasting Serum Glucose At	
	20 Minutes	30 Minutes
Islet cell tumor	17–50	40–60
Normal functional hyperinsulinism	50–80	60–76
Borderline diabetes	80–84	77–81
Probable diabetes	85–89	82–86
Diabetes	≧ 90	≧ 87

INSULIN TOLERANCE TEST
Administer 0.1 unit insulin/kg body weight intravenously. *Use smaller dose if hypopituitarism is suspected. Always keep IV glucose available to prevent severe reaction.*

Normal
Blood glucose falls to 50% of fasting level within 20–30 minutes; returns to fasting level within 90–120 minutes.

Increased Tolerance
Blood glucose falls <25% and returns rapidly to fasting level.
Hypothyroidism
Acromegaly
Cushing's syndrome
Diabetes mellitus (some patients; especially older, obese ones)

Decreased Tolerance
Increased sensitivity to insulin (excessive fall of blood glucose)
Hypoglycemic irresponsiveness (lack of response by glycogenolysis)

Pancreatic islet cell tumor
Adrenal cortical insufficiency
Adrenal cortical insufficiency secondary to hypopituitarism
Hypothyroidism
von Gierke's disease (some patients)
Starvation (depletion of liver glycogen)

INSULIN GLUCOSE TOLERANCE TEST

Administer simultaneously 0.1 unit insulin/kg body weight intrave-
nously and 0.8 gm glucose/kg body weight orally.
Insulin-sensitive diabetics show little change in blood sugar.
Insulin-resistant diabetics show a diabetic glucose tolerance curve.
Other changes parallel those in the insulin tolerance test.

INTRAVENOUS GLUCOSE PHOSPHORUS TOLERANCE TEST

This test is indicated in diabetes suspects who also show evidence
of liver disease. Liver disease and diabetes have a more prolonged decline than normal.
Normal. Serum phosphorus decreases to 60–90% (average = 75%)
of fasting level by 1 hour after IV glucose administration
Liver disease. Serum phosphorus decreases to average 63% of
fasting level. Minimum level occurs in 90 minutes.
Diabetes mellitus. Serum phosphorus decreases to average 88% of
fasting level. Minimum level occurs in 120 minutes.

CORTISONE GLUCOSE TOLERANCE TEST

Cortisone increases the sensitivity of the oral GTT, but its clinical
status is still uncertain.
Administer 50 mg cortisone acetate orally (62.5 mg if body weight
is >160 lb [72 kg]) at 8½ and 2 hours before test. Oral glucose of
1.75 gm/kg ideal weight is given as a 25% solution.
Upper limit of normal at 2 hours = 140 mg/100 ml.
Correct for age of patient: Add 18 mg for age 40 (158 mg/100 ml);
add an additional 18 mg/100 ml for each decade over 40.

ORAL DISACCHARIDE TOLERANCE TEST

Administer 1 gm/kg body weight of the test carbohydrate (disaccharide). Determine blood glucose at fasting, ½-, 1-, 2-, and
3-hour intervals.
Normal. Blood glucose increases >24 mg/100 ml above fasting
level.
Abnormal in disaccharide malabsorption. Blood glucose increases
0–21 mg/100 ml above fasting level. False abnormal test may be
due to delayed gastric emptying or delayed blood collection.
Confirm disaccharide malabsorption by
  Repeating tolerance test using constituent monosaccharides
  Testing stool for
    pH: ≦5 is abnormal.
    Sugar: >0.5% is abnormal; 0.25–0.5% is suspicious;
      0.25% is normal.
  Taking intestinal biopsy for histologic study and disac-
    charidase activity assay

D-XYLOSE TOLERANCE TEST

Give 25 gm D-xylose in water orally. Collect a total 5-hour urine specimen (normal is >5 gm in 5 hours). Blood may also be taken at fasting, ½-, 1-, and 2-hour intervals (normal is >25 mg/100 ml). The test reflects intestinal malabsorption.

Chief value is in distinguishing small intestinal malabsorption, which has decreased values, from pancreatic steatorrhea, which has normal values (see p. 199)

Decreased In

Malabsorption in jejunum (e.g., celiac disease, sprue, some patients with *Giardia lamblia* infestation, small-intestine bacterial overgrowth, viral gastroenteritis)—<4 gm in 5-hour urine

Elderly persons

Normal absorption but decreased urinary excretion (e.g., renal insufficiency, myxedema, vomiting, dehydration)

Patients with ascites (urine values are low)

Normal In

Steatorrhea due to pancreatic disease

Cirrhosis of liver

Postgastrectomy state

Malnutrition

GALACTOSE TOLERANCE TEST

Use an oral dose of 35 gm of galactose/sq m body area.

Normal. Serum galactose increases to 30–50 mg/100 ml; returns to normal within 3 hours.

Galactosemia. Serum increase is greater, and return to baseline level is delayed.

Heterozygous carrier. Response is intermediate.

The test is not specific or sensitive enough for genetic studies.

Beware of hypoglycemia in von Gierke's disease.

CAROTENE TOLERANCE TEST

Low values for serum carotene levels are usually associated with steatorrhea.

Measure serum carotene following daily oral loading of carotene for 3–7 days.

Normal

Increase of serum carotene by >35 μg/100 ml indicates previously low dietary intake of carotene and/or fat.

Decreased In

Steatorrhea. Serum carotene increases <30 μg/100 ml. Patients with sprue in remission with normal fecal fat excretion may still show low carotene absorption.

Mineral oil interferes with carotene absorption. On a fat-free diet only 10% is absorbed.

IODINE TOLERANCE TEST

A fasting patient who has received no iodine for 1 week is given 0.3–0.5 ml of strong iodine solution in milk. Blood iodine determinations are made every half-hour for 2½ hours.

Normal. Blood iodine increases from 10 to $\leqq$ 160 or 170 μg/100 ml in half an hour; by 2½ hours it decreases to only 150 μg.

Hyperthyroidism. Blood iodine increases from 15 μg to only 40 μg after 1 hour.

CREATINE TOLERANCE TEST
(ingestion of 1–3 gm creatine)

Normal. Creatine is not increased in blood or urine.

Decreased muscle mass. Blood and urine creatine increases in
    Neurogenic atrophy
    Polymyositis
    Addison's disease
    Hyperthyroidism
    Male eunuchoidism
    Other

TRYPTOPHAN TOLERANCE TEST

The test demonstrates pyridoxine deficiency. It may be positive in pyridoxine-responsive anemia or it may be normal.

A positive test produces abnormally large urinary excretion of xanthurenic acid.

ELLSWORTH-HOWARD TEST

Determine urinary phosphorus before and after injection of *potent* parathyroid extract.

Hypoparathyroidism. Urinary phosphorus is increased > 10 times.

Pseudohypoparathyroidism. Urinary phosphorus is increased < 2 times (i.e., poor or no response to parathormone injection).

Pseudo-pseudohypoparathyroidism. Response to parathormone injection is normal. Urinary phosphorus is increased 5–6 times.

Basal cell nevus syndrome. Decreased response to parathormone injection is often shown.

RESPONSE OF ELEVATED SERUM CALCIUM TO CORTICOIDS

Corticoids do not suppress elevated serum calcium in hyperparathyroidism.

Corticoid administration does suppress the elevated serum calcium level in
    Sarcoidosis
    Metastatic neoplasm
    Vitamin D excess
    Multiple myeloma
    Hyperthyroidism

CALCIUM TOLERANCE

Constant diet. Measure phosphorus in three 24-hour urines. On second day, administer calcium intravenously (15 mg/kg body weight)

Normal. Calcium infusion causes marked decrease in urine phosphorus on second day, followed by rebound increase on third day.

Hyperparathyroidism. Only slight changes appear in urine phosphorus.

PHOSPHATE DEPRIVATION

After a diet of 800 mg phosphate/day, determine serum phosphorus and BUN and 12-hour urine phosphorus.

Normal: 6–17 ml/minute

Hyperparathyroidism: higher (even with renal dysfunction)

Hypoparathyroidism: lower (e.g., <6 ml/minute), even when hypocalcemia has been corrected

TUBULAR REABSORPTION OF PHOSPHATE (TRP)

After a constant dietary intake of moderate calcium and phosphorus for 3 days, phosphorus and creatinine are determined in fasting blood and 4-hour urine specimens to calculate TRP.

$$TRP = 100 \left(1 - \frac{\text{urine phosphorus} \times \text{serum creatinine}}{\text{urine creatinine} \times \text{serum phosphorus}} \right)$$

Normal: TRP is >78% on normal diet; higher on low-phosphate diet (430 mg/day)

Hyperparathyroidism: TRP is <74% on normal diet; <85% on low-phosphate diet

False-positive result may occur in uremia, renal tubular disease (some patients), osteomalacia, sarcoidosis.

URINE CONCENTRATION TEST

Restrict water intake for 14–16 hours; then collect three urines at 1-, 2-, and 4-hour intervals and measure specific gravity.

Normal. Urine specific gravity is ≥ 1.025.

With decreased renal function, specific gravity is <1.020. As renal impairment is more severe, specific gravity approaches 1.010.

The test is sensitive for early loss of renal function, but a normal finding does not necessarily rule out active kidney disease.

The test is unreliable in the presence of any severe water and electrolyte imbalance (e.g., adrenal cortical insufficiency, edema formation), low-protein or low-salt diet, chronic liver disease, pregnancy, lack of patient cooperation.

Fluid deprivation may be contraindicated in heart disease or early renal failure.

VASOPRESSIN (PITRESSIN) CONCENTRATION TEST

The bladder is emptied and urine is collected 1 and 2 hours after subcutaneous injection of 10 units of vasopressin. Water intake is not restricted, but no diuretics should be administered.

Normal. The specific gravity should reach ≥ 1.020.

Interpretation is the same as in the urine concentration test.

In diabetes insipidus, urine specific gravity becomes normal after vasopressin administration but not after fluid restriction.

The test may be used in the presence of edema or ascites. It is contraindicated in coronary artery disease and pregnancy.

See Diabetes Insipidus, pp. 422–423.

URINE OSMOLALITY

Measurement of urine osmolality during water restriction is an accurate, sensitive test of decreased renal function.

The patient is on a high-protein diet for 3 days; has a dry supper and no fluids on the evening before the test; empties the bladder at 6 A.M., discards urine, and returns to bed. Test urine specimen is collected at 8 A.M.

Normal: concentration of >800 mOsm/kg

Minimal impairment of renal concentrating ability: 600–800 mOsm/kg

Moderate impairment: 400–600 mOsm/kg

Severe impairment: <400 mOsm/kg

Urine osmolality may be impaired when other tests are normal (Fishberg concentration test, BUN, PSP excretion test, creatinine clearance, IV pyelogram); may be especially useful in diabetes mellitus, essential hypertension, silent pyelonephritis.

It may be well also to measure serum osmolality and calculate urine-serum ratio (normal = >3).

See Diabetes Insipidus, pp. 422–423.

URINE DILUTION TEST

No breakfast is allowed; 1500 ml of water is taken within 30–45 minutes, and urine is collected every hour for 4 hours.

Normal. Urine volume is >80% of ingested amount (1200 ml). Specific gravity is 1.003 in at least one specimen.

With decreased renal function there is a smaller volume of urine. Specific gravity may not fall below 1.010.

Loss of dilution ability occurs later than loss of concentrating ability.

Water loading may be contraindicated in kidney and heart disease.

PHENOLSULFONPHTHALEIN (PSP) EXCRETION TEST

Administer an IV injection of 1 mg/kg body weight or usually 6 mg in 1 ml volume. Collect urine and (sometimes) blood samples at 15-, 30-, and 60-minute intervals.

The test is useful to detect slight to moderate decrease in renal function. It is not useful in chronic azotemia with fixed specific gravity (serum creatinine and creatinine clearance are more useful then).

It is hazardous in severe renal insufficiency or heart failure because adequate prior hydration is required to obtain sufficient urine volume. Using small urine volumes magnifies errors.

The test is distorted by residual bladder urine, abnormal drainage sites (e.g., fistulas), and interfering substances (e.g., hematuria).

Hepatic disease may give falsely elevated values (because 20% of the dye is normally removed by the liver). False results may also occur in multiple myeloma (because of excessive protein binding) and in hypoalbuminemia. Certain drugs may interfere with PSP excretion (e.g., salicylates, penicillin, some diuretic and uricosuric drugs, and some x-ray contrast media).

The 15-minute PSP excretion correlates with the glomerular filtration rate (GFR); a normal 15-minute value indicates normal GFR. Progressive decrease of 15-minute value is proportional to decreased GFR (e.g., 15% PSP excretion in 15 minutes approximates a 45% GFR). If the GFR is normal, the PSP test indicates renal blood flow or tubular function; there are better tests available for measuring these two functions, and the PSP test is now rarely used.

Increased dye excretion in later time periods compared to the initial 15-minute period suggests increased residual urine due to obstructive uropathy or incomplete bladder emptying; the latter can be ruled out by indwelling catheterization during the test.

PSP that is normal with increased BUN and serum creatinine and decreased GFR suggests acute glomerulonephritis. PSP parallels these parameters in most chronic renal diseases.

OTHER RENAL FUNCTION TESTS*
Glomerular filtration rate (GFR) is measured with urea clearance, creatinine clearance, or inulin clearance.

Renal plasma flow (RPF) is measured with para-aminohippurate (PAH) clearance or Diodrast clearance.

Filtration fraction (FF) $= \dfrac{GFR}{RPF}$ (normal = 0.2)

Urea clearance is normal until >50% of renal parenchyma is inactivated. With renal insufficiency, the clearance test parallels the parenchymal destruction.

Urinary acidification is impaired in chronic renal disease with azotemia. It is decreased without parallel impairment of GFR in renal tubular acidosis, some cases of Fanconi syndrome, and some cases of acquired nephrocalcinosis.

Proximal tubular malfunction is indicated by urinary excretion of substances normally reabsorbed by tubules: in renal glycosuria (blood glucose <180 mg/100 as in Fanconi syndrome, heavy-metal poisoning), aminoaciduria, phosphaturia.

See also Serum BUN (p. 40), Serum Creatinine (p. 41), PSP Excretion Test (preceding section), Urine Concentration Test (p. 93) and Urine Dilution Test (p. 94).

Serum creatinine and BUN are not useful in discovering early renal insufficiency because they do not become abnormal until 50% of renal function has been lost. The creatinine clearance test, particularly serial measurements, is the most reliable test of renal function. After baseline measurements have been obtained, serum creatinine levels can be evaluated.

If there is a discrepancy between these two tests, additional studies

---

*See standard laboratory texts for information on the technical performance of clearance tests.

Table 9. Laboratory Guide to Evaluation of Renal Impairment

Condition	Renal Clearance of Endogenous Creatinine[a] (glomerular filtration rate)	Urinary Excretion of IV PSP[b] in 15 Minutes (renal tubular transport mechanisms)
Normal	Men: 130–200 L/24 hours (90–139 ml/min) Women: 115–180 L/24 hours (80–125 ml/min)	≧ 25%
Slight impairment	75–90 L/24 hours (52.0–62.5 ml/min)	15–25%
Mild impairment	60–75 L/24 hours (42–52 ml/min)	10–15%
Moderate impairment	40–60 L/24 hours (28–42 ml/min)	5–10%
Marked impairment	<40 L/24 hours (<28 ml/min)	<5%

[a]Creatinine clearance is normally less in women than men, and it usually decreases with age, starting at age 20.
[b]Phenolsulfonphthalein.

may be performed (e.g., concentration and dilution tests, urinalyses, biochemical studies of serum and urine, urine cultures, renalgrams and scans, biopsy).

Impairment may be more severe than indicated by laboratory studies if signs and symptoms are more disabling.

SPLIT RENAL FUNCTION TESTS
(for aid in diagnosis of renal artery stenosis)
Affected kidney shows decreased urine volume and sodium excretion, and decreased urine concentration of creatinine, inulin, or PAH.

These tests are not useful in presence of urinary tract obstruction (e.g., in men over age 50).

RENAL BIOPSY
Electron microscopy and immunofluorescent microscopy should be available.

May Be Indicated In
Acute renal failure to differentiate
> Acute glomerulonephritis—to be treated with immunosuppressive agents and dialysis
> Drug-induced (e.g., methicillin) acute interstitial nephritis with eosinophilia—to be treated with prednisone
> Interstitial nephritis and papillary necrosis due to analgesic drug abuse—to be treated with dialysis and cessation of analgesics (see p. 526)
> Systemic lupus erythematosus (SLE), necrotizing angiitis, and Goodpasture's syndrome (to be treated with prednisone or hydrocortisone) are to be distinguished from ischemic or nephrotoxic renal failure (to be treated with dialysis; does not need drug therapy).

Lipoid nephrosis to differentiate
> Systemic lupus erythematosus (SLE)—to be treated with prednisone
> Amyloid nephropathy—to be treated by therapy of underlying infection
> Occult bacterial endocarditis—to be treated with antibiotics
> Renal vein thrombosis—to be treated with anticoagulants
> Characteristic lipoid nephrosis of children and young adults is prednisone-responsive.
> Diffuse generalized membranous glomerulonephritis is steroid-resistant.
> Proliferative glomerulonephritis (e.g., poststreptococcal, anaphylactoid purpura) is to be treated with immunosuppressive agents.

Fixed and persistent proteinuria that does not respond to trial of prednisone therapy; routine biopsy not indicated in children or adolescents.

In adults, corticosteroid treatment should not be instituted until a responsive disease has been diagnosed by biopsy.

Diagnosis of unsuspected disease (e.g., nephrocalcinosis of hyper-parathyroidism)
Diagnosis of renal disease of unknown etiology
Evaluation of therapeutic effect (e.g., SLE, polyarteritis nodosa)
Complete diagnosis prior to renal transplantation or chronic dialysis
Culture of organism in some cases of pyelonephritis
Other

Contraindicated In
Patient with bleeding tendencies
Patient with unilateral kidney
Uncooperative patient

CYTOLOGIC EXAMINATION OF VAGINAL SMEAR (PAPANICOLAOU SMEAR) FOR EVALUATION OF OVARIAN FUNCTION

Maturation index (MI) is the proportion of parabasal, intermediate, and superficial cells in each 100 cells counted.

Lack of estrogen effect shows predominance of parabasal cells (e.g., MI = 100/0/0).

Low estrogen effect shows predominance of intermediate cells (e.g., MI = 10/90/0).

Increased estrogen effect shows predominance of superficial cells (e.g., MI = 0/0/100), as in hormone-producing tumors of ovary, persistent follicular cysts.

Some Patterns of Maturation Index in Different Conditions

	Index
Childhood	
Normal	80/20/0
Cortisone therapy	0/98/2
Childbearing years	
Preovulatory (late follicular) phase	0/40/60
Premenstrual (late luteal) phase	0/70/30
Pregnancy (second month)	0/90/10
Cortisone therapy	0/85/15
Amenorrhea after ovarian irradiation	0/30/70
Surgical oophorectomy	0/80/20–0/90/10
Bilateral oophorectomy and adrenalectomy	0/98/2
Postmenopausal years, early (age 60)	65/30/5
Postmenopausal years, late (age 75)	
Untreated	100/0/0
Moderate estrogen treatment	0/50/50
High-dose estrogen treatment	0/0/100
Years after bilateral oophorectomy	100/0/0
Postadrenalectomy, bilateral	6/94/0

Karyopyknotic index (KI) is the percent of cells with pyknotic nuclei.

Increased estrogen effect (e.g., KI = >85%) is seen, as in cystic glandular hyperplasia of the endometrium.
Eosinophilic index is the percent of cells showing eosinophilic cytoplasm; it may also be used as a measure of estrogen effect.
Combined progesterone-estrogen effect. No quantitative cytologic criteria are available. Endometrial biopsy should be used for this purpose.

The pattern may be obscured by cytolysis (e.g., infections, excess bacilli), increased red or white blood cells, excessively thin or thick smears, or drying of smears before fixation (artificial eosinophilic staining)

HEMATOLOGY

CAUSES OF LEUKOPENIA
Infections, especially
    Bacterial (e.g., overwhelming bacterial infection, septicemia, miliary tuberculosis, typhoid, paratyphoid, brucellosis, tularemia)
    Viral (e.g., infectious mononucleosis, hepatitis, influenza, measles, rubella, psittacosis)
    Rickettsial (e.g., scrub typhus, sandfly fever)
    Other (e.g., malaria, kala-azar)
Drugs and chemicals, especially
    Sulfonamides
    Antibiotics
    Analgesics
    Marrow depressants
    Arsenicals
    Antithyroid drugs
    Many others
Ionizing radiation
Hematopoietic diseases
    Pernicious anemia
    Aleukemic leukemia
    Aplastic anemia and related conditions
    Hypersplenism
    Gaucher's disease
    Felty's syndrome
Anaphylactic shock
Cachexia
Miscellaneous
    Disseminated lupus erythematosus
    Severe renal injury
    Various neutropenias
Artifactual associated with automated WBC counters (artifact is corrected when manual WBC counts are performed)
    Leukocyte fragility due to immunosuppressive and antineoplastic drugs
    Lymphocyte fragility in lymphocytic leukemia
    Excessive clumping of leukocytes in monoclonal gam-

mopathies (e.g., multiple myeloma), cryofibrinogenemia (e.g., SLE), in presence of cold agglutinins

CAUSES OF LEUKOCYTOSIS
Acute infections
    Localized (e.g., pneumonia, meningitis, tonsillitis, abscess)
    Generalized (e.g., acute rheumatic fever, septicemia, cholera)
Intoxications
    Metabolic (uremia, acidosis, eclampsia, acute gout)
        Poisoning by chemicals, drugs, venoms, etc. (e.g., mercury, epinephrine, black widow spider)
        Parenteral foreign protein and vaccines
Acute hemorrhage
Acute hemolysis of red blood cells
Myeloproliferative diseases
Tissue necrosis
    Acute myocardial infarction
    Necrosis of tumors
    Burns
    Gangrene
    Bacterial necrosis, etc.
Physiologic conditions (e.g., exercise, emotional stress, menstruation, obstetrical labor)

CAUSES OF LYMPHOCYTOSIS
Infections
    Pertussis
    Infectious lymphocytosis
    Infectious mononucleosis
    Infectious hepatitis
    Mumps
    German measles
    Chronic tuberculosis
    Undulant fever
    Convalescence from acute infection
    Thyrotoxicosis (relative)
    Neutropenia with relative lymphocytosis
    Lymphatic leukemia

CAUSES OF ATYPICAL LYMPHOCYTES
Lymphatic leukemia
Viral infections
    Infectious lymphocytosis
    Infectious mononucleosis
    Infectious hepatitis
    Viral penumonia and other exanthems of childhood
    Mumps
    Chickenpox
    German measles
Pertussis
Brucellosis
Syphilis (in some phases)
Toxoplasmosis

Table 10. Some Common Causes of Leukemoid Reaction

Cause	Myelocytic	Lymphocytic	Monocytic

Infections	Endocarditis
	Pneumonia
	Septicemia
	Leptospirosis
	Other
		Infections mono-
		  nucleosis
		Infectious lympho-
		  cytosis
		Pertussis
		Chickenpox
		Tuberculosis
			Tuberculosis

Toxic
  conditions
	Burns
	Eclampsia
	Poisoning (e.g.,
	  mercury)		

Neoplasms	Carcinoma of colon
	Embryonal car-
	  cinoma of kidney
		Carcinoma of
		  stomach
		Carcinoma of breast	

Miscellaneous	Treatment of mega-
	  loblastic anemia
	  (of pregnancy,
	  pernicious anemia)
	Acute hemorrhage
	Acute hemolysis
	Recovery from
	  agranulocytosis
		Dermatitis
		  herpetiformis	

Myeloprolifera- tive diseases			

CLUES TO DIAGNOSIS OF ATYPICAL OR LEUKOPENIC LEUKEMIA
Peripheral monocytosis
Peripheral cytopenia with normoblasts
Hypercellular marrow with hyperplasia of myeloid and/or erythroid elements
Acquired Pelger-Huët anomaly (see p. 319).

BASOPHILIC LEUKOCYTES

Increased In
Chronic myelogenous leukemia
Polycythemia
Myeloid metaplasia
Hodgkin's disease
Postsplenectomy
Chronic hemolytic anemia (some patients)
Chronic sinusitis
Chickenpox
Smallpox
Myxedema
Nephrosis (some patients)
Foreign protein injection

Decreased In
Hyperthyroidism

Pregnancy
Period following irradiation, chemotherapy, and glucocorticoids
Acute phase of infection

CAUSES OF MONOCYTOSIS
(>10% of differential count; absolute count >500/cu mm)
Monocytic leukemia, other leukemias
Myeloproliferative disorders (myeloid metaplasia, polycythemia vera)
Hodgkin's disease and other malignant lymphomas
Lipid storage diseases (e.g., Gaucher's disease)
Tetrachlorethane poisoning
Recovery from agranulocytosis and subsidence of acute infection
Many protozoan infections (e.g., malaria, kala-azar, trypanosomiasis)
Some rickettsial infections (e.g., Rocky Mountain spotted fever, typhus)
Certain bacterial infections (e.g., subacute bacterial endocarditis, tuberculosis, brucellosis)
Chronic ulcerative colitis and regional enteritis
Sarcoidosis
Collagen diseases (e.g., rheumatoid arthritis, SLE)

PLASMA CELLS

Increased In
Plasma cell leukemia
Multiple myeloma
Serum reaction
Infectious mononucleosis
Rubella
Measles
Chickenpox
Benign lymphocytic meningitis

Decreased In
Not clinically significant

CAUSES OF EOSINOPHILIA
Allergic diseases (e.g., bronchial asthma, hay fever, urticaria, drug therapy)
Parasitic infestation, especially with tissue invasion (e.g., trichinosis, echinococcus disease) (see Pulmonary Infiltrations Associated with Eosinophilia, p. 186).
Some infectious diseases (e.g., scarlet fever, erythema multiforme)
Some skin diseases (e.g., pemphigus, dermatitis herpetiformis)
Some hematopoietic diseases (e.g., pernicious anemia, chronic myelogenous leukemia, polycythemia, Hodgkin's disease); postsplenectomy
Some gastrointestinal diseases (e.g., eosinophilic gastroenteritis, ulcerative colitis, regional enteritis)
Postirradiation
Miscellaneous conditions

Polyarteritis nodosa
Certain tumors (ovary, involvement of bone or serosal sur-
faces)
Sarcoidosis
Loeffler's parietal fibroplastic endocarditis (see p. 178).
Familial condition
Poisoning (e.g., phosphorus, black widow spider bite)

LEUKOCYTE ALKALINE PHOSPHATASE STAINING REACTION
(in untreated diseases)

Usually Increased In
Leukemoid reaction
Polycythemia vera
Lymphoma (including Hodgkin's, reticulum cell sarcoma)
Acute and chronic lymphatic leukemia
Multiple myeloma
Myelosclerosis
Aplastic anemia
Agranulocytosis
Bacterial infections
Cirrhosis
Obstructive jaundice
Pregnancy and immediate postpartum period
Administration of Enovid
Mongolism (trisomy 21)
Klinefelter's syndrome (XXY)

Usually Decreased In
Chronic myelogenous leukemia
Paroxysmal nocturnal hemoglobinuria
Hereditary hypophosphatasia
Nephrotic syndrome
Progressive muscular dystrophy
Refractory anemia (siderotic)
Sickle cell anemia

Usually Normal In
Secondary polycythemia
Hemolytic anemia
Infectious mononucleosis
Viral hepatitis
Lymphosarcoma

Usually Variable In
Pernicious anemia
Idiopathic thrombocytopenic purpura
Iron-deficiency anemia
Acute myelogenous leukemia
Acute undifferentiated leukemia

This test is clinically most useful in differentiating chronic myelogenous leukemia from leukemoid reaction.

NITROBLUE TETRAZOLIUM (NBT) REDUCTION IN NEUTROPHILS

Increased In
Bacterial infections, including miliary tuberculosis and tuberculous meningitis
Nocardia and other systemic fungal infections
Various parasitic infections
Malaria
Chédiak-Higashi syndrome
Idiopathic myelofibrosis
Normal infants up to age 2 months
Pregnancy
Patients taking birth control pills
Some patients with lymphoma suppressed by chemotherapy

Decreased or Normal (in absence of bacterial infection)
Normal persons
Postpartum state
Postoperative state (after 7–10 days)
Cancer
Tissue transplantation
Other conditions with fever or leukocytosis not due to bacterial infection (e.g., rheumatoid arthritis)

Decreased or Normal (in presence of bacterial infection)
Antibiotic therapy—effectiveness of treatment indicated by reduction of previous elevation, sometimes in <6 hours
Localized infection
Administration of corticosteroids and immunosuppressive drugs (contrary findings with corticosteroids have also been reported)
Miscellaneous conditions, probably involving metabolic defects of neutrophil function
    Chronic granulomatous disease
    Neutrophilic deficiency of glucose-6-phosphate dehydrogenase or myeloperoxidase
    SLE
    Sickle cell disease
    Chronic myelogenous leukemia
    Lipochrome histiocytosis
    Congenital and acquired agammaglobulinemia
    Other

Increased (from previously determined normal level)
May be used before other clinical parameters to monitor development of infection in chronically ill patients
    Development of wound sepsis in burn patients
    Development of infection in uremic patients on chronic hemodialysis
    Other

Usual normal values reported are <10% but there is considerable variation (≦14%), and each laboratory should establish its own normal range.

NBT test has been used principally in differentiating untreated bacterial infection from other conditions that may simulate it and for the diagnosis of poor neutrophilic function, particularly in chronic granulomatous disease. In many studies, few patients are included, considerable variation in technical performance occurs, or inadequate data are presented for comparison. Further evaluation of the clinical usefulness of the test in many of the conditions in which contradictory findings have been reported must await more definitive studies.

PLATELET COUNT

May Be Increased In (>500,000/cu mm)
Malignancy, especially disseminated, advanced, or inoperable
Myeloproliferative disease (e.g., polycythemia vera, chronic myelogenous leukemia)
Patients recently having surgery, especially splenectomy
Collagen disorders, usually rheumatoid arthritis
Iron deficiency anemia
Miscellaneous disease states (e.g., acute infection, cardiac disease, cirrhosis of the liver, chronic pancreatitis)

Approximately 50% of patients with "unexpected" increase of platelet count are found to have a malignancy.

Decreased In
See Thrombocytopenic Purpura (p. 333).

ERYTHROCYTE SEDIMENTATION RATE (ESR)
(see Table 11)
ESR is useful to
> Detect occult disease (e.g., screening program)
> Follow course of a certain disease (e.g., tuberculosis, rheumatic fever, myocardial infarction)
> Confirm a diagnosis or a differential diagnosis (e.g., acute myocardial infarction as opposed to angina pectoris; early acute appendicitis versus ruptured ectopic pregnancy or acute pelvic inflammatory disease; rheumatoid arthritis as opposed to osteoarthritis)

Decreased In
Sickle cell anemia
Polycythemia
Hyperviscosity syndrome should be suspected in patients with hyperproteinemia (e.g., multiple myeloma, Waldenström's macroglobulinemia) with rouleaux formation but no increase of ESR.

SERUM C-REACTIVE PROTEIN (CRP)
Normally CRP is not detected in serum.

Increased In
Any acute inflammatory change or necrosis. CRP precedes the rise in ESR; with recovery, disappearance of CRP precedes the

Table 11. Changes in Erythrocyte Sedimentation Rate[a]

Disease	Increased In	Not Increased In
Infectious	Tuberculosis (especially) Acute hepatitis	Typhoid fever Undulant fever Malarial paroxysm Infectious mononucleosis Uncomplicated viral diseases
Cardiac	Acute myocardial infarction Active rheumatic fever Postcommissurotomy syndrome	Angina pectoris Active renal failure with heart failure
Abdominal	Acute pelvic inflammatory disease Ruptured ectopic pregnancy Pregnancy—third month to about 3 weeks postpartum Menstruation	Acute appendicitis (first 24 hours) Unruptured ectopic pregnancy Early pregnancy
Joint	Rheumatoid arthritis Pyogenic arthritis	Degenerative arthritis
Miscellaneous	Significant tissue necrosis especially neoplasms (most frequently malignant lymphoma, cancer of colon and breast) Increased serum globulins (e.g., myeloma, cryoglobulinemia, macroglobulinuria) Decreased serum albumin Hypothyroidism Hyperthyroidism Acute hemorrhage Nephrosis, renal disease with azotemia Arsenic and lead intoxication Dextran and polyvinyl compounds in blood	Peptic ulcer Acute allergy Polycythemia vera Secondary polycythemia Sickle cell anemia, spherocytosis, anisocytosis

[a]Extreme elevation of ESR is found particularly in association with malignancy (most frequently malignant lymphoma, carcinomas of colon and breast), hematologic diseases (most frequently myeloma), collagen diseases (e.g., rheumatoid arthritis, SLE), renal diseases (especially with azotemia), infections, and other conditions (e.g., cirrhosis). Westergren method is more accurate; Wintrobe method is more convenient.

return to normal of the ESR. CRP disappears when inflammatory process is suppressed by steroids or salicylates.

Acute myocardial infarction. CRP appears within 24–48 hours, begins to fall by third day and becomes negative after 1–2 weeks.

Acute rheumatic fever. CRP reflects rheumatic activity more
promptly than ESR.
Bacterial infections
Neoplasm with widespread metastases

Increased Inconsistently In
Active tuberculosis
Viral infections
Rheumatoid arthritis

PERIPHERAL BLOOD SMEAR IN DIFFERENTIAL DIAGNOSIS OF ANEMIAS

The smear may also indicate leukemia, other conditions.
Confirm the RBC indices.
Basophilic or polychromatophilic macrocytes—shows increased
erythropoiesis in hemorrhage or hemolysis
Oval macrocytes with increased number of lobules of polynuclear
leukocytes—in megaloblastic anemia
Target cells—in hemoglobinopathies (especially Hb C); also
thalassemia, iron deficiency anemia, liver disease
Abnormally shaped RBCs—ovalocytes, sickle cells, spherocytes,
poikilocytes, schistocytes
Microcytes with stippling—in thalassemia, lead poisoning

CONDITIONS ASSOCIATED WITH RBC INCLUSIONS

Reticulocytes*	Any condition with increased reticulocyte count
Basophilic stippling (multiple dark dots)	Lead poisoning, heavy metal poisoning, and severe anemia
Cabot's rings	Occasionally seen in severe hemolytic anemias and pernicious anemia
Howell-Jolly bodies (dark purple spherical bodies)	Occasionally seen in severe hemolytic anemias and pernicious anemia
	Occasionally seen in leukemia, thalassemia, postsplenectomy
Pappenheimer bodies (siderotic granules) (purple coccoid granules at periphery)	Anemias with defect of incorporating iron into hemoglobin; show hypochromic microcytic anemia with increased serum iron and total iron-binding capacity (e.g., thalassemia, lead poisoning, di Gugliel-mo's disease, pyridoxine-responsive anemia, pyridoxine-unresponsive anemia)

*Not seen with Wright's stain; requires supravital cresyl violet stain.

Heinz-Ehrlich bodies*	Congenital G-6-PD deficiencies; other drug-induced hemolytic anemias
Plasmodium trophozoites	Malaria

RETICULOCYTES

Increased In
After blood loss of increased RBC destruction: normal response is three- to sixfold increase
After iron therapy for iron deficiency anemia
After specific therapy for megaloblastic anemias

Increase indicates effective RBC production mechanisms. It is a useful index of therapeutic response in these diseases.

Possibly other hematologic conditions (e.g., polycythemia, metastatic carcinoma in bone marrow, di Guglielmo's disease)

Decreased In
Ineffective erythropoiesis or decreased RBC formation
    Severe autoimmune type of hemolytic disease
    Aregenerative crises

SICKLING OF RBCs

Occurs In
Sickle cell disease
Sickle cell trait

False Positive In
First 4 months after transfusion with RBCs having sickle cell trait
Mixture on slide with fibrinogen, thrombin, gelatin (glue)
Excessive concentration of sodium metabisulfite (e.g., $\geqq 4\%$ instead of 2%)
Drying of wet coverslip preparation
Poikilocytosis

False Negative In
First 4 months after transfusion with normal RBCs
Heating, bacterial contamination, or prolonged washing with saline of RBCs
Newborn

Sickling should be confirmed with hemoglobin electrophoresis and genetic studies.

SEVERELY DISTORTED RBCs (BURR, HELMET, TRIANGLE, ACANTHOID FORMS) IN PERIPHERAL BLOOD SMEARS
These cells may be found in some acquired hemolytic disorders (some patients with mechanical factors that cause RBC damage

*Not seen with Wright's stain; requires supravital cresyl violet stain.

and distortion with secondary hemolysis; some patients with consumption coagulopathy [defibrination syndrome]):
  Prosthetic heart valves
  Severe rheumatic valvular disease
  Hemolytic anemia in uremia
  Thrombotic thrombocytopenic purpura
  Gastric carcinoma and peptic ulcer with bleeding
  Microangiopathic hemolytic anemia
  Cirrhosis with hemolytic anemia (associated with thrombocytopenia, reticulocytosis, increased serum indirect bilirubin)
  Hereditary acanthocytosis, pyruvate kinase deficiency, hexokinase deficiency
  Snakebite (see p. 532)

OSMOTIC FRAGILITY

Increased In
Hereditary spherocytic anemia (*This disease can be ruled out if there is a normal fragility after 24-hour sterile incubation.*)
Hereditary nonspherocytic hemolytic anemia
Acquired hemolytic anemia (*usually normal in paroxysmal nocturnal hemoglobinuria*)
Hemolytic disease of newborn due to ABO incompatibility
Some cases of secondary hemolytic anemia (usually normal)
After thermal injury
Symptomatic hemolytic anemia in some cases of
    Malignant lymphoma
    Leukemia
    Carcinoma
    Pregnancy
    Cirrhosis
    Infection (e.g., tuberculosis, malaria, syphilis)

Decreased In
Early infancy
Iron deficiency anemia
Thalassemia
Sickle cell anemia
Homozygous hemoglobin C disease
Nutritional megaloblastic anemia
Postsplenectomy
Liver disease
Jaundice

SERUM IRON

Increased In
Idiopathic hemochromatosis
Hemosiderosis of excessive iron intake (e.g., repeated blood transfusions, iron therapy)
Decreased formation of RBCs (e.g., thalassemia, pyridoxine-deficiency anemia, pernicious anemia in relapse)
Increased destruction of RBCs (e.g., hemolytic anemias)

Acute liver damage (degree of increase parallels the amount of hepatic necrosis); some cases of chronic liver disease
Progesteronal birth control pills

Decreased In
Iron deficiency anemia
Normochromic (normocytic or microcytic) anemias of infection and chronic diseases (e.g., neoplasms, active collagen diseases)
Nephrosis (due to loss of iron-binding protein in urine)
Pernicious anemia at onset of remission

SERUM TOTAL IRON-BINDING CAPACITY (TIBC)

Increased In
Iron deficiency anemia
Acute and chronic blood loss
Hepatitis
Late pregnancy

Decreased In
Hemochromatosis
Cirrhosis of the liver
Thalassemia
Anemias of infection and chronic diseases (e.g., uremia, rheumatoid arthritis, some neoplasms)
Nephrosis

SERUM TRANSFERRIN SATURATION

Increased In
Hemochromatosis
Hemosiderosis
Thalassemia

Decreased In
Iron deficiency anemia
Anemias of infection and chronic diseases (e.g., uremia, rheumatoid arthritis, some neoplasms)

SERUM FERRITIN
Chief iron-storage protein in the body
Reflects reticuloendothelial storage of iron

Decreased In
Iron deficiency anemia

Increased In
Iron overload, e.g., hemosiderosis, normal idiopathic hemochromatosis (*can be used to monitor therapeutic removal of excess storage iron*)
Anemias other than iron deficiency, e.g., inflammation
Many patients with various acute and chronic liver diseases
Leukemias and Hodgkin's disease

STAINABLE IRON (HEMOSIDERIN) IN BONE MARROW

Increased In
Hemolytic anemias (decrease or absence may signify acute hemolytic crisis)
Megaloblastic anemias in relapse
Hemochromatosis and hemosiderosis
Uremia (some patients)
Chronic infection (some patients)
Chronic pancreatic insufficiency

Decreased In
Iron deficiency anemia (e.g., inadequate dietary intake, chronic bleeding, malignancy, acute blood loss)
Polycythemia vera (usually absent in polycythemia vera but usually normal or increased in secondary polycythemia)
Pernicious anemia in early phase of therapy
Collagen diseases (especially rheumatoid arthritis, systemic lupus erythematosus)
Infiltration of marrow (e.g., malignant lymphomas, metastatic carcinoma, myelofibrosis, miliary granulomas)
Uremia
Chronic infection (e.g., pulmonary tuberculosis, bronchiectasis, chronic pyelonephritis)
Miscellaneous conditions (e.g., old age, diabetes mellitus)

The absence of iron in marrow is the most reliable index of iron deficiency; its presence almost invariably rules out iron deficiency anemia. Only individuals with decreased marrow iron are likely to benefit from iron therapy.

Marrow iron disappears before the peripheral blood changes. It rapidly disappears after hemorrhage.

One may have a normal serum iron and TIBC in iron deficiency anemia, especially if Hb is <9 gm/100 ml.

EXCESSIVE IRON DEPOSITION IN DISEASES ASSOCIATED WITH IRON OVERLOAD
Idiopathic hemochromatosis
Hemochromatosis secondary to
    Increased intake (e.g., Bantu siderosis, excessive medicine ingestion)
    Anemias with increased erythropoiesis (especially thalassemia major; also thalassemia minor, some other hemoglobinopathies, paroxysmal nocturnal hemoglobinuria, "sideroachrestic" anemias, refractory anemias with hypercellular bone marrow, etc.)
    Liver injury (e.g., following portal shunt surgery)
    Atransferrinemia

SERUM CERULOPLASMIN

Decreased In
Wilson's disease (deficient or absent in early stages) (*may be normal in 2–5% of patients*)
Moderate transient deficiencies in some patients with
   Nephrosis
   Sprue
   Kwashiorkor
Normal infants

Increased In
Pregnancy
Patients taking estrogen or birth control pills
Rheumatoid arthritis (may cause green color of plasma)
Thyrotoxicosis
Cancer
Cirrhosis
Infection

*Measure ceruloplasmin in any patient under age 30 with hepatitis,
   hemolysis, or neurologic symptoms to allow early diagnosis and
   treatment of Wilson's disease.*

SERUM COPPER

Increased In
Anemias
   Pernicious anemia
   Megaloblastic anemia of pregnancy
   Iron deficiency anemia
   Aplastic anemia
Leukemia, acute and chronic
Infection, acute and chronic
Malignant lymphoma
Hemochromatosis
Collagen diseases (including SLE, rheumatoid arthritis, acute
   rheumatic fever, glomerulonephritis)
Hypothyroidism
Hyperthyroidism
Frequently associated with increased C-reactive protein

Decreased In
Nephrosis (ceruloplasmin lost in urine)
Wilson's disease
Acute leukemia in remission
Some iron deficiency anemias of childhood (that require copper as
   well as iron therapy)
Kwashiorkor

SERUM VITAMIN B_{12}

Increased In
Leukemia—acute and chronic myelogenous; about one-third of the

cases of chronic lymphatic; some cases of monocytic. Normal in stem cell leukemia, multiple myeloma, Hodgkin's disease.
Leukocytosis
Polycythemia vera
Some cases of carcinoma (especially with liver metastases)
Liver disease (acute hepatitis, chronic hepatitis, cirrhosis, hepatic coma)

Decreased In
Inadequate absorption
    Lack of intrinsic factor
        Pernicious anemia
        Loss of gastric mucosa (e.g., gastrectomy, cancer of stomach)
        Primary hypothyroidism (Almost 50% of patients have serum achlorhydria with intrinsic factor failure and low vitamin B_{12}; rarely megaloblastic anemia develops.)
    Malabsorption (e.g., sprue, celiac disease, idiopathic steatorrhea, regional ileitis, fistulas, resection of bowel)
    Loss of ingested vitamin B_{12}; fish tapeworm (*Diphyllobothrium latum*) infestation
    Inadequate intake due to severe dietary restrictions
Pregnancy—progressive decrease during pregnancy (*normal serum B_{12} level in megaloblastic anemia of pregnancy*)

SERUM FOLIC ACID

Decreased In
Inadequate intake (e.g., megaloblastic anemia of pregnancy, megaloblastic anemia of infancy, nutritional megaloblastic anemia, some cases of liver disease)
Malabsorption (e.g., sprue, celiac disease, idiopathic steatorrhea)
Folic acid antagonist drugs (e.g., Aminopterin for treatment of leukemia, anticonvulsant drugs)
Excessive utilization due to marked cellular proliferation (e.g., hemolytic anemias, myeloproliferative diseases, carcinomas)

Serum folic acid activity <3 ng/ml is associated with a positive formiminoglutamic acid (FIGLU) test and positive hematologic findings.
Serum folic acid activity 3–6 ng/ml is associated with a variable FIGLU test and variable hematologic findings.
Serum folic acid activity >6 ng/ml is associated with a normal FIGLU test and normal hematologic findings.

Increased In
Period following folic acid administration
Vegetarians
Some cases of blind loop syndrome (due to folate synthesis by bacteria in intestine)
A few patients with pure vitamin B_{12} deficiency anemia

FETAL HEMOGLOBIN
(alkali denaturation method; confirmed by examination of hemoglobin bands on electrophoresis)

Normal
<2% over age 2
>50% at birth; gradual decrease to $\cong$ 5% by age 5 months

Increased In
Various hemoglobinopathies (see Table 42, pp. 298–299). $\cong$ 50% of patients with thalassemia minor have high levels of HbF; even higher levels are found in virtually all patients with thalassemia major. In sickle cell disease, Hb F > 30% protects the cell from sickling; therefore, even infants with homozygous S have few problems before age 3 months.

Hereditary persistence of fetal hemoglobin

Nonhereditary refractory normoblastic anemia (one-third of patients)

Pernicious anemia (50% of untreated patients); increases after treatment and then gradually decreases during next 6 months; some patients still have slight elevation thereafter. Minimal elevation occurs in $\cong$ 15% of patients with other types of megaloblastic anemia.

Some patients with leukemia, especially juvenile myeloid leukemia with Hb F of 30–60%, absence of Philadelphia chromosome, rapid fatal course, more pronounced thrombocytopenia, and lower total WBC count

Multiple myeloma

Molar pregnancy

Patients with an extra D chromosome (trisomy 13–15, D_1 trisomy) or an extra G chromosome (trisomy 21, Down's syndrome, mongolism)

Acquired aplastic anemia (due to drugs, toxic chemicals, or infections, or idiopathic); returns to normal only after complete remission and therefore is reliable indicator of complete recovery. Better prognosis in patients with higher initial level.

Decreased In
A rare case of multiple chromosome abnormalities (probably C/D translocation)

SERUM HEMOGLOBIN

Slight Increase In
Sickle cell thalassemia
Hemoglobin C disease

Moderate Increase In
Sickle cell–hemoglobin C disease
Sickle cell anemia
Thalassemia major
Acquired (autoimmune) hemolytic anemia

Marked Increase In
Any rapid intravascular hemolysis

SERUM HAPTOGLOBINS

Increased In
One-third of patients with obstructive biliary disease
Conditions associated with increased ESR and alpha$_2$ globulin (infection; inflammation; trauma; necrosis of tissue; collagen diseases such as rheumatic fever, rheumatoid arthritis, and dermatomyositis, scurvy, amyloidosis; nephrotic syndrome; disseminated neoplasms such as Hodgkin's disease, lymphosarcoma)
Therapy with steroids or androgens

Decreased In
Parenchymatous liver disease (especially cirrhosis)
Hemoglobinemia (related to the duration and severity of hemolysis)
Due To
    Intravascular hemolysis
    Extravascular hemolysis (e.g., large retroperitoneal hemorrhage, hereditary spherocytosis with marked hemolysis, pyruvate kinase deficiency, autoimmune hemolytic anemia, some transfusion reactions)
    Intramedullary hemolysis (e.g., thalassemia, megaloblastic anemias, sideroblastic anemias)
Genetically absent in 1% of general population

Haptoglobin determinations are useful
    When splenectomy is being considered. Patients with chronic hemolysis (e.g., hereditary spherocytosis, pyruvate kinase deficiency) should not have splenectomy when serum haptoglobin is >40 mg/100 ml if infection and inflammation have been ruled out. Increased haptoglobin level following splenectomy for these conditions indicates success of surgery; haptoglobin reappears at 24 hours and becomes normal in 4–6 days in hereditary spherocytosis treated with splenectomy.
    In diagnosis of transfusion reaction by comparison of pretransfusion and posttransfusion levels. Posttransfusion reaction serum haptoglobin level decreases in 6–8 hours; at 24 hours it is <40 mg/100 ml or <40% of pretransfusion level.
    In paternity studies. May aid by determination of haptoglobin phenotypes.

BONE MARROW ASPIRATION

May Be Useful In
Nonhematologic diseases
    Metastatic tumor
    Parasitic infestations (e.g., malaria, kala-azar, histoplasmosis)
    Infections (e.g., tuberculosis, brucellosis)

Granulomas (e.g., sarcoidosis, Hodgkin's disease)
Histiocytoses (Gaucher's disease, Niemann-Pick disease)
Hemosiderin staining of bone marrow
Hematologic diseases
With normal myeloid-erythyroid ratio (in normal adult it is
3 : 1–4 : 1)
Aplastic anemia
Myelosclerosis
Multiple myeloma
Diseases of megakaryocytes
With increased myeloid-erythyroid ratio
Most infections
Leukemoid reaction
Myeloid leukemias
Decreased number of nucleated red cells
With decreased myeloid-erythyroid ratio
Decreased number of myeloid cells (agranulocytosis)
Hyperplasia of erythyroid cells
Megaloblastic anemias (see, e.g., pernicious anemia,
sprue, steatorrhea)
Normoblastic anemias (see, e.g., iron deficiency
anemia, hemorrhage, hemolysis, thalassemia)
Normoblastic hyperplasia (e.g., polycythemia vera)

NEEDLE ASPIRATION OF SPLEEN

May Be Useful In
Differential diagnosis of
Lymphocytic leukemia (>90% lymphocytes, many of which
are abnormal and have increased number of mitoses)
Myelocytic leukemia (20–60% of cells are myelocytes)
Myeloid metaplasia of spleen with myelofibrosis (50–60% of
cells are lymphocytes that still persist)
Chronic inflammatory splenomegaly (myelocytes are <5% of
cells)
Leukemoid reaction and leukemia
Parasitic infestations (e.g., malaria, leishmaniasis)
Infections (e.g., tuberculosis, brucellosis)
Histiocytoses
Hodgkin's disease

See Some Causes of Splenomegaly, p. 320–321.

SMEARS OF LYMPH NODE PUNCTURE

May Be Useful In Diagnosis Of
Metastatic carcinoma
Acute and chronic lymphatic leukemia
Lymphosarcoma
Hodgkin's disease
Lymphadenitis

COAGULATION

DUKE BLEEDING TIME
Normal is 1–4 minutes; ≤ 5.5 minutes is not necessarily pathologic. The test is useful as part of a coagulation workup.

Usually Prolonged In
Thrombocytopenia
Defective platelet function (thrombocytopathies)
von Willebrand's disease (2 hours after dose of 10 grains of aspirin; bleeding time is variable without this aspirin tolerance test)
Other coagulation defects—variable results

Usually Normal In
Hemophilia
Severe hereditary hypoprothrombinemia
Severe hereditary hypofibrinogenemia
Scurvy
Other

COAGULATION (CLOTTING) TIME (CT) ("LEE-WHITE CLOTTING TIME")

Prolonged In
Severe deficiency of any known plasma clotting factors except Factors XIII (fibrin-stabilizing factor) and VII
Afibrinogenemia
Marked hyperheparinemia

Normal In
Thrombocytopenia
Deficiency of Factor VII
von Willebrand's disease
Mild coagulation defects due to any cause

This is the routine method for control of heparin therapy. It is not a reliable screening test for bleeding conditions because it is not sensitive enough to detect mild conditions but will only detect severe ones. Normal CT does not rule out a coagulation defect. There are many variables in the technique of performing the test.

TOURNIQUET TEST

Positive In
Thrombocytopenic purpuras
Nonthrombocytopenic purpuras
Thrombocytopathies
Scurvy

PROTHROMBIN TIME (PT)

Prolonged by Defect In
Factor I (fibrinogen)
Factor II (prothrombin)
Factor V (labile factor)
Factor VII (stable factor)
Factor X (Stuart-Prower factor)

Prolonged In
Inadequate vitamin K in diet
    Premature infants
    Newborn infants of vitamin K–deficient mothers (hemorrhagic
      disease of the newborn)
Poor fat absorption (e.g., obstructive jaundice, fistulas, sprue,
    steatorrhea, celiac disease, colitis, chronic diarrhea)
Severe liver damage (e.g., poisoning, hepatitis, cirrhosis)
Drugs (e.g., coumarin-type drugs for anticoagulant therapy, salicy-
    lates)
Idiopathic familial hypoprothrombinemia
Circulating anticoagulants
Hypofibrinogenemia (acquired or inherited)

The test is very useful for control of long-term oral anticoagulant
    therapy.

PARTIAL THROMBOPLASTIN TIME (PTT)

Prolonged by Defect In
Factor I (fibrinogen)
Factor II (prothrombin)
Factor V (labile factor)
Factor VIII
Factor IX
Factor X (Stuart-Prower)
Factor XI
Factor XII (Hageman)

Normal In
Thrombocytopenia
Platelet dysfunction
von Willebrand's disease (may be prolonged in some patients)
Isolated defects of Factor VII

PTT is the best *single screening* test for disorders of coagulation; it
    is abnormal in 90% of patients with coagulation disorders when
    properly performed.
The test may not detect mild clotting defects (25–40% of normal
    levels), which seldon cause significant bleeding.

PROTHROMBIN CONSUMPTION
Impaired by any defect in phase I or phase II of blood coagulation
    Thrombocytopathies
    Thrombocytopenia

Hypoprothrombinemia
Hemophilias
Circulating anticoagulants
Other

THROMBOPLASTIN GENERATION TEST (TGT)
(Table 12)

This test uses 3 components ($BaSO_4$-adsorbed plasma, serum, washed platelets) that are individually substituted in turn to mixtures of patient's blood to localize the defect in thromboplastin generation. It can be used to localize coagulation defects due to
Factor VIII
Factor IX (may not detect mild deficiencies)
Factor X
Factor V
Factor VII
Thrombasthenia
Circulating anticoagulant

It may not detect disease after recent blood or plasma transfusion.

Table 12. Thromboplastin Generation Test

Components	Mixtures			
$BaSO_4$-adsorbed plasma (Factors V, VIII present; VII, IX, X absent) from	P	P	N	N
Serum (VII, IX, X present; V, VII absent) from	P	N	P	N
Washed platelets from	N	N	N	P
Abnormality				
Normal	+	+	+	+
Thrombocytopenia, thrombocytasthenia	+	+	+	0
von Willebrand's disease	0	0	+	+
Factor V deficiency (severe)	0	0	+	+
Factor VII deficiency	+	+	+	+
Factor VIII deficiency (hemophilia)	0	0	+	+
Factor IX deficiency (Christmas disease)	0	+	0	+
Factor X deficiency	0	+	0	+
Factor XI (PTA) deficiency	0	+	+	+
Factor XII deficiency	0	+	+	+
Circulating anticoagulant	0	0	0	+

P = patient; N = normal control; + = thromboplastin is generated (i.e., fibrin clot forms); O = thromboplastin is not generated (i.e., fibrin clot does not form).

POOR CLOT RETRACTION
Various thrombocytopenias
Thrombasthenia

COAGULATION TESTS
See Hematologic Diseases, Table 46, pp. 330–332, for specific diseases and altered test results.

SEROLOGY

"PREGNANCY" TEST
(immunoassay detection of human chorionic gonadotropin [HCG] in urine, serum, plasma)

Positive In

Pregnancy. Test becomes positive as early as 4 days after expected date of menstruation; it is >95% reliable by 10th–14th day. HCG increases to peak at 60th–70th day, then drops progressively.

Hydatidiform mole, choriocarcinoma. Test negative 1 or more times in >60%, and negative at all times in >20%, of these patients, for whom more sensitive methods (e.g., radioimmunoassay) should be used. Quantitative titers should be performed for diagnosis and for following the clinical course of patients with these conditions.

False negative results may occur with dilute urine or in cases of missed abortion, dead fetus syndrome, ectopic pregnancy. False positive results may occur with bacterial contamination or protein or blood in urine or in patients on methadone therapy.

With the latex agglutination type of test, only urine should be used if patient has rheumatoid arthritis.

Older techniques used animals (e.g., mouse, rat, frog, toad, rabbit) for injection of specimen (usually concentrated urine) followed by examination of the ovaries after specific periods of time. These methods are more cumbersome and more subject to false positive reactions (e.g., due to high titers of pituitary gonadotropin or high titers of follicle-stimulating hormone in menopause or primary ovarian failure; aspirin, chlorpromazine, phenothiazides within 48 hours) and false negative reactions due to toxic substances in urine (e.g., drugs, such as barbiturates and salicylates, excess electrolytes, such as potassium, and bacterial contamination).

Leukocyte alkaline phosphatase scoring may also be used as a test for pregnancy (see p. 103).

See also Urinary Chorionic Gonadotropins, p. 140.

HETEROPHIL AGGLUTINATION
(agglutination of sheep RBCs by serum of patients with infectious mononucleosis)

Titers $\leq$ 1:56 may occur in normal persons and in patients with other illnesses.

A titer of $\geq$ 1:224 is presumptive evidence of infectious mononucleosis but may also be caused by recent injection of horse serum or horse immune serum. Therefore a differential absorption test should be performed using guinea pig kidney and beef cell antigens.

Guinea pig absorption will not reduce the titer in infectious mononucleosis to <25% of the original value; most commonly the titer is not reduced by more than 1 or 2 tube dilutions.

Table 13. Sample Titers in Heterophil Agglutination

Presumptive Test	After Guinea Pig Kidney Absorption	After Beef RBC Absorption	Interpretation of Diagnosis of Infectious Mononucleosis
1:224	1:112	0	+
1:224	1:56	0	+
1:224	1:28	0	+
1:224	1:14 or less	0	−
1:224	1:56	1:56	−
1:224	0	1:112	−
1:56	1:56 to 1:7	0	+
1:56	1:56	1:28	−
1:28	1:28 to 1:7	0	+

SEROLOGIC TESTS FOR SYPHILIS

	% Reactive Patients with Syphilis in Different Stages				
	Primary	*Secon-dary*	*Late*	*Latent*	*Presumably Normal*
Fluorescent treponemal antibody absorbed (FTA-ABS)—most sensitive and specific cases. Test of choice for confirmation of diagnosis	85	99	95	95	1
Treponema pallidum immobilization (TPI—specific but somewhat less sensitive than FTA-ABS. Antibodies appear later so test is less sensitive in early syphilis. Is being replaced by microhemagglutination technique that can be automated and quantitated and is more sensitive and more easily performed.	56	94	92	94	0
Veneral Disease Research Laboratory (VDRL)—simple test for routine screening at local level; frequent local requirement for premarital and prenatal serology. Does not become positive until 7–10 days after appearance of chancre. Reactive and weakly reactive tests should be confirmed with FTA-ABS.	78	97	77	74	0

If >90% of the agglutination is removed by guinea pig adsorption, the test is considered negative.

Beef red cell absorption takes most (90%) or all of the sheep agglutinations and does reduce the titer in infectious mononucleosis; failure to reduce the titer is evidence against a diagnosis of infectious mononucleosis.

Heterophil agglutination may be negative when positive hematologic and clinical findings are present; a second heterophil agglutination in 1–2 weeks may become positive later in the course of the disease. The heterophil agglutination may have become negative even though some residual hematologic findings are still present.

False positive tests are very rare and occur in relatively low titers.

Results of these tests are positive in presence of antibodies of related treponematoses (e.g., yaws, pinta, bejel). Once antibodies develop, the tests may thereafter remain positive despite therapy. (This is the mechanism for one type of BFP.) If therapy is given before antibodies develop, these tests may never be positive.

Biologic false positive (BFP) tests should be confirmed with FTA-ABS.

≦ 20% of reactive screening tests may be BFP. Two-thirds of these revert to normal within 6 months; patients have usually had recent infections or immunizations. The remaining third that do not become nonreactive in 6 months have serious underlying disease (e.g., SLE) in 25% or are shown to have syphilis in 50%. BFP occurs in 20–25% of narcotics addicts. ≦ 10% of patients over age 70 may show BFP. >20% of patients with BFP also show positive tests for RA, antinuclear antibodies, antithyroid antibodies, cryoglobulins, elevated serum gamma globulins.

IgM-FTA-ABS may become available. It is valuable for early detection of congenital syphilis and detection of untreated, inadequately treated, recently treated, or reinfected patients. Test becomes negative 2 years after therapy.

See Syphilis, pp. 471–473.

ANTISTREPTOCOCCAL ANTIBODY TITERS (ASOT)

A high or rising titer is indicative only of current or recent streptococcal infection.

    Direct diagnostic value in
        Scarlet fever
        Erysipelas
        Streptococcal pharyngitis and tonsillitis
    Indirect diagnostic value in
        Rheumatic fever
        Glomerulonephritis

Antibody appears about 2 weeks after infection; titer rises for 4–6 weeks and may remain elevated for months.

Serial determinations are most desirable since individual determinations depend upon various factors (e.g., duration and severity of infection, antigenicity). Even in severe streptococcal infection, there will be an elevated ASO titer in only 70–80% of patients.

Conditions	Usual ASO Titer (Todd Unit)
Normal persons	12–166
Active rheumatic fever	500–5000
Inactive rheumatic fever	12–250
Rheumatoid arthritis	12–250
Acute glomerulonephritis	500–5000
Streptococcal upper respiratory tract infections	100–333
Collagen diseases	12–250

Other streptococcal antigens may be tested:
> Antistreptococcal hyaluronidase (ASH) (significant titer > 128)
> Antideoxyribonuclease (ADNase) (significant titer > 10)

Useful In
Detecting subclinical streptococcal infection
Differential diagnosis of joint pains of rheumatic fever and rheumatoid arthritis

LUPUS ERYTHEMATOSUS (LE) CELL TEST
LE cells occur in
> 75% of patients with systemic lupus erythematosus (SLE)
> 10% of patients with rheumatoid arthritis (only half of these have multisystem disease)
> 10% of patients with scleroderma
> 100% of patients with lupoid hepatitis
> Patients with drug-induced lupuslike syndrome (e.g., due to procainamide, hydralazine, isoniazid, various anticonvulsants)
> Some infections

The test becomes negative in ≧4–6 weeks in 60% of patients treated successfully. It is not useful as a guide to therapy; it is not correlated with the clinical picture.

The test is positive when 2 typical LE cells are found; it may be repeated for verification. Because of gradual changes in LE cell factor, repetition in < 3 weeks is not useful; instead a more sensitive technique or a serologic test for antinuclear or anti-DNA antibodies should be used.

Rosettes (clusters of polynuclear leukocytes surrounding an extracellular hematoxylin body) are usually found in association with LE cells.

Hematoxylin bodies (homogeneous round extracellular material) may be found in SLE, rheumatoid arthritis, multiple myeloma, cirrhosis. In SLE they may be found without LE cells in the same sample.

See Systemic Lupus Erythematosus pp. 516–517.

SEROLOGIC TESTS FOR SYSTEMIC LUPUS ERYTHMATOSUS (SLE)

The Hyland "LE test" using latex nucleoprotein is quite specific but positive in only 30% of patients with LE.

Anti-DNA antibody is usually present only in SLE and correlates with activity of the disease; it is absent during sustained remission. It may be absent in SLE, in which case doubts should be raised about the diagnosis. It may be found in $\cong$ 50% of patients with systemic sclerosis, dermatomyositis, and polyarteritis nodosa; 10% of patients with rheumatoid arthritis; variable number of patients with discoid lupus; 4–17% of patients with liver disease, thyroiditis, ulcerative colitis, myasthenia gravis.

Antinucleoprotein antibody is present in high titer in almost all patients in the active stage of SLE and sometimes during remission. Therefore a negative test is useful to rule out SLE. But the SLE test is positive in somewhat lower titers in other diseases more frequently than is the LE cell test (e.g., rheumatoid arthritis, drug reactions) or when the LE cell test is usually negative (e.g., infection, lymphoma). Significant titer is 1:32 or greater; low levels can be found in old age and most of the connective tissue diseases. In SLE, titers are particularly high, often >1:256.

See Systemic Lupus Erythematosus pp. 516–517.

TEST FOR RHEUMATOID FACTOR (RA TEST)

The test is negative in one-third of patients with definite rheumatoid arthritis. It gives useful objective evidence of rheumatoid arthritis, but a negative RA test does not rule out rheumatoid arthritis.

It is positive in 5% of rheumatoid variants (arthritis associated with psoriasis, ulcerative colitis, regional enteritis, Reiter's syndrome, juvenile rheumatoid arthritis, rheumatoid spondylitis).

It is positive in $\leqq$ 5% of normal persons; progressive increase with age $\leqq$ 25% of persons over age 70.

It may be positive in up to one-third of patients with SLE.

It may be positive in syphilis, chronic infections, viral infections, scleroderma, sarcoidosis, chronic liver disease, subacute bacterial endocarditis, chronic pulmonary interstitial fibrosis, etc.

Use slide test only for screening; confirm positive test with tube dilution. Significant titer is $\geqq$ 1:80. In rheumatoid arthritis, titers are often 1:640 to 1:5120 and sometimes $\leqq$ 1:320,000. Titers in conditions other than rheumatoid arthritis are usually < 1:80.

See Rheumatoid Arthritis pp. 276–277.

COOMBS' (ANTIGLOBULIN) TEST

Positive Direct Coombs' Test (using patient's RBCs coated with antibody)

Erythroblastosis fetalis

Most cases of autoimmune hemolytic anemia, including $\leqq$ 15% of certain systemic diseases, especially acute and chronic leukemias, malignant lymphomas, collagen diseases

75% of patients receiving cephalothin therapy (blood level of 333–666 ug/ml), especially if azotemia is present
The test is negative in hemolytic anemias due to intrinsic defect in RBCs (e.g., G-6-PD deficiency, hemoglobinopathies).

Positive Indirect Coombs' Test (using patient's serum which contains antibody)
Specific antibody—usually isoimmunization from previous transfusion
"Nonspecific" autoantibody in acquired hemolytic anemia
Incompatible crossmatched blood prior to transfusion

Beware of false positive and false negative results due to poor quality test serum, not using fresh blood (must have complement), etc.

FLUORESCENT ANTIBODY TESTS
Antimitochondrial antibodies are found in $\cong 85\%$ of patients with primary biliary cirrhosis but almost never in diffuse extrahepatic biliary obstruction; therefore antibodies are useful in differentiating these two conditions.
May also be found in two other liver disorders associated with autoimmune disease: active chronic hepatitis and cryptogenic cirrhosis.
Smooth muscle antibodies may be found in $\cong 80\%$ of patients with chronic active hepatitis (lupoid hepatitis) and in patients with biliary cirrhosis.
Antibodies against the cross-striations of skeletal muscle are present in 30–40% of patients with myasthenia gravis; a changing titer may indicate response to treatment or thymectomy.

COLD AUTOHEMAGGLUTINATION
Increased In
Primary atypical (virus) pneumonia (30–90% of patients). Titer of $\geqq 1:14-1:224$. Negative titer does not rule out primary atypical pneumonia (see pp. 483, 485).

Atypical hemolytic anemia
Paroxysmal hemoglobinuria
Raynaud's disease
Cirrhosis of the liver
Trypanosomiasis
Malaria
Infectious mononucleosis
Adenovirus infections
Influenza
Psittacosis
Mumps
Measles
Scarlet fever
Rheumatic fever

HEPATITIS B SURFACE ANTIGEN (HB$_s$Ag) (FORMERLY, AUSTRALIA ANTIGEN; HEPATITIS-ASSOCIATED ANTIGEN—Au; HAA; SH)

Occurs In

0.1% of normal Americans

3–20% of the population in many tropical parts of the world and Southeast Asia

63% of patients with acute viral hepatitis with a history of parenteral exposure

30% of patients with acute viral hepatitis without a history of parenteral exposure

2% of habitual drug users

Patients with chronic active hepatitis (10–30% of Americans) and persistent viral hepatitis

Patients with certain chronic diseases with impaired immune mechanisms; 30% of patients with Down's syndrome kept in large institutions (who also show mild abnormalities of SGPT, BSP retention, thymol turbidity, cephalin flocculation, liver biopsy evidence of hepatitis); patients with lymphocytic leukemia, Hodgkin's disease, lepromatous leprosy; patients undergoing hemodialysis therapy for chronic renal disease

Appears in blood during incubation period a variable time after apparent infection (usually 2 weeks to 4 months) but precedes signs and symptoms and elevation of SGOT. Disappears within days or weeks of first detection.

Transfusion of blood containing HB$_s$Ag-caused hepatitis or appearance of HB$_s$Ag in blood in >50% of recipients. Transfusion of blood not containing HB$_s$Ag-caused anicteric hepatitis in 16% of recipients and icteric hepatitis in 2%.

HB$_s$Ag is probably responsible for ≅25% of cases of posttransfusion hepatitis.

Hepatitis following transfusion of HB$_s$Ag-negative blood tends to be clinically mild, and tests for HB$_s$Ag are negative. Hepatitis following transfusion of HB$_s$Ag-positive blood tends to be clinically severe, and tests for HB$_s$Ag are positive in acute phase. Disappears during recovery, but in 20–30% of patients persists for months to years, indicating a carrier state. This is a marker of infectivity and patient should be considered potentially infectious regardless of clinical state; carriers tend to have mild or anicteric hepatitis. Patients with severe, icteric hepatitis tend to revert to HB$_s$Ag-negative state.

Positive test for HB$_s$Ag indicates Type B hepatitis, but negative test is inconclusive, since antigen may have already disappeared or patient may have Type A hepatitis.

Screening of blood donors for HB$_s$Ag will reduce posttransfusion hepatitis by 25% using counterimmunoelectrophoresis and by 30–40% using RIA, but latter produces some false positive results.

When HB$_s$Ag carrier is discovered (e.g., in screening program), 60–80% show some evidence of hepatic damage.

Persons with a positive test for HB$_s$Ag should never be permitted to donate blood or plasma.

SOME DISEASES ASSOCIATED WITH HL-A ANTIGENS (HISTOCOMPATIBILITY COMPLEX)*

Certain Associations
Ankylosing spondylitis
Reiter's syndrome
Acute anterior uveitis
Juvenile rheumatoid arthritis
Psoriatic arthritis
Yersinia arthritis
Gluten-sensitive enteropathy and celiac disease
Graves' disease
Myasthenia gravis
Dermatitis herpetiformis
Chronic active hepatitis
Insulin-dependent diabetes mellitus
Multiple sclerosis
Psoriasis vulgaris

Probable Associations
SLE
Pemphigus
Idiopathic autoimmune hemolytic anemia
Poliomyelitis
Behçet's disease

Possible Associations
Acute lymphoblastic leukemia
Chronic glomerulonephritis
Infectious mononucleosis
Leprosy
Hodgkin's disease in patients over age 45
Periodontitis (decreased risk)
Chronic myelocytic leukemia (decreased risk)

OTHER PROCEDURES
See Chap. 34, Infectious Diseases, for specific serologic tests (e.g., complement fixation, hemagglutination, neutralizing antibody, precipitin antibody, latex particle agglutination, flocculation) that are applicable in the diagnosis of diseases due to various organisms (e.g., bacteria, viruses, *Rickettsia*, protozoa).

*For further information see S. Ritzman, HL-A patterns and disease associations. *J.A.M.A.* 236:2305, 1976; F. Bach and J. van Rood, The major histocompatibility complex: Genetics and biology. *N. Engl. J. Med.* 295:927, 1976.

16

URINE

DETECTION OF BACTERIURIA

A colony count is significant if there are > 100,000 bacteria/cu mm under the following conditions: Periurethral area has first been thoroughly cleaned with soap, a midstream, clean-catch first morning specimen is submitted in a sterilized container, and the specimen is refrigerated until the colony count is performed. A positive result in a single specimen containing gram-negative rods has an 85% chance of being the same in the next specimen (i.e., 15% error in a single specimen determination). Colony counts < 10,000/cu mm in the absence of therapy largely rule out bacteriuria. False low colony counts may occur with a high rate of urinary flow, low urine specific gravity, low urine pH, presence of antibacterial drugs, or inappropriate cultural techniques (e.g., tubercle bacilli, Mycoplasma, L-forms, anaerobes).

Direct microscopical examination of uncentrifuged urine unstained or gram-stained has 80–95% of the reliability of a colony count. It may show > 10% false positive results. Microscopic detection of pus cells is less sensitive and produces more false positive results than detection of bacteria. ≦ 50% of patients with bacteriuria may not show significant numbers of WBC on urine microscopic examination; however, ≧ 10 WBC/field is associated with bacteriuria in ≅ 90% of cases. Maximum sensitivity is obtained with microscopic detection of both bacteria and pus cells. "Sterile" pyuria (i.e., pyogenic infection is absent) may occur in renal tuberculosis, chemical inflammation, mechanical inflammation (e.g., calculi, instrumentation), early acute glomerulonephritis prior to appearance of hematuria or proteinuria, extreme dehydration, hyperchloremic renal acidosis, nonbacterial gastroenteritis and respiratory tract infections, and after administration of oral polio vaccine.

Dye tests (bacterial reduction of nitrate to nitrite; tetrazolium reduction) do not detect 10–50% of infections. Bacteria show great variability in rate of dye reduction; some important bacteria do not reduce dye at all. Dye tests are not to be recommended.

Decreased glucose in urine (< 2 mg/100 ml) in properly collected first morning urine (no food or fluid intake after 10 P.M., no urination during night) correlates well with colony count.

A culture should be performed for identification of the organism and determination of sensitivity when these screening tests are positive. If culture shows a common gram-positive saprophyte, it should be repeated because the second culture is often negative. Causative bacteria are usually enteric organisms; < 10% are gram-positive cocci (see Table 15, pp. 150–151). If culture shows mixed flora, contamination should be suspected and culture should be repeated; but true mixed infections may occur after instrumentation or with chronic infection. *If* Pseudomonas *or* Proteus *is found, the patient may have an anatomic abnormality. If organism other than* Escherichia coli *is found, patient probably has chronic pyelonephritis even if this is the first clinical episode of infection.*

Bacteriuria may be found in
    10% of patients who are pregnant
    15% of patients with diabetes mellitus
    20% of patients with cystocele
    70% of patients with prostatic obstruction
    95% of patients (untreated) with an indwelling catheter for >4
        days

URINE SPECIFIC GRAVITY

Moderate increase of urine specific gravity results from
    Refrigeration of the urine
    Excretion of protein in urine
Marked increase of specific gravity results from
    Excretion of radiographic contrast medium (frequently
        ≦ 1.040–1.050)
    Sucrosuria (see pp. 365–366)
None of these affect urinary osmolality.

See also urine concentration and dilution tests, pp. 93, 94.

DIFFERENTIATION OF URINARY PROTEINS
Precipitated by 5% Sulfosalicylic Acid

On boiling, precipitate remains	Albumin
	Globulin
	Pseudo–Bence Jones protein
On boiling, precipitate disappears	Bence Jones protein
	A "proteose"

Precipitated at 40–60°C
Resuspend precipitate in normal urine
and an equal volume of 5%
sulfosalicylic acid and boil:

Precipitate dissolves	Bence Jones protein
Precipitate does not dissolve	Pseudo–Bence Jones protein

BENCE JONES PROTEINURIA

About 20% of tests will be false positive (i.e., urine electrophoresis does not show a spike and immunoelectrophoresis does not show a monoclonal light chain) due to
    Connective tissue diseases (e.g., rheumatoid arthritis, polymyositis, Wegener's granulomatosis)
    Chronic renal insufficiency
    Lymphoma and leukemia
    Metastatic carcinoma
80% of tests are true positive due to
    Myeloma (70% of all positive tests)
    Amyloidosis
    Adult Fanconi syndrome
    Hyperparathyroidism
    Benign monoclonal gammopathy (see p. 322)

Positive test for Bence Jones proteinuria by heat test should al-

ways be confirmed by electrophoresis and immunoelectro-phoresis of concentrated urine.

"Dip-stick" test for albumin does not detect Bence Jones protein.

POSITIVE BENEDICT REACTIONS IN URINE
Glycosuria
> Hyperglycemia
>> Endocrine (e.g., diabetes mellitus, pituitary, adrenal, thyroid disease)
>> Nonendocrine (e.g., liver, CNS diseases)
>> Due to administration of hormones (e.g., ACTH, corticosteroids, thyroid, adrenalin) or drugs (e.g., morphine, anesthetic drugs, tranquilizers)
> Renal tubular origin (low Tm_G)
>> Renal diabetes
>> Toxic renal tubular disease (e.g., due to lead, mercury, degraded tetracycline)
>> Associated with defective amino acid transport
>> Inflammatory renal disease (e.g., acute glomerulonephritis, nephrosis)
> Idiopathic
Melituria*
> Hereditary (e.g., galactose, fructose, pentose, lactose)
> Neonatal (e.g., physiologic lactosuria, sepsis, gastroenteritis, hepatitis)
> Lactosuria during lactation
Non-sugar-reducing substances (e.g., ascorbic acid, glucuronic acid, homogentisic acid, salicylates)

Galactosuria (in galactosemia) shows a positive urine reaction with Clinitest but negative with Clinistix and Tes-Tape.

False negative tests for glucose may occur in presence of ascorbic acid using glucose oxidase paper test (Labstix); found in >1% of routine urine analyses in hospital.

KETONURIA
(ketone bodies—acetone, beta-hydroxybutyric acid, acetoacetic acid—appear in urine)

Occurs In
Metabolic conditions
> Diabetes mellitus
> Renal glycosuria `
> Glycogen storage disease
Dietary conditions
> Starvation
> High-fat diets

---

*5% of cases of melituria in the general population are due to renal glycosuria (incidence is 1:100,000), pentosuria (incidence is 1:50,000), essential fructosuria (incidence is 1:120,000).

Increased metabolic requirements
  Hyperthyroidism
  Fever
  Pregnancy and lactation
  Other

False positive results may occur after injection of Bromsulphalein (BSP test).

SUBSTANCES AND CONDITIONS THAT MAY CAUSE ABNORMAL COLOR OF URINE

Porphyrins (see p. 132)

Sickle cell crises produce a characteristic dark-brown color independent of volume or specific gravity that becomes darker on standing or on exposure to sunlight. Increase in total porphyrins, coproporphyrins, and uroporphyrins is routinely shown; increase in the porphyrin precursors (delta-aminolevulinic acid and porphobilinogen) is occasionally shown.

Hemoglobin (see p. 132)

Myoglobin (see p. 132)

Melanin (see p. 133)

Red urine may be caused by ingestion of beets, blackberries, certain cold-drink and food dyes, certain drugs (e.g., phenolphthalein in laxatives); presence of urates and bile may also cause red urine.

Darkening of urine on standing, alkalinization, or oxygenation is nonspecific and may be due to melanogen, hemoglobin, indican, urobilinogen, porphyrins, phenols, salicylate metabolites (e.g., gentisic acid), homogentisic acid (due to alkaptonuria; *if acid pH, may not darken for hours*), and may appear in tyrosinosis. Darkened urine may follow administration of metronidazole (Flagyl).

Biliverdin. Blue or green color is due to oxidation of bilirubin in poorly preserved specimens. *Gives negative diazo tests for bilirubin (Ictotest), but oxidative tests (Harrison spot test) may still be positive.*

Methylene blue ingestion may cause a similar urine color. Blue urine occurs very rarely in *Pseudomonas* infection.

Blue diaper syndrome results from indigo blue in urine due to familial metabolic defect in tryptophan absorption associated with idiopathic hypercalcemia and nephrocalcinosis.

Red diaper syndrome is due to a nonpathogenic chromobacterium *(Serratia marcescens)* that produces a red pigment when grown aerobically at 25–30°C.

White cloud is due to excessive oxalic acid and glycolic acid in urine; occurs in oxalosis (primary hyperoxaluria).

Chyluria (see p. 133)

Lipuria (see p. 133)

URINE UROBILINOGEN

Increased In

Increased hemolysis (e.g., hemolytic anemias)

Hemorrhage into tissues (e.g., pulmonary infarction, severe bruises)

Hepatic parenchymal cell damage (e.g., cirrhosis, acute hepatitis in early and recovery stages)

Cholangitis

Decreased In
Complete biliary obstruction

PORPHYRINURIA
(due mainly to coproporphyrin)
Lead poisoning
Cirrhosis
Infectious hepatitis
Passive in newborn of mother with porphyria; lasts for several days
Porphyria

HEMOGLOBINURIA
Renal threshold is 100–140 mg/100 ml plasma.

Infarction of kidney
Hematuria with hemolysis in urine
Intravascular hemolysis due to
    Parasites (e.g., malaria, Oroya fever due to *Bartonella bacilliformis*)
    Fava bean sensitivity
    Antibodies (e.g., transfusion reactions, acquired hemolytic anemia, paroxysmal cold hemoglobinuria, paroxysmal nocturnal hemoglobinuria)
    Hypotonicity (e.g., transurethral prostatectomy with irrigation of bladder with water)
    Chemicals (e.g., napthalene, sulfonamides)
    Thermal burns injuring RBCs
    Strenuous exercise and march hemoglobinuria

False positive (Occultest) results may occur in the presence of pus, iodides, bromides.

MYOGLOBINURIA
Renal threshold is 20 mg/100 ml plasma.

Hereditary
    Phosphorylase deficiency (McArdle syndrome)
    Metabolic defects (e.g., associated with muscular dystrophy)
Sporadic
    Ischemic (e.g., arterial occlusion) (in acute myocardial infarction, levels of >5 mg/ml often occur within 48 hours and sometimes within 1 hour; may precede ECG and serum enzyme changes)
    Crush syndrome
    Exertional (e.g., exercise, some cases of march hemoglobinuria, electric shock, convulsions, and seizures)

Metabolic myoglobinuria (e.g., Haff disease, alcoholism, seasnake bite, carbon monoxide poisoning, diabetic acidosis, hypokalemia, fever and systemic infection, barbiturate poisoning)

In $\leqq 50\%$ of patients with progressive muscle disease (e.g., dermatomyositis, polymyositis, SLE, others) in active stage

MELANOGENURIA

In some patients with malignant melanoma, when the urine is exposed to air for several hours, colorless melanogens are oxidized to melanin and urine becomes deep brown and later black.

Is also said to occur in some patients with Addison's disease or hemochromatosis and in intestinal obstruction in negroes.

Confirmatory tests
    Ferric chloride test
    Thormählen's test
    Ehrlich test

None of these is consistently more reliable or sensitive than observation of urine for darkening.

Melanogenuria occurs in 25% of patients with malignant melanoma; it is said to be more frequent with extensive liver metastasis. It is not useful for judging completeness of removal or early recurrence.

Beware of false positive red-brown or purple suspension due to salicylates.

CHYLURIA

Milky urine is due to chylomicrons recognized as fat globules by microscopy (this is almost entirely neutral fat). Protein is normal or low. Hematuria is common. Specific gravity is low and reaction is acid.

A test meal of milk and cream may cause chyluria in 1–4 hours.

Chyluria is due to obstruction of the lymphochylous system, usually filariasis.

Microfilariae appear in the urine for 6 weeks after acute infection, then disappear unless endemic.

Laboratory findings are due to the pyelonephritis that is usually present.

LIPURIA

Lipids in the urine include all fractions. Double refractile (cholesterol) bodies can be seen. There is a high protein content.

May Occur In
Nephrotic syndrome
Severe diabetes mellitus
Severe eclampsia
Phosphorus poisoning
Carbon monoxide poisoning

URINE ELECTROLYTES

Usually of limited value because of the wide range of normal values (due to wide range of dietary intake of water and electrolytes), failure to obtain 24-hour excretion levels rather than random samples, or recent administration of diuretics; clinical problem may be more easily diagnosed if other tests are used.

Occasionally urinary electrolyte determination is useful in determining the cause of the problems listed in column 1.

Metabolic Problems	Causes	Urine Electrolytes
Volume depletion	Extrarenal sodium loss	Sodium <10 mEq/L
	Adrenal insufficiency or renal salt wasting	Sodium >10 mEq/L
Acute oliguria	Prerenal azotemia	Sodium <10 mEq/L
	Acute tubular necrosis	Sodium >30 mEq/L
Hyponatremia	Severe volume depletion: edematous states	Sodium <10 mEq/L
	Inappropriate antidiuretic hormone secretion; adrenal insufficiency	Sodium ≥ dietary intake
Hypokalemia	Extrarenal potassium loss	Potassium <10 mEq/L
	Renal potassium loss	Potassium >10 mEq/L
Metabolic alkalosis	Chloride-responsive alkalosis	Chloride <10 mEq/L
	Chloride-resistant alkalosis	Chloride parallels dietary intake

URINE CALCIUM

Increased In

Hyperparathyroidism
Idiopathic hypercalciuria
High-calcium diet
　　Excess milk intake
Immobilization (especially in children)
Lytic bone lesions
　　Metastatic tumor
　　Multiple myeloma
　　Osteoporosis (primary or secondary to hyperthyroidism, Cushing's syndrome, acromegaly)
Excess vitamin D ingestion
Drug therapy
　　Mercurial diuretics
　　Ammonium chloride
Fanconi's syndrome
Renal tubular acidosis

Decreased In

Hypoparathyroidism
Rickets, osteomalacia

Steatorrhea
Renal failure
Metastatic carcinoma of prostate

URINE CREATINE

Increased In
Physiologic states
    Growing children
    Pregnancy
    Puerperium (2 weeks)
    Starvation
    Raw meat diet
Increased formation
    Myopathy
        Amyotonia congenita
        Muscular dystrophy
        Poliomyelitis
        Myasthenia gravis
        Crush injury
        Acute paroxysmal myoglobinuria
    Endocrine diseases
        Hyperthyroidism
        Addison's disease
        Cushing's syndrome
        Acromegaly
        Diabetes mellitus
        Eunuchoidism
        Therapy with ACTH, cortisone, or DOCA
Increased breakdown
    Infections
    Burns
    Fractures
    Leukemia
    Disseminated lupus erythematosus

Decreased In
Hypothyroidism

FERRIC CHLORIDE TEST OF URINE
(to be used as screening test)

Positive In
Phenylketonuria (unreliable for diagnosis)
Tyrosinuria—transient elevation in newborns
Maple syrup urine disease
Alkaptonuria
Histidinemia
Tyrosinosis
Oasthouse urine disease

A positive test should always be followed by chromatography of blood and urine.

TYROSINE CRYSTALS IN URINE
Massive hepatic necrosis (acute yellow atrophy)

URINARY LACTIC DEHYDROGENASE (LDH) ACTIVITY

Increased In
Carcinoma of kidney, bladder, and prostate (high proportion of cases—useful for detection of asymptomatic lesions or screening of susceptible population groups, and differential diagnosis of renal cysts)
Other renal diseases
 Active glomerulonephritis, SLE with nephritis, nephrotic syndrome, acute tubular necrosis, diabetic nephrosclerosis, malignant nephrosclerosis, renal infarction
 Active pyelonephritis (25% of patients), cystitis, and other inflammations
Instrumentation of the GU tract (especially cystoscopy with retrograde pyelography) (transient increase—< 1 week)
Myocardial infarction and other conditions with considerably increased serum levels.
Other

Normal In
Benign nephrosclerosis
Pyelonephritis (most patients)
Obstructive uropathy
Renal stones
Polycystic kidneys
Renal cysts

The test is not useful in routine screening for malignancy of kidney, renal pelvis, and bladder; increased values usually precede clinical symptoms. Increased levels suggest GU tract disease but do not indicate its nature.

Precautions: 8-hour overnight urine collection, clean voided to prevent bacterial and menstrual contamination. Refrigerate until analysis is begun. Specimen must be dialyzed to remove inhibitors in urine. Microscopic examination of urine should be performed first since false positive LDH may occur if there are > 10 bacteria/hpf or if RBCs or hemolyzed blood is present.

URINARY EXCRETION OF FIGLU (FORMIMINOGLUTAMIC ACID)
Histidine loading is followed after 3 hours by a 5-hour urine collection.

Increased In
Folic acid deficiency occurring in
 Idiopathic steatorrhea ($\leqq 80$ mg/hour)
 Pregnancy, especially with toxemia and increased age, parity, and multiple pregnancy
 Administration of folic acid antagonists

Malnutrition (some patients), chronic liver disease, use of anticonvulsant drugs, congenital hemolytic anemia

Normal is <2 mg/hour or 3 mg/100 ml

URINARY 5-HYDROXYINDOLEACETIC ACID (5-HIAA)

Increased In
Carcinoid syndrome
Ingestion of bananas, tomatoes, avocados, red plums, walnuts, eggplant, reserpine (Serpasil), mephenesin carbamate, phenothiazine derivatives, Lugol's solution, etc.

Normal is 2–9 mg/day; carcinoid syndrome is >40 mg/day, often 300–1000 mg/day.

URINARY ALDOSTERONE

Increased In
Primary and secondary aldosteronism (see pp. 405–407)

Decreased In
Hypoadrenalism
Panhypopituitarism

URINARY CATECHOLAMINES (NOREPINEPHRINE, NORMETANEPHRINE)*

Increased In
Pheochromocytoma
Neural crest tumors (neuroblastoma, ganglioneuroma, ganglioblastoma)
Progressive muscular dystrophy and myasthenia gravis (some patients)
May also be increased by vigorous exercise prior to urine collection (≦7 times)
False increase may be due to drugs that produce fluorescent urinary products (e.g., tetracyclines, Aldomet, epinephrine and epinephrine-like drugs, large doses of vitamin B complex. See p. 543). *Avoid such medications for 1 week before urine collection.*

URINE VANILLYLMANDELIC ACID (VMA)
VMA is the urinary metabolite of both epinephrine and norepinephrine.

Increased In
Pheochromocytoma
Neuroblastoma, ganglioneuroma, ganglioblastoma

Beware of false positive results due to certain foods (e.g., coffee, tea, chocolate, vanilla, some fruits and vegetables, especially

---

*Not all methods include dopamine in determination of total catecholamines.

*bananas); certain drugs (e.g., vasopressor drugs), some an-
tihypertensive drugs (e.g., methyldopa). Monamine oxidase inhibitors may increase metanephrine and decrease VMA. See p.
543.*

URINARY 17-KETOSTEROIDS (17-KS)

Increased In
Adrenal cortical hyperplasia (causing Cushing's syndrome, ad-
    renogenital syndrome)
Adrenal cortical adenoma or carcinoma
Arrhenoblastoma and lutein cell tumor of ovary (if androgenic)
Interstitial cell tumor of testicle
Pituitary tumor or hyperplasia
ACTH administration
Severe stress
Third trimester of pregnancy
Testosterone administration
Nonspecific chromagens in urine

Decreased In
Addison's disease
Panhypopituitarism
Hypothyroidism (myxedema)
Generalized wasting diseases
Nephrosis
Hypogonadism in men (castration)
Primary ovarian agenesis

*Urinary 17-KS may have a daily variation of 100% in the same
    individual.*

URINARY 17-KETOSTEROIDS BETA FRACTION

Increased In
Adrenal carcinoma

URINARY 17-KETOSTEROIDS BETA-ALPHA RATIO
(Beta fraction is largely dehydroepiandrosterone; alpha fraction is
    mostly androsterone and etiocholanolone.)
Normal. Beta-alpha ratio is usually <0.2.
Adrenal cortical hyperplasia. Ratio is usually normal; even when it
    is increased it is rarely >0.3.
Adrenal carcinoma. Ratio is usually 0.28–0.4. In adults some pa-
    tients may have a ratio >0.2 but the ratio is increased in most
    cases in children. The ratio is most helpful if it is >0.4 when it is
    most indicative of carcinoma.
Unless the total 17-KS are increased, the beta-alpha ratio is not
    likely to be abnormal.

BLOOD AND URINARY CORTICOSTEROIDS
(17-KETOGENIC STEROIDS)

Increased In
Adrenal hyperplasia

Adrenal adenoma
Adrenal carcinoma
ACTH therapy
Stress

Decreased In
Addison's disease
Panhypopituitarism
Cessation of corticosteroid therapy
General wasting disease

URINARY PORTER-SILBER REACTION
This reaction measures only OH at C-17 and C-21 and O=at C-20; does not measure pregnanetriol and other C-20 OH compounds.

Increased In
Cushing's syndrome (sometimes markedly)
Severe stress (e.g., eclampsia, pancreatitis [may be marked], infection, burns, surgery)
Third trimester of pregnancy (moderately)
Early pregnancy (slightly)
Severe hypertension (slightly)
Virilism (slightly)

Decreased or Normal In
Addison's disease
Hypopituitarism

Certain drugs (e.g., paraldehyde) interfere with determination.

URINARY DEHYDROISOANDROSTERONE (ALLEN BLUE TEST)

Increased In
Adrenal carcinoma

URINARY PREGNANEDIOL

Increased In
Luteal cysts of ovary
Arrhenoblastoma
Hyperadrenocorticism

Decreased In
Toxemia of pregnancy
Fetal death
Threatened abortion (some patients)
Amenorrhea

URINARY PREGNANETRIOL

Increased In
Adrenogenital syndrome (congenital adrenal hyperplasia)

URINARY ESTROGENS

Increased In
Granulosa cell tumor of ovary
Theca cell tumor of ovary
Luteoma of ovary
Interstitial cell tumor of testis
Pregnancy
Hyperadrenalism
Liver disease

Decreased In
Primary hypofunction of ovary
Secondary hypofunction of ovary

URINARY CHORIONIC GONADOTROPINS
(see also "Pregnancy" Test, p. 120)

Increased In
Normal pregnancy
Hydatidiform mole (sometimes markedly)
Chorionepithelioma (sometimes markedly)
  Of uterus
  Of testicle

Normal In
Nonpregnant state
Fetal death

URINARY PITUITARY GONADOTROPINS
This is a practical assay only for combined follicle-stimulating hormone and interstitial cell–stimulating hormone.

Increased In
Menopause
Male climacteric
Primary hypogonadism
Hyperpituitarism, early

Decreased In
Secondary hypogonadism
Simmonds' disease
Hyperpituitarism, late

Because of small amounts present in 24-hour urine, a 5–10 day continuous collection must be concentrated.

OTHER PROCEDURES
Urine findings in various diseases (see Table 66, pp. 427–429)
Urine amylase (p. 234)
See also specific tests on urine in various chapters (e.g., Endocrine Diseases, Metabolic and Hereditary Diseases, Gastrointestinal Diseases, Hematologic Diseases).

17

OCCULT BLOOD IN STOOL

Chief usefulness is for screening for asymptomatic ulcerated lesions of gastrointestinal tract, especially carcinoma of the colon that is beyond the reach of routine sigmoidoscopy.

QUALITATIVE SCREENING TEST FOR STOOL FAT

Microscopic examination for neutral fat (ethyl alcohol + Sudan III) and free fatty acids (acetic acid + Sudan III + heat) is made.

Random specimen is taken, on diet of >60 gm of fat daily.

4+ fat in stool means excessive fecal fat loss.

Increased neutral fat
  Mineral and castor oil ingestion
  Dietetic low-calorie mayonnaise ingestion
  Rectal suppository use
  Steatorrhea

CHEMICAL DETERMINATION OF FECAL FAT

A 3-day stool sample is taken, on diet of 100 gm of fat daily.

Determination parallels but is more sensitive than triolein ^{131}I test in chronic pancreatic disease.

Normal is <6 gm/24 hours.

In chronic pancreatic disease fecal fat is >10 gm/24 hours.

UROBILINOGEN IN STOOL

Increased In
Hemolytic anemias

Decreased In
Complete biliary obstruction
Severe liver disease
Oral antibiotic therapy altering intestinal bacterial flora
Decreased hemoglobin turnover (e.g., aplastic anemia, cachexia)

MICROSCOPIC EXAMINATION OF DIARRHEAL STOOLS FOR FECAL LEUKOCYTES

Primarily polynuclear leukocytes in
  Shigellosis
  Salmonellosis
  Invasive *Escherichia coli* colitis
  Ulcerative colitis
Primarily mononuclear leukocytes in
  Typhoid
Leukocytes absent in
  Cholera
  Viral diarrheas
  Noninvasive *E. coli* diarrhea
  "Nonspecific" diarrheas
  Normal persons

OTHER PROCEDURES

Examination for ova and parasites
Isotopic studies (pp. 153–154)
Trypsin digestion (see Cystic Fibrosis of Pancreas, p. 236)
Microscopic examination (see Laboratory Diagnosis of Malabsorption, p. 199)
Other

18

GASTRIC AND DUODENAL FLUIDS

GASTRIC ANALYSIS

1-hour basal acid

<2 mEQ	Normal, gastric ulcer, or carcinoma
2–5 mEq	Normal, gastric or duodenal ulcer
>5 mEq	Duodenal ulcer
>20 mEq	Zollinger-Ellison syndrome

1-hour after stimulation (histamine or betazole hydrochloride)

0 mEq	Achlorhydria, gastritis, gastric carcinoma
1–20 mEq	Normal, gastric ulcer, or carcinoma
20–35 mEq	Duodenal ulcer
35–60 mEq	Duodenal ulcer, high normal, Zollinger-Ellison syndrome
>60 mEq	Zollinger-Ellison syndrome

Ratio of basal acid to poststimulation outputs

20%	Normal, gastric ulcer, or carcinoma
20–40%	Gastric or duodenal ulcer
40–60%	Duodenal ulcer, Zollinger-Ellison syndrome
>60%	Zollinger-Ellison syndrome

Serum gastrin levels are indicated with any of the following:

Basal acid secretion >10 mEq/hour in patients with intact stomachs

Ratio of basal to poststimulation output >40% in patients with intact stomachs

All patients with recurrent ulceration after surgery for duodenal ulcer

All patients with duodenal ulcer for whom elective gastric surgery is planned

When basal serum gastrin level is equivocal, serum gastrin level should be measured following stimulation with infusion of secretin or calcium.

Achlorhydria

Gastric carcinoma (50% of patients) even following histamine or betazole stimulation. Hypochlorhydria occurs in 25% of patients with gastric carcinoma; hydrochloric acid is normal in 25% of patients with gastric carcinoma; hyperchlorhydria is rare in gastric carcinoma.

Pernicious anemia (virtually all patients)

Adenomatous polyps of stomach (85% of patients)

Gastric atrophy

Achlorhydria occurs in normal persons: in 4% of children, increasing to 30% of adults over age 60.
  True achlorhydria excludes duodenal ulcer.
Tubeless gastric analysis (Diagnex Blue) is useful to rule out achlorhydria, as in pregnant patients with macrocytic anemia or in screening for gastric carcinoma.
If no free acid is demonstrated with Diagnex Blue test or examination of gastric juice, further examination (e.g., stimulation with histamine or betazole) is required to prove the absence of free HCl.
Measure acid output after IV insulin to demonstrate adequacy of vagotomy (see below, Insulin Test Meal).
Hyperchlorhydria and hypersecretion
    Duodenal ulcer
    Zollinger-Ellison syndrome (see pp. 396–397). Twelve-hour night secretion shows acid of >100 mEq/L and volume of >1500 ml. Basal secretion is >60% of secretion caused by histamine or betazole stimulation.

INSULIN TEST MEAL
Aspirate gastric fluid every 15 minutes for 2 hours after IV administration of sufficient insulin (usually 15–20 units) to produce blood sugar of <50 mg/100.ml.
Normal. Hypoglycemia increases free HCl.
Successful vagotomy produces achlorhydria.

PANCREOZYMIN-SECRETIN TEST
The test measures the effect of IV administration of pancreozymin and secretin on (1) volume, bicarbonate concentration, and amylase output of duodenal contents and (2) increase in serum lipase and amylase.

Normal duodenal contents
    Volume of 95–235 ml/hour
    Bicarbonate concentration of 74–121 mEq/L
    Amylase output of 87,000–267,000 mg

This is the most sensitive and reliable test of chronic pancreatic disease; avoid gastric contamination.
Normally serum lipase and amylase do not rise above normal limits.

19

SEROUS FLUIDS
(PLEURAL, PERICARDIAL, AND ASCITIC)

Table 14. Comparison of "Typical"[a] Findings in Transudates and Exudates

Finding	Transudates (e.g., heart failure, nephrosis, cirrhosis)	Exudates (e.g., neoplasm, tuberculosis, infection)
Specific gravity	<1.016	>1.016
Protein (gm/100 ml)	<3.0	>3.0
Clot (fibrinogen)	Absent	Present
Cells		
WBCs	Few lymphocytes	Many WBCs; may be grossly purulent
RBCs	Few	Variable; few or may be grossly bloody
Glucose	Equivalent to serum	May be decreased because of bacteria or many WBCs

[a]"Typical" means ≅67–75% of patients.

Culture is positive in about 67% of cases due to tuberculosis.

Pleural fluid eosinophilia frequently occurs with pneumothorax and militates against the diagnosis of tuberculosis or malignant neoplasm.

Repeat cytology is positive in more than 90% of cases due to neoplasm. Pleural or ascitic effusion occurs in 20–30% of patients with malignant lymphoma; cytology establishes the diagnosis in ≅50% of patients.

LDH in nonpurulent, nonhemolyzed, and nonbloody effusions is generally low in cirrhosis and heart failure but increased in malignancy.

Increased amylase level in ascitic fluid occurs in acute pancreatitis, perforated peptic ulcer, necrosis of small intestine (e.g., mesenteric vascular occlusion), and in some cases of pleural and peritoneal metastases (including those originating from nonpancreatic primary sites).

See also Rheumatoid Pleurisy with Effusion, pp. 189, 192.

See also Pulmonary Embolism and Infarction, pp. 188–189.

20

SWEAT

SWEAT ELECTROLYTES

Increased In
Cystic fibrosis of pancreas
   Chloride: 50–120 mEq/L (mean = 97); normal: 4–60 mEq/L
      (mean = 18)
   Sodium: 50–140 mEq/L (mean = 103); normal: 0–40 mEq/L in
      children and 0–60 mEq/L in adults
   Potassium (mean = 15 mEq/L); normal (mean = 9 mEq/L)
Untreated adrenal insufficiency (Addison's disease)
Some unusual disease syndromes (e.g., glucose-6-phosphatase
   deficiency, glycogen-storage disease, vasopressin-resistant dia-
   betes insipidus)

*Sweat sodium is reduced by administration of mineralocorticoids
(e.g., aldosterone) by ≅50% in normal subjects and 10–20% in
cystic fibrosis patients whose final sodium concentration remains abnormally high.*

BACTERIA COMMONLY CULTURED FROM VARIOUS SITES

Table 15. Most Common Bacteria Isolated in Cultures from Various Sites

Site	Normal Flora	Pathogens
External ear	*Staphylococcus epidermidis* Alpha-hemolytic streptococci Coliform bacilli Aerobic corynebacteria *Corynebacterium acnes* *Candida* species *Bacillus* species	*Pseudomonas* species *Staphylococcus aureus* Coliform bacilli Alpha-hemolytic streptococci · *Proteus* species *Streptococcus (Diplococcus) pneumoniae* *Corynebacterium diphtheriae*
Middle ear	Sterile	<u>Acute Otitis Media</u> *Haemophilus influenzae* Beta-hemolytic streptococci Pneumococci <u>Chronic Otitis Media</u> *Staphylococcus aureus* *Proteus* species *Pseudomonas* species Other gram-negative bacilli Alpha-hemolytic streptococci Beta-hemolytic streptococci
Nasal passages	*Staphylococcus epidermidis* *Staphylococcus aureus* Diphtheroids Pneumococci Alpha-hemolytic streptococci Nonpathogenic *Neisseria* species Aerobic corynebacteria	<u>Acute Sinusitis</u> *Staphylococcus aureus* Pneumococci *Klebsiella-Enterobacter* species Alpha-hemolytic streptococci Beta-hemolytic streptococci <u>Chronic Sinusitis</u> *Staphylococcus aureus* Alpha-hemolytic streptococci Pneumococci Beta-hemolytic streptococci
Pharynx and tonsils	Alpha-hemolytic streptococci *Neisseria* species *Staphylococcus epidermidis* *Staphylococcus aureus* (small numbers) Pneumococci	Beta-hemolytic streptococci *Corynebacterium diphtheriae* *Bordetella pertussis* *Neisseria meningitidis* *Haemophilus influenzae* Group B

Table 15 (Continued)

Site	Normal Flora	Pathogens
	Nonhemolytic (gamma) streptococci Diphtheroids Coliforms Beta-hemolytic streptococci (not Group A) *Actinomyces israelii* *Haemophilus* species *Marked predominance of one organism may be clinically significant even if it is a normal inhabitant.*	*Staphylococcus aureus* *Candida albicans*
Gastrointestinal tract		
Mouth	Alpha-hemolytic streptococci Enterococci Lactobacilli Staphylococci Fusobacteria *Bacteroides* species Diphtheroids	*Candida albicans* *Borrelia vincentii* with *Fusobacterium fusiforme*
Stomach	Sterile	
Small intestine	Sterile in one-third Scant bacteria in others *Escherichia coli* *Klebsiella-Enterobacter* Enterococci Alpha-hemolytic streptococci *Staphylococcus epidermidis* Diphtheroids	
Colon	Abundant bacteria *Bacteroides* species *Escherichia coli* *Klebsiella-Enterobacter* Paracolons *Proteus* species Enterococci (Group D streptococci) Yeasts	Enteropathogenic *Escherichia coli* *Candida albicans* Various amebae and parasites *Aeromonas* species *Salmonella* species *Shigella* species
Gallbladder Sterile		*Escherichia coli* Enterococci *Klebsiella-Enterobacter-Serratia* Occasionally Coliforms *Proteus* species *Pseudomonas* species

Table 15 (Continued)

Site	Normal Flora	Pathogens
		Salmonella species
Blood	Sterile	Staphylococci (coagulase positive and negative)
		Coliform and related bacilli
		Alpha- and beta-hemolytic streptococci
		Pneumococci
		Enterococci
		Haemophilus influenzae
		Clostridium perfringens
		Pseudomonas species
		Proteus species
		Bacteroides and related anaerobes
		Neisseria meningitidis
		Brucella species
		Pasteurella tularensis
		Listeria monocytogenes
		Achromobacter (Herellea) species
		Streptobacillus moniliformis
		Leptospira species
		Vibrio fetus
		Opportunistic fungi (e.g., *Candida* species, *Nocardia* species, *Blastomyces dermatitidis, Histoplasma capsulatum*)
		Salmonella species
Eye	Usually sterile	*Staphylococcus aureus*
	Occasionally small numbers of diphtheroids and coagulase-negative staphylococci	*Haemophilus* species
		Streptococcus (Diplococcus) pneumoniae
		Neisseria gonorrhoeae
		Alpha- and beta-hemolytic streptococci
		Achromobacter (Herellea) species
		Coliform bacilli
		Pseudomonas aeruginosa
		Other enteric bacilli
		Morax-Axenfeld bacillus
		Bacillus subtilis (occasionally)
Spinal fluid	Sterile	*Haemophilus influenzae*
		Neisseria meningitidis
		Streptococcus pneumoniae
		Mycobacterium tuberculosis
		Staphylococci, streptococci
		Cryptococcus neoformans
		Coliform bacilli

Table 15 (Continued)

Site	Normal Flora	Pathogens
		Pseudomonas and *Proteus* species
		Bacteroides species
Urethra, male	*Staphylococcus aureus*	*Neisseria gonorrhoeae*
	Staphylococcus epidermidis	Enterococci
	Enterococci	Beta-hemolytic streptococci (usually Group B)
	Diphtheroids	Anaerobic and microaerophilic streptococci
	Achromobacter wolffi (Mima)	
	Haemophilus vaginalis	*Bacteroides* species
	Bacillus subtilis	*Escherichia* and *Klebsiella-Enterobacter*
		Staphylococcus aureus
Urethra, female, and vagina	*Lactobacillus* (large numbers)	Yeasts and *Candida albicans*
	Coli-aerogenes	*Clostridium perfringens*
	Staphylococci	*Listeria monocytogenes*
	Streptococci (aerobic and anaerobic)	*Haemophilus vaginalis*
	Candida albicans	*Trichomonas vaginalis*
	Bacteroides species	*Neisseria gonorrhoeae*
	Achromobacter wolffi (Mima)	(See also entries under Urethra, male)
	Haemophilus vaginalis	
Prostate	Sterile	*Streptococcus faecalis*
		Staphylococcus epidermidis
		Escherichia coli
		Proteus mirabilis
		Pseudomonas species
		Klebsiella species
Uterus		Anaerobic and microanaerophilic streptococci (alpha, beta, and gamma types)
		Bacteroides species
		Enterococci
		Beta-hemolytic streptococci (usually Group B)
		Staphylococci
		Proteus species
		Clostridium perfringens
		Escherichia coli and *Klebsiella-Enterobacter-Serratia*
		Listeria monocytogenes
Urine	Staphylococci, coagulase negative	*Escherichia coli, Klebsiella-Enterobacter-Serratia*
	Diphtheroids	*Proteus* species
	Coliform bacilli	*Pseudomonas* species
	Enterococci	Enterococci

Table 15 (Continued)

Site	Normal Flora	Pathogens
	Proteus species Lactobacilli Alpha- and beta-hemolytic streptococci	Staphylococci, coagulase positive and negative *Alcaligenes* species *Achromobacter (Herellea)* species *Candida albicans* Beta-hemolytic streptococci *Neisseria gonorrhoeae* *Mycobacterium tuberculosis* *Salmonella* and *Shigella* species
Wound		*Staphylococcus aureus* *Streptococcus pyogenes* Coliform bacilli *Bacteroides* species; other gram-negative rods *Proteus* species *Pseudomonas* species *Clostridium* species Enterococci *Achromobacter (Herellea)* species *Serratia* species
Pleura	Sterile	*Staphylococcus aureus* *Streptococcus pneumoniae* *Haemophilus influenzae* *Mycobacterium tuberculosis* Anaerobic streptococci *Streptococcus pyogenes*
Peritoneum	Sterile	*Escherichia coli* Enterococci *Streptococcus pneumoniae* *Bacteroides* species; other gram-negative rods Anaerobic streptococci *Clostridium* species
Bones	Sterile	*Staphylococcus aureus* *Haemophilus influenzae* Beta-hemolytic streptococci *Neisseria gonorrhoeae* *Mycobacterium tuberculosis*
Joints	Sterile	*Staphylococcus aureus* Beta-hemolytic streptococci Pneumococci Gram-negative pathogens in newborns *Salmonella* species in sickle cell disease

RADIOISOTOPE STUDIES

SCHILLING TEST

The fasting patient is given 0.5 μc of ^{60}Co B$_{12}$ (or ^{57}Co) as radiocyanocobalamin orally followed in 1 hour by a "flushing dose" of 1000 μg of intramuscular B$_{12}$ (nonradioactive). Radioactivity is measured in total urine collection for the next 24 hours and compared to the amount of radioactivity ingested.

Normal is $\geq 7\%$ of ingested radioactivity.
In pernicious anemia, 0–3% of the administered radioactivity appears in 24-hour urine.

If $< 7\%$ appears in the urine, the test is repeated with the addition of 60 μg of intrinsic factor orally.

In pernicious anemia, 24-hour urine radioactivity becomes normal.
In malabsorption, 24-hour urine radioactivity remains low.

BLOOD VOLUME

Blood volume determination is usually done using albumin tagged with ^{125}I or ^{131}I; red cell mass may be measured by labeling RBCs with ^{51}Cr.

May Be Useful To

Determine the most appropriate blood component (whole blood, plasma, or packed cells) for replacement therapy. For example, normal total blood volume and decreased red cell mass indicate the need for packed red cell transfusion.

Evaluate the clinical course. For example, immediately after acute severe hemorrhage, the hemoglobin concentration, hematocrit value, and RBC may be normal and not indicate the severity of blood loss whereas appropriate measurements will show decreased blood volume, plasma volume, and red cell mass. After hemorrhage, the subsequent fluid shift from extravascular to intravascular space may produce a "falling" value for hemoglobin concentration, hematocrit, and RBC and falsely suggest continuing hemorrhage.

Assess the real degree of anemia in chronic conditions in which other mechanisms may disguise or accentuate the extent of RBC deficiency. For example, anemia and hemoconcentration together may produce an apparently normal hemoglobin concentration, hematocrit reading, and RBC. Hemodilution in uremia may make the anemia more marked and apparently more severe.

Alert the surgeon who compares the preoperative and postoperative values in surgical patients to

Unexpected blood loss

Need for replacement of the appropriate blood component, which may vary with the surgical procedure (e.g., in thoracoplasty the blood loss may be 900 ml, representing

approximately equal red cell and plasma losses; in gastrectomy the blood loss may be 1800 ml, representing an RBC
loss of 400 ml and a plasma loss of 1400 ml)

Differentiate polycythemia vera (increased total blood volume,
plasma volume, red cell mass) and secondary polycythemia
(normal or decreased total blood volume and plasma volume) in
most cases.

*Radioisotopes should not be administered to children or pregnant
women. In the presence of active hemorrhage, the isotope is lost
via the bleeding site, and a false value will be produced.*

THYROID UPTAKE OF RADIOACTIVE IODINE (^{131}I OR ^{125}I)

A tracer dose of radioactive iodine is administered (usually orally),
and the radioactivity over the thyroid is measured at specific
intervals (e.g., 1, 2, 6, or 24 hours). The test may also measure
radioactivity in urine, saliva, etc.

The test is contraindicated in pregnant or lactating women, infants,
and children. It is invalidated for 2–4 weeks after administration
of antithyroid drugs, thyroid, or iodides; the effect of organic
iodine (e.g., x-ray contrast media) may persist for a much longer
time.

	Thyroid Uptake of ^{131}I[a]			*24-Hour Excretion*
	1 hour	*6 hours*	*24 hours*	*of* ^{131}I *in Urine*
Normal	9–19%	7–25%	10–50%	40–70%
Hyperthyroid	20%	25%	50%	5–40%
Hypothyroid	9%	7%	15%	70–90%

[a]Increase in dietary iodine in the United States has caused a progressive
decrease of ^{131}I values, markedly diminishing its value for primary diagnosis of hyperthyroidism or hypothyroidism. Principal use is for the T-3
suppression test (see below) and for scanning.

The test was considered most valuable in the diagnosis of hyperthyroidism. Uptake is usually greater in diffuse toxic goiter than
in toxic nodules or recurrent hyperthyroidism following surgery
or radioactive iodine treatment.

T-3 suppression test: Administration of triiodothyronine (75 or 100
μg/day for 1 week) causes less suppression in the hyperthyroid
patient than in the normal person. Failure to suppress uptake to
<65% after antithyroid drug treatment often means the patient
will relapse.

*Very low uptake associated with a very high serum PBI probably
means ingestion of iodine. Low uptake associated with a
moderately high serum PBI suggests thyroiditis.*

TRIOLEIN ^{131}I ABSORPTION TEST

The patient fasts overnight after taking 30 drops of Lugol's iodine
solution on the previous day.

Administer 15–20 μc of triolein ^{131}I. Collect blood every 1–2 hours
for the next 6–8 hours.

Collect stools for 48–72 hours until radioactivity disappears.

Normal: $\geqq$ 10% of administered radioactivity appears in the blood within 6 hours; < 5% appears in the feces.

The test is useful for screening patients with steatorrhea. Normal values indicate that digestion of fat in the small bowel and absorption of fat in the small bowel are normal.

If results are abnormal, do an oleic acid ^{131}I absorption test.

OLEIC ACID ^{131}I ABSORPTION TEST

Methodology and normal values are the same as for the triolein absorption test.

An abnormal result indicates a defect in small bowel mucosal absorption function (e.g., sprue, Whipple's disease, regional enteritis, tuberculous enteritis, collagen diseases involving the small bowel, extensive resection). Abnormal pancreatic function does not affect the test.

POLYVINYLPYRROLIDONE (PVP)- [131]I

Give 15–25 μc of PVP-^{131}I intravenously and collect all stools for 4–5 days.

Normal: < 2% is excreted in feces when the mucosa of the GI tract is intact.

In protein-losing enteropathy > 2% of administered radioactivity appears in the stool.

[51]Cr TEST FOR GASTROINTESTINAL BLEEDING

Tag 10 ml of the patient's blood with 200 μc of ^{51}Cr and administer it intravenously. Collect daily stools for radioactivity measurement and also measure simultaneous blood samples.

Radioactivity in the stool establishes GI blood loss. Comparison with radioactivity measurements of 1 ml of blood indicates the amount of blood loss.

The test is useful in ulcerative diseases (e.g., ulcerative colitis, regional enteritis, peptic ulcer).

RBC UPTAKE OF RADIOACTIVE IRON (^{59}Fe)

[59]Fe is injected intravenously, and blood samples are drawn in 3, 7, and 14 days for measurement of radioactivity.

In pure red cell anemia the rate of uptake of ^{59}Fe is markedly decreased.

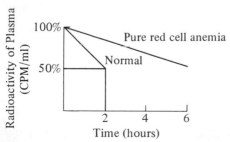

Fig. 3.   RBC uptake of radioactive iron (^{59}Fe).

PLASMA IRON ^{59}Fe CLEARANCE

^{59}Fe is injected intravenously, and blood samples are drawn in 5, 15, 30, 60, and 120 minutes for measurement of radioactivity.

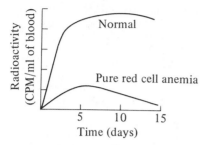

Fig. 4. Plasma iron (^{59}Fe) clearance.

ERYTHROCYTE SURVIVAL IN HEMOLYTIC DISEASES (^{51}Cr)

Increased In
Thalassemia minor

Decreased In
Idiopathic acquired hemolytic anemia
Paroxysmal nocturnal hemoglobinuria
Association with chronic lymphatic leukemia
Association with uremia
Congenital nonspherocytic hemolytic anemia
Hereditary spherocytosis
Elliptocytosis with hemolysis
Hemoglobin C disease
Sickle cell–hemoglobin C disease
Sickle cell anemia
Pernicious anemia
Megaloblastic anemia of pregnancy
In the normal person, half of the radioactivity of plasma disappears in 1–2 hours.
In pure red cell anemia, half of the plasma radioactivity may not disappear for 7–8 hours.

Normal In
Sickle cell trait
Hemoglobin C trait
Elliptocytosis without hemolysis or anemia

EVALUATION OF RENAL TRANSPLANT FUNCTION BY SODIUM IODOHIPPURATE ^{131}I CLEARANCE

Blood samples taken 20 and 30 minutes after IV hippuran ^{131}I
This test is useful for early detection of renal function impairment

due to rejection of renal transplant, especially in the first 24 hours when other tests of renal function are less useful.

THYROID SCAN WITH RADIOACTIVE IODINE

Useful To
Differentiate "hot" nodule from "cold" nodule
Detect presence and localization of functioning metastases
Differentiate mediastinal tumors from substernal thyroid (use ^{131}I rather than ^{125}I); first stimulate uptake with TSH
Differentiate tongue mass from lingual thyroid
Diagnose subacute thyroiditis
> Differentiates inflammatory transient cold nodules from cancer since inflammatory nodule may disappear after prednisone treatment
> Shows migration of focal thyroiditis
> Differentiates diffuse and focal types of thyroiditis

LIVER SCANNING
(radioactive technetium —^{99m}Tc)

Indications
Assess hepatic size, shape, location in abdomen
Differentiation of abdominal mass as being part of liver or extrahepatic
Focal lesions (primary or secondary tumors, abscess, cyst, hematoma)—minimal size to be visualized is 2.5 cm; must be located within range of instrument focus (30% of patients with metastatic carcinoma of liver have lesions too small to visualize)
Location of focal lesions prior to needle biopsy
Subphrenic abscess (combine with lung scan or chest x-ray to locate diaphragm)
Cirrhosis of liver—mottled appearance of small liver and isotope uptake in reticuloendothelial system of vertebrae; enlarged spleen that may have a density equal to or greater than that of liver

Beware of variability in porta hepatis region.
A diffuse pattern may occur with hepatitis or diffuse metastases.
False negative diagnosis is made in $\leqq$ 12% of patients; false positive in $\leqq$ 5%.

LUNG SCANNING
(macroaggregates of radioactive iodinated serum albumin (RISA); 150–300 μc ^{131}I and 0.6 mg albumin—after first blocking thyroid gland)

Useful In
Demonstration of pulmonary blood flow (i.e., detects regional pulmonary ischemia), down to vessels 1–2 mm in size. May demonstrate emboli too small for angiographic demonstration.
Evaluation of pulmonary function of individual lungs (instead of bronchospirometry) in preoperative evaluation of candidates for pulmonary resection

BRAIN SCANNING

99mTc has wider application and repeatability than 197Hg or 203Hg. The scan is safe, nontoxic, easy to administer intravenously or orally, and painless; patient must remain quiet.

It is most accurate with meningiomas and malignant glioblastomas; least accurate with slow-growing astrocytomas. At present, it is more accurate in scanning cerebral hemispheres than midline or posterior fossa and more accurate for supratentorial (80%) than infratentorial lesions (70%)—somewhat less precise, that is, than angiography or positive contrast ventriculography.

A positive scan is not specific for tumor (scan may also be positive in infarct, contusion, abscess, subdural hematoma, granuloma, arteriovenous malformation, scalp hematomas, and fluid accumulations).

A negative scan does not rule out tumor or other structural lesions.

The scan does not reveal type of tumor, blood supply, or ventricular system.

RENAL SCANNING

Use of 99mTc-iron complex may be the best at present.

Useful To

Detect renal masses (not as useful as renal arteriogram, which provides higher resolution and distinguishes benign from malignant lesions by vascular patterns)

Localize kidney prior to needle biopsy in children (permits greater frequency of successful biopsy)

Localize functioning renal parenchyma (e.g., extent of the bridge in horseshoe kidney)

The scan represents renal plasma flow in each kidney. If total renal plasma flow is measured by PAH clearance, individual renal plasma flow can be determined without ureteral catheterization.

CARDIAC BLOOD POOL SCANNING (99mTc)

Useful In

Pericardial effusion or tumor (halo area around heart)

Ventricular aneurysm (appears as tumor in vicinity of left ventricle that contains tracer isotope)

Aortic aneurysm (differentiated from mediastinal tumors)

Localization of other aneurysms in body

Localization of placenta

Demonstration of cardiac dilatation

SPLEEN SCANNING

Method 1

Use patient's RBCs which have been damaged (by heat or chemicals) after tagging with isotope such as 51Cr, 197Hg, or 81Rb; these damaged RBCs are preferentially sequestered in splenic sinusoids. This method is indicated for

Demonstration of ectopic spleen location

Demonstration that functional splenic tissue is absent
Demonstration of accessory spleens after splenectomy
Detecting rejection of splenic transplant
Demonstrating spleen size quantitatively or detecting some cases of minimal splenomegaly

Method 2

Use radioactive colloids such as ^{198}Au, ^{99m}Tc, or ^{113m}In which are phagocytosed by the reticuloendothelial cells in the spleen (and other organs). This method is preferred (because of lower irradiation dose) in the differential diagnosis of left upper quadrant abdominal masses or delineation of space-occupying lesions of the spleen. This is the only method that visualizes spleen and liver simultaneously in cases of diffuse hepatic disease and splenomegaly.

BONE SCANNING

Sodium fluoride ^{18}F is superior to the formerly used ^{47}Ca and ^{85}Sr.
The scan is used for detection of bone metastases (both osteolytic and osteoblastic). Diagnosis prior to definite x-ray evidence of these lesions is its chief clinical usefulness.
It may also be positive in primary bone tumors (e.g., Ewing's sarcoma, osteogenic sarcoma).
It is not useful in soft-tissue sarcomas.
Since ^{18}F is indicator of increased bone metabolism, nonneoplastic reparative bone activity may cause positive scan in patients with Paget's disease, osteomyelitis, fractures, healing postoperative areas, osteoarthritis, rheumatoid spondylitis, and osteoporosis. For these cases, roentgenograms are essential to establish diagnosis and rule out tumor.

PAROTID GLAND SCANNING
(using ^{99m}Tc)

Preliminary Findings

"Hot" nodule in Warthin's tumor (papillary cystadenoma lymphomatosum); probably will also be found in other ductal tumors (oncocytoma, mucoepidermoid tumor)
"Cold" nodules (> 2 cm in size)
    Benign tumors or cysts—smooth, sharply defined outlines
    Adenocarcinoma—ragged irregular outlines

SCANNING OF THE PANCREAS
(using selenomethionine —^{75}Se)

The liver may also be scanned with ^{198}Au to delineate the medial border of the liver.
Inability to demonstrate the pancreas is the most reliable sign of pancreatic disease. Distortion of pancreatic shape is not always indicative of abnormality.
Radioactivity in the upper jejunum is a sign of pancreatic normality.
Diagnosis of normal pancreas is correct in 90% of patients.
Diagnosis of abnormal pancreas is correct in < 60% of patients.

SCANNING OF THE PARATHYROID GLANDS
(using ^{75}Se)
Useful in consistently visualizing adenomas larger than 2 gm
Not useful for detecting adenomas smaller than 1 gm or mediastinal
   lesions or parathyroid hyperplasia

SCANNING OF THE ADRENAL GLANDS
(using [131]I-19-iodocholesterol)
In Cushing's syndrome that persists or recurs after total adrenalectomy, photoscanning demonstrates residual adrenal tissue.
In primary aldosteronism, localizes site of adrenal adenoma and
   distinguishes unilateral from bilateral tumor. May become useful
   to distinguish adenoma from bilateral hyperplasia (photoscanning before and after administration of dexamethasone shows
   suppression of adrenal uptake in hyperplasia but no suppression
   in adenoma).

SCANNING IN CANCER DIAGNOSIS
(using ^{67}Ga)
Appears to be most sensitive in detecting bronchogenic carcinoma
   irrespective of cell type (93%) and malignant lymphoma, especially Hodgkin's disease (87%), in which it may also be useful for
   determining the stage of the disease.

SCANNING IN CARDIOVASCULAR DISEASE

Peripheral Vascular Disease
[125]I fibrinogen is injected intravenously (after thyroid uptake is
blocked with iodide), and then legs are scanned at different sites
to detect increased radioactivity. This test is most valuable for
determining active venous thrombosis, but it is still awaiting
FDA approval. The disadvantages of the test are that it cannot
detect inactive disease, it is not sensitive to disease proximal to
midthigh, and it often detects clinically insignificant disease in
the calf, especially in postoperative patients.

Acute Myocardial Infarction
[99m]Tc-pyrophosphate imaging 60–90 minutes after administration in
different projections is sensitive for the detection of infarcts 12
hours to 6 days old. The drawbacks of this technique are that it is
less dependable for subendocardial infarcts than for transmural
infarcts and that it may be positive following electrical shock and
in the presence of ventricular aneurysm without acute infarction.
It may be particularly useful in certain patients, e.g., those with
chest pain in the presence of left bundle-branch block, in which
enzyme elevation has occurred for other reasons (such as postoperative status); a negative scan is useful to rule out acute
infarction during the preceding 6 days.

23

NUCLEAR SEX CHROMATIN AND KARYOTYPING

NUCLEAR SEXING

Epithelial cells from buccal smear (or vaginal smear, etc.) are stained with cresyl violet and examined microscopically.

A dense body (Barr body) on the nuclear membrane represents one of the X chromosomes and occurs in 30–60% of female somatic cells. The maximum number of Barr bodies is 1 less than the number of X chromosomes.

If there are < 10% of the cells containing Barr bodies in a patient with female genitalia, karyotyping should be done to delineate probable chromosomal abnormalities.

A normal count does not rule out chromosomal abnormalities.

2 Barr bodies may be found in
    47 XXX female
    48 XXXY male (Klinefelter's syndrome)
    49 XXXYY male (Klinefelter's syndrome)

3 Barr bodies may be found in
    49 XXXXY male (Klinefelter's syndrome)

EVALUATION OF SEX CHROMOSOME IN LEUKOCYTES

Presence of a "drumstick" nuclear appendage in $\cong 3\%$ of leukocytes in normal females indicates the presence of 2 X chromosomes in the karyotype. It is not found in males.

It is absent in the XO type of Turner's syndrome.

There is a lower incidence of drumsticks in Klinefelter's syndrome (XXY) as opposed to the extra Barr body. *(Mean lobe counts of neutrophils are also decreased.)*

Incidence of drumsticks is decreased and mean lobe counts are lower also in mongolism.

Double drumsticks are exceedingly rare and diagnostically impractical.

SOME INDICATIONS FOR CHROMOSOME ANALYSIS (KARYOTYPING)

Suspected Autosomal Syndromes
    Down's (mongolism)
    E_{18} Trisomy
    D_{13} Trisomy
    Cri du chat syndrome

Suspected Sex-Chromosome Syndromes
    Klinefelter's XXY, XXXY
    Turner's XO
    "Superfemale" XXX, XXXX
    "Supermale" XYY

"Funny-looking kid" syndromes, especially with multiple anomalies including mental retardation and low birth weight

Possible myelogenous leukemia to demonstrate Philadelphia chromosome (22)

Ambiguous genitalia
Infertility (some patients)
Repeated miscarriages
Primary amenorrhea or oligomenorrhea
Mental retardation with sex anomalies
Hypogonadism
Delayed puberty
Abnormal development at puberty
Disturbances of somatic growth

SOME INDICATIONS FOR DIAGNOSTIC AMNIOCENTESIS FOR CHROMOSOME STUDIES
(should be performed between 14 and 16 weeks' gestation; should always be preceded by ultrasound studies)

Chromosomal Disorders

With advanced maternal age, risk of chromosome disorder in off-spring is 2.2% for women aged 35–39, 3.4% for women aged 40–44, 10% for women aged 45 and over.

When one parent is carrier of a chromosomal translocation (particularly D/G and D/D), risk of chromosome disorder in offspring is 9% when mother is carrier and 4% when father is carrier.

Previous child with trisomy 21 (Down's syndrome)

Sex-Linked Disorders (usually carried by females and found in 50% of their male children)

Only Lesch-Nyhan syndrome, Hunter syndrome, and Fabry's disease are specifically diagnosable. When the mother is a known carrier, sex prediction and abortion of male fetuses prevent two-thirds of these disorders.

Hereditary Biochemical Disorders

Lipidoses
Mucopolysaccharidoses
Disorders of amino acid or carbohydrate metabolism
Other

See p. 349ff.

Congenital Malformations

Increased level of alpha-fetoprotein allows prenatal diagnosis of 90% of cases of open neural tube defects (e.g., anencephaly, spina bifida) but may also indicate fetal distress or death or other disorders. Risk of neural tube defects is greater when it has occurred in a sibling or a parent.

Table 16. Chromosome Number and Karyotype in Various Clinical Conditions

Clinical Condition	Chromosome Number and Karyotype	Incidence
Normal male	46 XY	
Normal female	46 XX	
Turner's syndrome	45 XO	1 in 3,000 live female births
	46 XX	Rare
	Mosaics	Infrequent
Klinefelter's syndrome	47 XXY	1 in 600 live male births
	48 XXXY 48 XXYY 49 XXXXY 49 XXXYY	Rare
	Mosaics	Infrequent
Superfemale	47 XXX	1 in 1–2,000 live female births
	48 XXXX 49 XXXXX Mosaics	Rare
Supermale	47 XYY	1 in 1,000 live male births
	48 XYYY	Rare
	Mosaics	Rare
Down's syndrome (mongolism; trisomy 21)	47 XX, G+ or 47 XY, G+	1 in 700 live births (2% are 46 count due to translocation and have 10% risk of Down's syndrome in subsequent pregnancies; 2% are 46/47 mosaics)
D_1 trisomy	47 XX, D+ or 47 XY, D+	1 in 5,000 live births
	Translocations	Rare
	Mosaics	
E_{18} trisomy	47 XX, E+ or 47 XY, E+	1 in 3,000 live births
	Translocations	Rare
	Mosaics	Rare
Cri du chat syndrome	46 with partial B deletion	1 in 30,000 live births

DISEASES OF ORGAN SYSTEMS

CARDIOVASCULAR DISEASES

HYPERTENSION
(present in 20% of adults in the United States)
Laboratory findings due to the primary disease. *These conditions are often occult or unsuspected and should always be carefully ruled out since many of them represent curable causes of hypertension.* (See Plasma Renin Activity, pp. 80–81.)

Systolic hypertension
Hyperthyroidism
Chronic anemia with hemoglobin <7 gm/100 ml
Arteriovenous fistulas—advanced Paget's disease of bone; pulmonary arteriovenous varix
Beriberi
Systolic and diastolic hypertension
Essential (primary) hypertension (causes 90% of cases of hypertension)
Secondary hypertension (causes <10% of cases of hypertension)
Endocrine diseases
Adrenal
Pheochromocytoma (0.5% of cases of hypertension)
Aldosteronism (1% of cases of hypertension)
Cushing's syndrome
Pituitary disease
Signs of hyperadrenal function
Acromegaly
Hyperthyroidism
Hyperparathyroidism
Renal diseases
Vascular (4% of cases of hypertension)
Renal artery stenosis (usually due to atheromatous plaque in elderly patients and to fibromuscular hyperplasia in younger patients)
Nephrosclerosis
Embolism
Arteriovenous fistula
Aneurysm
Parenchymal
Glomerulonephritis
Pyelonephritis
Polycystic kidneys
Kimmelstiel-Wilson syndrome
Amyloidosis
Collagen diseases
Renin-producing renal tumor (Wilms' tumor; renal hemangiopericytoma)
Miscellaneous

Urinary tract obstructions
Central nervous system diseases
Cerebrovascular accident
Brain tumors
Poliomyelitis
Other
Toxemia of pregnancy
Polycythemia

Laboratory findings indicating the functional renal status (e.g., urinalysis, BUN, creatinine, uric acid, serum electrolytes, PSP, creatinine clearance, Addis count, radioisotope scan of kidneys, renal biopsy)

Laboratory findings due to complications of hypertension (e.g., congestive heart failure, uremia, cerebral hemorrhage, myocardial infarction)

Laboratory findings due to administration of some antihypertensive drugs

Oral diuretics (e.g., benzothiadiazines)
Increased incidence of hyperuricemia (to 65–75% of hypertensive patients from incidence of 25–35% in untreated hypertensive patients)
Hypokalemia
Hyperglycemia or aggravation of preexisting diabetes mellitus
Less commonly, bone marrow depression, aggravation of renal or hepatic insufficiency by electrolyte imbalance, cholestatic hepatitis, toxic pancreatitis

Hydralazine
Long-term dosage of >200 mg/day may produce syndrome not distinguishable from systemic lupus erythematosus (SLE). Usually regresses after drug is discontinued. Antinuclear antibody may be found in ≦50% of asymptomatic patients.

Methyldopa
≦20% of patients may have positive direct Coombs' test, but relatively few have hemolytic anemia. When drug is discontinued, Coombs' test may remain positive for months but anemia usually reverses promptly.

Abnormal liver function tests indicate hepatocellular damage without jaundice associated with febrile influenzalike syndrome.
RA and LE tests may occasionally be positive.
Rarely, granulocytopenia or thrombocytopenia may occur.

Monoamine oxidase inhibitors (e.g., pargyline hydrochloride)
Wide range of toxic reactions, most serious of which are
Blood dyscrasias
Hepatocellular necrosis

Diazoxide
Sodium and fluid retention
Hyperglycemia (usually mild and manageable by insulin or oral hypoglycemic agents)

When hypertension is associated with decreased serum potassium, rule out
Primary aldosteronism
Pseudoaldosteronism (due to excessive ingestion of licorice)
Secondary aldosteronism (e.g., malignant hypertension)
Hypokalemia due to diuretic administration
Potassium loss due to renal disease
Cushing's syndrome

CORONARY HEART DISEASE
Beware of coronary heart disease in presence of
Increased serum cholesterol (>260 mg/100 ml)
Increased serum triglyceride (>250 mg/100 ml)
Abnormal lipoprotein electrophoresis (see Table 50, pp. 352–355
Hyperglycemia (fasting blood sugar >120 mg/100 ml; postprandial blood sugar >180 mg/100 ml)
Decreased glucose tolerance
Significant glycosuria
Increased serum uric acid (>8.5 mg/100 ml)
Laboratory findings due to hypertension (see preceding section)

ACUTE MYOCARDIAL INFARCTION

Laboratory Determinations Required
Because ECG changes may be inconclusive (e.g., masked by bundle-branch block or Wolff-Parkinson-White syndrome or may not reveal intramural or diaphragmatic infarcts)
For differential diagnosis (e.g., angina pectoris, pulmonary infarction). Normal serum enzyme levels during 48 hours after onset of clinical symptoms indicate no myocardial infarction.
To follow the course of the patient with acute myocardial infarction
To estimate prognosis (e.g., marked elevation of serum enzyme [4–5 times normal] correlates with increased incidence of ventricular arrhythmia, shock, heart failure, and with higher mortality)

Blood should be drawn promptly after onset of symptoms. Repeat determinations should be performed at appropriate intervals (see Fig. 5, p. 172) and also if symptoms recur or new signs or symptoms develop. Changes may indicate additional myocardial infarction or other complications (e.g., pulmonary infarction).

Specific Findings
Serum creatine phosphokinase (CPK) is particularly valuable for the following reasons
Increased levels occur in >90% of the patients when blood is drawn at the appropriate time.
It allows early diagnosis because increased levels appear within 3–6 hours after onset and peak levels in 24–36 hours.
It is a more sensitive indicator than other enzymes because

increased the CPK level shows a larger amplitude of change (6–12 times normal).

Less diagnostic confusion occurs because CPK is not increased by many diseases that may be associated with myocardial infarction (e.g., liver damage due to congestion, drug therapy, etc., may increase SGOT) or that may be difficult to distinguish from myocardial infarction (e.g., pulmonary infarction may increase LDH).

It returns to normal by third day; a poorer prognosis is suggested if the increase lasts more than 3–4 days. Reinfarction is indicated by an elevated level after the fifth day that had previously returned to normal.

It is useful in differential diagnosis of diseases with normal enzyme level (e.g., angina pectoris) or from those with increased levels of other enzymes (e.g., increased LDH in pulmonary infarction).

Serum Creatine Phosphokinase (CPK) Isoenzymes

MB isoenzyme is increased in acute myocardial infarction, cardiac surgery, and muscular dystrophy; it is not increased by cardiac catheterization or transvenous pacemakers even though total serum CPK may be increased. In acute myocardial infarction, MB isoenzyme is evident at 4–8 hours, peaks at 24 hours, and is present in 100% of patients within the first 48 hours. By 72 hours, two-thirds of patients still show some increase in MB isoenzyme. CPK isoenzyme studies provide the best laboratory discrimination between the presence or absence of myocardial necrosis.

Serum SGOT is useful for the following reasons:

It is increased in >95% of the patients when blood is drawn at the appropriate time.

It allows early diagnosis because increased levels appear within 6–8 hours and peak levels in 24 hours. Usually returns to normal in 4–6 days.

Peak level is usually $\cong$ 200 units (5 times normal). A higher level >300 units), along with a more prolonged increase, suggests a poorer prognosis.

Reinfarction is indicated by a rise following a return to normal.

Serum SGPT is usually not increased unless there is liver damage due to congestive heart failure, drug therapy, etc.

Serum LDH is almost always increased, beginning in 10–12 hours and reaching a peak in 48–72 hours (of about 3 times normal). The prolonged elevation of 10–14 days is particularly useful for late diagnosis when the patient is first seen after sufficient time has elapsed for CPK and SGOT to become normal. Levels >2000 units suggest a poorer prognosis. Because many other diseases may increase the LDH, isoenzyme studies should be performed. Increased serum LDH with an LDH_1-LDH_2 ratio >1 ("flipped" LDH) occurs in acute renal infarction and hemolysis associated with hemolytic anemia or prosthetic heart valves, as well as in acute myocardial infarction. In acute myocardial infarction, flipped LDH usually appears between 12–24 hours and is present within 48 hours in 80% of patients; after 1

Table 17. Summary of Increased Serum Enzyme Levels After Acute Myocardial Infarction[a]

Serum Enzymes	Earliest Increase (hours)	Maximum Level (hours)	Return to Normal by (days)	Amplitude of Increase × Normal	Comment[b]
CPK	3–6	24–36	3	7	Recommended for early diagnosis
MDH	4–6	24–48	5	4	Early use parallels CPK; no advantage over other enzymes; technically difficult to do
SGOT	6–8	24–48	4–6	5	Most commonly used
LDH	10–12	48–72	11	3	See α-HBD; isoenzyme determination to differentiate pulmonary infarction, congestive heart failure, etc.
α-HBD	10–12	48–72	13	3–4	Particularly useful for later diagnosis (in 2nd week) when other enzymes have returned to normal, because of longer duration of increased activity; more specific than LDH
ALD	6–8	24–48	4	4	
SGPT	Usually normal unless liver damage due to congestive heart failure, shock, drug therapy (e.g., Coumadin)				
ICD	Usually normal				

[a]The time periods all represent average values.
[b]Least number of false positive results occur with tests of CPK, α-HBD, heat-stable LDH.

169

Table 18. Triad of Laboratory Tests Suggested for Differential Diagnosis of Acute Myocardial Infarction[a]

Serial Tests Done Within 2 Days of Onset	Acute Myocardial Infarction	Angina Pectoris	Pulmonary Embolism or Infarction[b]	Pneumonia or Atelectasis	Congestive Heart Failure	Pulmonary Embolism and Myocardial Infarction
SGOT	I	N	Usually N	N	N	I
LDH	I	N	I	N	N	I
Serum bilirubin	N	N	I ≅ 20% of patients	N	May be slightly I	I

I = increased; N = normal.

[a]Not useful in presence of severe liver disease.

[b]"Triad" of increased LDH and serum bilirubin associated with normal SGOT is found in ≅15% of patients.

week it is still present in < 50% of patients even though total serum LDH may still be elevated. Flipped LDH never appears before CPK MB isoenzyme. LDH_1 may remain elevated after total LDH has returned to normal; with small infarcts, LDH_1 may be increased while total LDH remains normal.

Serum Isoenzymes. In patients with suspected acute myocardial infarction, blood samples should be taken on admission and at 24 and 48 hours, and isoenzyme determinations should be performed when CPK or LDH is increased. If increased CPK MB isoenzyme and flipped LDH both occur in any of the blood specimens (not necessarily at the same time), it is virtually certain that the patient has acute myocardial infarction and there is no need for further diagnostic testing; if these criteria are not met within 48 hours, the diagnosis is considered not to be acute myocardial necrosis and enzyme measurement can be terminated.

Serum α-HBD parallels increase of fast-moving LDH with peak (3–4 times normal) in 48 hours and persistent elevation for up to 2 weeks.

Serum MDH is useful because an early increase (4–6 hours) parallels changes in CPK.

Serum ICD is normal.

Leukocytosis is almost invariable; commonly detected by second day but may occur as early as 2 hours. Usually the WBC count is 12,000 to 15,000; up to 20,000 is not rare; sometimes it is very high. Usually there are 75–90% neutrophilic leukocytes with only a slight shift to the left. Leukocytosis is likely to develop before fever.

Sedimentation rate (ESR) is increased, usually by second or third day (may begin within a few hours); peak rate is in 4–5 days, persists for 2–6 months. Increased ESR is sometimes more sensitive than WBC as it may occur before fever and it persists after temperature and WBC have returned to normal. Degree of increase of ESR does not correlate with severity or prognosis.

Glycosuria and hyperglycemia occur in $\leqq 50\%$ of patients.

Glucose tolerance is decreased.

Myoglobinuria often occurs (see p. 132).

Differential Diagnosis

Serum enzymes not elevated in angina pectoris; increased levels mean myocardial infarction or another condition.

Serum enzymes usually show little or no increase in inflammatory myocardial lesions (e.g., rheumatic fever) unless disease is severe. (Salicilates may cause some increase of SGOT and SGPT due to liver damage.)

Little or no change occurs in chronic heart failure.

Some increase of SGOT and SGPT may occur in acute heart failure due to liver congestion; it is quickly reversed with appropriate therapy. There may be marked increase in cardiac tamponade due to pericardial effusion.

SGPT is higher than SGOT (which is only slightly increased) in pulmonary infarction and upper abdominal disease (e.g., liver injury).

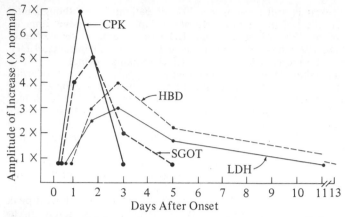

Fig. 5.   Sequential changes in serum enzymes after acute myocardial infarction. (From J. H. Wilkinson, The diagnostic value of LDH isoenzymes in clinical medicine. *Clinical Profile* 1:1, 1968.)

CONGESTIVE HEART FAILURE

Renal changes. Urine—slight albuminuria (<1 gm/day) is common. There are isolated RBCs and WBCs, hyaline and (sometimes) granular casts. Urine is concentrated, with specific gravity >1.020. Oliguria is a characteristic feature of right-sided failure. PSP excretion and urea clearance are usually depressed. Moderate azotemia (BUN usually <60 mg/100 ml) is evident with severe oliguria; may increase with vigorous diuresis. *(Primary renal disease is indicated by proportionate increase in serum creatinine and low specific gravity of urine despite oliguria.)*

ESR may be decreased because of decreased serum fibrinogen.

Plasma volume is increased. Serum albumin and total protein are decreased, with increased gamma globulin. Hematocrit reading is slightly decreased but red cell mass may be increased.

Liver function changes (see p. 223).

Laboratory findings due to underlying disease (e.g., rheumatic fever, viral myocarditis, bacterial endocarditis, chronic severe anemia, hypertension, hyperthyroidism, Hurler's disease).

Fluid and electrolytes

Urine sodium is decreased. Plasma sodium and chloride tend to fall but may be normal before treatment. Total body sodium is markedly increased. Plasma potassium is usually normal or slightly increased (because of shift from intracellular location); may be somewhat reduced with hypochloremic alkalosis due to some diuretics. Total body potassium is decreased. Saliva sodium and chloride is decreased and potassium is increased.

Acidosis (reduced blood pH) occurs when renal insufficiency is associated or there is CO_2 retention due to pulmonary insufficiency, low plasma sodium, or ammomium chloride toxicity.

Alkalosis (increased blood pH) occurs in uncomplicated heart failure itself, hyperventilation, alveolar-capillary block due to associated pulmonary fibrosis, after mercurial diuresis that causes hypochloremic alkalosis, because of potassium depletion.

Alkalosis (with normal or increased blood pH) showing increased plasma bicarbonate and moderately increased pCO_2 after acute correction of respiratory acidosis is due to CO_2 retention when there is chloride deficit and usually decreased potassium.

ACUTE RHEUMATIC FEVER

Antistreptolysin O titer increase indicates recent hemolytic streptococcus infection and indirectly corroborates clinical findings of rheumatic fever. Increased titer develops only after second week and reaches a peak in 4–6 weeks. Increasing titer is more significant than a single determination. Titer is usually >250 units; more significant if >400–500 units. A normal titer helps to rule out clinically doubtful rheumatic fever. Sometimes ASO is not increased even when other titers (antifibrinolysin, antihyaluronidase) are increased. Increased titer is found in 80% of patients within the first 2 months. Height of titer is not related to severity; rate of fall is not related to course of disease.

Antihyaluronidase titer of 1000–1500 follows recent streptococcus A disease and ≤ 4000 with rheumatic fever. Average titer is higher in early rheumatic activity than in subsiding or inactive rheumatic fever or nonrheumatic streptococcal disease or nonstreptococcal infections. Antihyaluronidase titer is increased as often as ASO and antifibrinolysin titers.

Antifibrinolysin (antistreptokinase) titer is increased in rheumatic fever and in recent hemolytic streptococcus infections.

One of the above three titers is elevated in 95% of patients with acute rheumatic fever; if all are normal, a diagnosis of rheumatic fever is less likely.

Sedimentation rate (ESR) increase is a sensitive test of rheumatic activity; returns to normal with adequate treatment with ACTH or salicylates. It may remain increased after WBC becomes normal. It is said to become normal with onset of congestive heart failure even in the presence of rheumatic activity. It is normal in uncomplicated chorea alone.

C-reactive protein (CRP) parallels ESR.

Serum proteins are altered, with decreased serum albumin and increased alpha$_2$ and gamma globulins. (*Streptococcus A infections do not increase alpha$_2$ globulin.*) Fibrinogen is increased.

White blood count may be normal but usually is increased (10,000–16,000/cu mm) with shift to the left; increase may persist for weeks after fever subsides. Count may decrease with salicylate and ACTH therapy.

Anemia (hemoglobin usually 8–12 gm/100 ml) is common; gradually improves as activity subsides; microcytic type. Anemia may be related to increased plasma volume that occurs in early phase of acute rheumatic fever.

Urine. There is a slight febrile albuminuria. Often mild abnormality of Addis count (protein, casts, RBC, WBC) indicates mild focal nephritis. Concomitant glomerulonephritis appears in $\leqq 2.5\%$ of cases.

Blood cultures are usually negative. Occasional positive culture is found in 5% of patients (bacteria usually grow only in fluid media, not on solid media), in contrast to bacterial endocarditis.

SGOT may be increased, but SGPT is normal unless the patient has cardiac failure with liver damage.

Determine clinical activity: follow ESR, CRP, and WBC. Return to normal should be seen in 6–12 weeks in 80–90% of patients; it may take $\leqq 6$ months. Normal findings do not prove inactivity if patient is receiving hormone therapy. When therapy is stopped after findings have been suppressed for 6–8 weeks, there may be a mild rebound for 2–3 days and then a return to normal. Relapse after cessation of therapy occurs within 1–8 weeks.

CHRONIC RHEUMATIC VALVULAR HEART DISEASE
Laboratory findings due to complications
    Congestive heart failure
    Rheumatic activity
    Bacterial endocarditis
    Embolic phenomena

CHRONIC NONRHEUMATIC VALVULAR HEART DISEASE
Laboratory findings due to associated or underlying disease
    Syphilis
    Carcinoid syndrome
    Marfan's syndrome
    Genetic disease of mucopolysaccharide metabolism (Hurler's syndrome, Schei's syndrome, Morquio-Ulrich syndrome)
    Rheumatoid arthritis
    Congenital defect (e.g., Ebstein's abnormality of tricuspid valve, bicuspid aortic valve)
    Calcific aortic stenosis
    Endocardial fibroelastosis
    Nonbacterial thrombotic endocarditis (see next section)
Laboratory findings due to complications
    Heart failure
    Bacterial endocarditis
    Embolic phenomena

NONBACTERIAL THROMBOTIC ENDOCARDITIS (TERMINAL ENDOCARDITIS; MARANTIC ENDOCARDITIS)
Laboratory findings due to underlying or predisposing conditions
    Rheumatic valvular disease
    Congenital valvular heart disease
    Terminal systemic neoplasms
    Other
Laboratory findings due to complications

Systemic emboli (e.g., cerebral, renal)
Bacterial endocarditis

BACTERIAL ENDOCARDITIS

Blood culture is positive in 80–90% of patients. Streptococcus viridans, enterococcus, or staphylococcus causes 95% of cases. Other causes may be gram-negative bacteria (e.g., *Haemophilus influenzae*), gram-positive bacteria (e.g., hemolytic streptococcus), fungi (e.g., *Candida, Histoplasma, Cryptococcus*).

Progressive normochromic normocytic anemia is a characteristic feature; in 10% of patients hemoglobin is <7 gm/100 ml. Rarely there is a hemolytic anemia with a positive Coombs' test. Serum iron is decreased. Bone marrow contains abundant hemosiderin. White blood count is normal in ≅ 50% of patients and elevated ≦ about 15,000/cu mm in the rest, with 65–86% neutrophils. Higher WBC indicates presence of a complication (e.g., cerebral, pulmonary). Occasionally there is leukopenia. Monocytosis may be pronounced. Large macrophages may occur in peripheral blood.

Platelet count is usually normal but occasionally it is decreased; rarely purpura occurs.

Serum proteins are altered, with an increase in gamma globulin; therefore positive cephalin flocculation, thymol turbidity, ESR, cryoglobulins, rheumatoid factor (RA test), etc., are found.

Hematuria (usually microscopic) occurs at some stage in many patients due to glomerulitis or renal infarct or focal embolic glomerulonephritis. Albuminuria is almost invariable even without these complications. Renal insufficiency with azotemia and fixed specific gravity is infrequent now. Nephrotic syndrome is rare.

Cerebrospinal fluid findings in various complications. See sections on meningitis, brain abscess, mycotic aneurysm.

Proper blood cultures require adequate volume of blood, at least 5 cultures taken during a period of several days with temperature 101°F or more (preferably when highest), anaerobic as well as aerobic growth, variety of enriched media, prompt incubation, prolonged observation (growth is usual in 1–4 days but may require 2–3 weeks). Beware of negative culture due to recent antibiotic therapy. Beware of transient bacteremia following dental procedures, tonsillectomy, etc., which does not represent bacterial endocarditis (in these cases, streptococci usually grow only in fluid media; in bacterial endocarditis, many colonies also occur on solid media). Blood culture is also negative in bacterial endocarditis due to *Rickettsia burnetii,* but Phase 1 complement fixation test is positive.

Positive blood cultures may be more difficult to obtain in prosthetic valve endocarditis (due to unusual and fastidious organisms), right-sided endocarditis, uremia, and long-standing endocarditis. A single positive culture must be interpreted with extreme caution. Aside from the exceptions noted in this paragraph, the diagnosis should be based on 2 or more cultures positive for the *same* organism.

Serum bactericidal test measures ability of serial dilutions of *pa-*

tient's serum to sterilize a standardized inoculum of *his* infecting organisms; it is sometimes useful to demonstrate inadequate antibiotic levels or to avoid unnecessary drug toxicity.

Laboratory findings due to underlying or predisposing diseases
Rheumatic heart disease
Congenital heart disease
Infection of genitourinary system
Other

MYXOMA OF LEFT ATRIUM OF HEART

Anemia which is hemolytic in type and mechanical in origin (due to local turbulence of blood) is to be looked for and may be severe. Bizarre poikilocytes may be seen in blood smear. Reticulocyte count may be increased. Other findings may reflect effects of hemolysis or compensatory erythroid hyperplasia. The anemia is recognized in $\cong 50\%$ of patients with this tumor. Increased serum LDH reflects hemolysis.

Serum gamma globulin is increased in $\cong 50\%$ of patients. IgG may be increased.

Increased ESR is a reflection of abnormal serum proteins.

Platelet count may be decreased (possibly the cause here also is mechanical) with resultant findings due to thrombocytopenia.

Negative blood cultures differentiate this tumor from bacterial endocarditis.

Occasionally WBC is increased, and CRP may be positive.

Laboratory findings due to complications
Emboli to various organs (*Increased SGOT may reflect many small emboli to striated muscle.*) (see next section)
Congestive heart failure

These findings are reported much less frequently in myxoma of the right atrium, which is more likely to be accompanied by secondary polycythemia than anemia.

EMBOLIC LESIONS

See separate sections for laboratory findings due to infarction of kidney, intestine, brain, etc.

Laboratory findings due to underlying causative disease
Bacterial endocarditis
Nonbacterial thrombotic vegetations on heart valves
Chronic rheumatic mitral stenosis with mural thrombi
Chronic atrial fibrillation (*rule out underlying hyperthyroidism*)
Mural thrombus due to underlying myocardial infarction
Myxoma of left atrium (see preceding section)

POSTCOMMISSUROTOMY SYNDROME

This condition occurs after cardiac surgery (e.g., commissurotomy, correction of pulmonary stenosis with atrial septal defect); it is the same as the postcardiac injury syndrome.

WBC is increased.

ESR is increased.

CRP is present by the second day.
SGOT is increased to 4–7 times normal by the second day.

COR PULMONALE
Secondary polycythemia
Increased blood CO_2 when cor pulmonale is secondary to chest deformities or pulmonary emphysema
Laboratory findings of the primary lung disease (e.g., chronic bronchitis and emphysema, multiple small pulmonary emboli, pulmonary schistosomiasis)

TETRALOGY OF FALLOT
Secondary polycythemia is present. Mortality for complete surgical correction is higher in patients with Hb >18 gm/100 ml than in those with Hb <18 gm/100 ml. Surgical risk is decreased if polycythemia is first reduced by a preliminary systemic-pulmonary anastomosis.
Laboratory findings due to complications (see next section)

COMPLICATIONS OF CONGENITAL HEART DISEASE
Laboratory findings due to
Congestive heart failure
Bacterial endocarditis
Pulmonary tuberculosis, especially with pulmonary stenosis
Paradoxical embolism—with right-to-left communication, especially patent foramen ovale
Brain abscess, especially with interventricular septal defect, particularly in tetralogy of Fallot; also in atrial septal defect
Rupture of aorta
Secondary polycythemia

COBALT-BEER CARDIOMYOPATHY
(bizarre syndrome of fulminating heart failure in drinkers of large amounts of beer of a brand that contains cobalt)
Polycythemia
Lactic acidosis and shock
Increased SGOT, CPK, and LDH, often to extremely high levels; these may rise even further after recovery from shock
Laboratory findings due to pericardial effusion and, less frequently, pleural effusion

ACUTE PERICARDITIS

Due To
Active rheumatic fever (40% of patients)
Bacterial infection (20% of patients)
Uremia (11% of patients)
Benign nonspecific pericarditis (10% of patients)
Neoplasms (3.5% of patients)
Collagen disease (e.g., disseminated lupus erythematosus, polyarteritis nodosa) (2% of patients)
Also acute myocardial infarction, postcardiac injury syndrome

Findings
See appropriate sections for laboratory findings of primary disease.
Radioisotope scan of cardiac pool
WBC—usually increased in proportion to fever; normal or low in
viral disease and tuberculous pericarditis; markedly increased in
suppurative bacterial pericarditis
Examination of aspirated pericardial fluid (see Table 14, p. 145)
Smears and cultures for pyogenic bacteria and tubercle bacilli
Cytologic examination for LE cells and neoplastic cells

CHRONIC PERICARDIAL EFFUSION
See appropriate sections for primary diseases and sections (Table
14, p. 145) on body fluids.

Due To
Tuberculosis
Myxedema
Metastatic tumor
Disseminated lupus erythematosus

Rarely Due To
Severe anemia
Scleroderma
Polyarteritis nodosa
Rheumatoid arthritis
Irradiation therapy
Mycotic infections
Endomyocardial fibrosis of Africa
Idiopathic causes

CHRONIC CONSTRICTIVE PERICARDITIS
Altered liver function tests
BSP retention increased
Thymol turbidity increased (some patients)
Other abnormalities as occur in congestive heart failure
Decreased serum albumin with normal total protein

LOEFFLER'S PARIETAL FIBROPLASTIC ENDOCARDITIS
Eosinophilia $\leq 70\%$; may be absent at first but appears sooner or
later
WBC frequently increased
Laboratory findings due to frequently occurring
Mural thrombi in heart and embolization of spleen and lung
Mitral and tricuspid regurgitation

AORTIC ARCH SYNDROME (TAKAYASU'S SYNDROME; PULSELESS DISEASE)
WBC usually normal
Serum proteins abnormal with increased gamma globulins (mostly
composed of IgM)
Increased ESR

Women patients have a continuous high level of urinary total estrogens (rather than the usual rise during luteal phase after a low excretion during follicular phase)

SYPHILITIC AORTITIS
Laboratory findings due to associated lesions
> Syphilitic aortic insufficiency, with congestive heart failure
> Myocardial infarction due to coronary ostial stenosis

Laboratory findings due to complications
> Hemorrhage (into pericardium, esophagus, bronchial tree, etc.)
> Pressure or erosion or obstruction of adjacent structures in mediastinum

Laboratory evidence of syphilis (see Serologic Tests for Syphilis, p. 121)

Serologic tests for syphilis (e.g., VDRL, Kolmer complement-fixation) are negative in >25% of patients with syphilitic aortitis at autopsy.

DISSECTING ANEURYSM OF AORTA
If patient survives the immediate episode
> Increased WBC
> Increased ESR
> Laboratory findings due to hemorrhage
> Normal serum CPK, SGOT, SGPT, LDH, α-HBD, unless complications occur

Laboratory findings due to complications
> Hemopericardium
> Interference with blood supply to heart, brain, kidney, intestine, etc.

Laboratory findings due to underlying disease
> Marfan's syndrome

ARTERIOSCLEROTIC ANEURYSM OF ABDOMINAL AORTA
Laboratory findings due to complications
> Hemorrhage, especially retroperitoneal; rarely into duodenum, etc.
> Obstruction of branches (e.g., renal arteries)

MYOCARDIAL DISEASE ASSOCIATED WITH MARKED EOSINOPHILIA

Due To
Trichinosis
Polyarteritis nodosa
Eosinophilic leukemia with infiltration of heart
Loeffler's fibroplastic endocarditis

MYOCARDIAL INVOLVEMENT IN SYSTEMIC DISEASES
Laboratory findings due to primary disease
> Infections (vital, rickettsial [e.g., scrub typhus], bacterial [e.g., diphtheria], protozoan [e.g., trypanosomiasis], parasitic [e.g., trichinosis])
> Hyperthyroidism
> Myxedema

Chronic anemias (with Hb <7 gm/100 ml)
Beriberi (alcoholism)
Arteriovenous fistulas (e.g., Paget's disease of bone, pulmonary arteriovenous fistula)
Acute glomerulonephritis
Collagen diseases (polyarteritis nodosa, SLE, scleroderma, rheumatoid arthritis)
Hypokalemia
Sarcoidosis
Amyloidosis
Muscular dystrophy
Mucopolysaccharidoses
Glycogen-storage disease
Leukemia and metastatic tumor
Idiopathic causes (e.g., hypertrophic subaortic stenosis)
Other
Laboratory findings due to complications
Systemic emboli
Pulmonary emboli
Heart failure
Pericardial effusion

Serum LDH, SGOT, SGPT, etc., show variable mild increase.

SHOCK
Leukocytosis is common, especially with hemorrhage. There may be leukopenia when shock is severe, as in gram-negative bacteremia. Circulating eosinophils are decreased.

Hemoconcentration (e.g., dehydration, burns) or hemodilution (e.g., hemorrhage, crush injuries, and skeletal trauma) takes place.

Hyperglycemia occurs early.

Acidosis appears when shock is well developed, with increased blood lactate, low serum sodium, low CO_2-combining power with decreased alkaline reserve. Serum potassium may be increased. Blood pH is usually relatively normal but may be decreased. BUN may be increased.

Oliguria with low specific gravity (unless due to dehydration) or anuria is seen, as are decreased renal blood flow and glomerular filtration.

PHLEBOTHROMBOSIS OF LEG VEINS
Staphylococcal clumping test measures breakdown products of fibrin in serum; these indicate the presence of a clot that has begun to dissolve.

Serial dilution protamine sulfate test measures the presence of a fibrin monomer that is one of the polymerization products of fibrinogen. It is less sensitive than the staphylococcal clumping test but indicates clotting earlier.

Tests indicate recent extensive clotting of any origin (e.g., postoperative surgical status).

Laboratory findings of pulmonary infarction (see p. 188) should be sought as evidence of embolization.

RECURRENT THROMBOPHLEBITIS
Laboratory findings will be due to the underlying disease, which is often occult and may be without other manifestations.

Due To
Carcinoma, especially of pancreas; also bronchus, ovary, others
Kaposi's disease
Polycythemia
Vibrio fetus infection

SEPTIC THROMBOPHLEBITIS
Laboratory findings due to associated septicemia
> Increased WBC (often >20,000/cu mm) with marked shift to left and toxic changes in neutrophils
> Disseminated intravascular coagulation may be present (see pp. 337–338).
> Respiratory alkalosis due to ventilation-perfusion abnormalities with hypoxia. Significant acidosis indicates shock.
> Azotemia
> Positive blood culture

Laboratory findings due to complications (e.g., septic pulmonary infarction)
Laboratory findings due to underlying disease

CONGENITAL ANGIOMATOUS ARTERIOVENOUS FISTULAS
Platelet count may be decreased.

RAYNAUD'S PHENOMENON

May Occur With
High titer of cold agglutinins
Presence of cryoglobulins (e.g., in multiple myeloma, leukemia)
Scleroderma
Other diseases without specific laboratory findings

LABORATORY FINDINGS OF HEART TRANSPLANT REJECTION AS GUIDE TO IMMUNOSUPPRESSIVE TREATMENT
Increasing ESR
Increasing WBC
Increased isoenzyme LDH_1 as amount (>100 IU) and percent (35%) of total LDH during first 4 weeks after surgery

These findings are reversed with effective immunosuppressive therapy. Total LDH continues to be increased even when LDH_1 becomes normal.

RESPIRATORY DISEASES

CERVICAL LYMPHADENITIS
Diagnostic tests for specific causative agents (see appropriate separate sections)

Beta-hemolytic streptococci cause 75–90% of cases.

Staphylococcus aureus

Mycobacterium tuberculosis

Atypical mycobacteria

Cat-scratch fever

Infectious mononucleosis

Viruses (e.g., rubella, measles, herpes simplex, adenoviruses)

Occasionally biopsy may be indicated to rule out malignancy.

DISEASES OF LARYNX
Culture and smears for specific organisms (e.g., tubercle bacilli, fungi)

Biopsy for diagnosis of visible lesions (e.g., leukoplakia, carcinoma)

CROUP (EPIGLOTTITIS, LARYNGOTRACHEITIS)
Cultures, smears, and tests for specific causative agents

Group-B *Hemophilus influenzae* causes >90% of cases of epiglottitis; other bacteria include beta-hemolytic streptococci and pneumococci.

Clinical picture in infectious mononucleosis or diphtheria may resemble epiglottitis.

Laryngotracheitis is usually viral (especially parainfluenza) but rarely bacterial in origin.

Blood cultures should be taken at the same time as throat cultures.

Neutrophilic leukocytosis is present.

CHRONIC SINUSITIS
Laboratory findings due to infection

Laboratory findings of underlying disease that may be present

Cystic fibrosis of pancreas

Mucopolysaccharidosis

Allergy

Hypothyroidism

CHRONIC BRONCHITIS
WBC normal or increased

Eosinophil count increased if there is allergic basis or component

ESR normal or increased

Sputum bacterial smears and cultures (most common pathogens: pneumococcus, *Hemophilus influenzae;* occasionally *Staphylococcus aureus* or gram-negative rods)

Smears and cultures of bronchoscopic secretions

Laboratory findings due to associated or coexisting diseases (e.g., emphysema, bronchiectasis)

ACUTE BRONCHITIS (ASTHMATIC BRONCHITIS)
WBC may be increased.
ESR may be increased.

BRONCHIAL ASTHMA
Sputum is white and mucoid without blood or pus (unless infection
is present). Eosinophils, crystals (Curschmann's spirals), and
mucus casts of bronchioles may be found.
Eosinophilia may be present.
Blood CO_2 may be decreased in early stages and may be increased
in later states.
With severe respiratory distress, rapid deterioration of patient's condition may be associated with precipitous fall in arterial pO_2 and rise in pCO_2. When patient requires hospitalization,
arterial blood gases should be measured frequently to assess his
status.
Laboratory findings due to underlying diseases that may be primary and that should be ruled out, especially
    Polyarteritis nodosa
    Parasitic infestation
    Bronchial carcinoid
    Drug reaction (especially aspirin)
    Poisoning (especially cholinergic drugs and pesticides)
    Hypogammaglobulinemia

BRONCHIECTASIS
WBC usually normal unless pneumonitis is present
Mild to moderate normocytic normochromic anemia with chronic
severe infection
Sputum abundant, and mucopurulent (often contains blood);
sweetish smell
Sputum bacterial smears and cultures
Laboratory findings due to complications (pneumonia, pulmonary
hemorrhage, brain abscess, sepsis, cor pulmonale)

*Rule out cystic fibrosis of the pancreas and hypogammaglobu-
linemia or agammaglobulinemia.*

BRONCHIOLITIS

Due To
Usually virus, especially respiratory syncytial virus (see p. 485).
When recurrent, especially in young infants, rule out cystic fibrosis
(see pp. 235–236).

OBSTRUCTIVE PULMONARY EMPHYSEMA
Laboratory findings of underlying disease that may be primary
(e.g., pneumoconiosis, tuberculosis, sarcoidosis, kyphoscoliosis, marked obesity, fibrocystic disease of pancreas,
$alpha_1$ antitrypsin deficiency)
Laboratory findings of associated conditions, especially duodenal
ulcer

Laboratory findings due to decreased lung ventilation
  Arterial blood oxygen decreased and CO_2 increased
  Ultimate development of respiratory acidosis
  Secondary polycythemia
  Cor pulmonale

PULMONARY DISEASES OF THE NEWBORN

Respiratory Distress Syndrome
Laboratory findings of hypoxemia with moderately severe respiratory acidosis (CO_2 tension may range from 50–90 mm Hg). Metabolic acidosis secondary to hypoxia may also occur.

Transient Tachypnea of the Newborn
Normal arterial blood gases and pH

Pulmonary Dysmaturity (Wilson-Mikity Syndrome)
Infants usually weigh < 1500 gm.
Arterial pCO_2 increased with cyanosis in 20–40% oxygen therapy.
Normal CBC.

ATELECTASIS
No specific laboratory findings

Rule out underlying lesions (e.g., tumor, tuberculosis, cystic fibrosis of pancreas).

PNEUMONIA

Due To
Bacteria—pneumococcus, staphylococcus, *Klebsiella pneumoniae, Hemophilus influenzae,* streptococcus, enterobacteria, tularemia, plague, tubercle bacilli

Organism(s)	Isolated in % of Patients	Mortality[a]
Diplococcus pneumoniae	62%	19%
Gram-negative bacilli	20%	79%
(e.g., *K. pneumoniae*		
Enterobacteria		
Escherichia coli		
Proteus mirabilis		
Pseudomonas aeruginosa)		
Staphylococcus	10%	41%
H. influenzae	8%	14%

[a]Mortality is much greater in persons over age 40.

Mycoplasma pneumoniae
Viruses—influenza, parainfluenza, adenoviruses, respiratory syncytial virus, echovirus, coxsackievirus, reovirus, cytomegalic inclusion virus, viruses of exanthems, herpes simplex

Rickettsiae—Q fever, typhus
Fungi—*Histoplasma* and *Coccidioides* in particular
Protozoans—*Toxoplasma, Pneumocystis carinii*

Laboratory Findings

WBC is frequently normal or slightly increased in nonbacterial pneumonias; considerable increase in WBC is more common in bacterial pneumonia. *In severe bacterial pneumonia, WBC may be very high or low or normal. Since individual variation is considerable, there is limited value in distinguishing bacterial and nonbacterial pneumonia.*

In the urine, protein, WBCs, hyaline and granular casts in small amounts are common. Ketones may occur with severe infection. *Check for glucose to rule out underlying diabetes mellitus.*

A blood culture should be taken before antibiotic therapy is started.

Sputum reveals abundant WBCs in bacterial pneumonias. Gram stain shows abundant organisms in bacterial pneumonias (e.g., pneumococcus, staphylococcus). Culture sputum for appropriate bacteria.

Acute-phase serum should be stored at onset. If etiologic diagnosis is not established, a convalescent-phase serum should be taken. A fourfold increase in antibody titer establishes the etiologic diagnosis.

Serologic tests determine whether pneumonia is due to *Histoplasma, Coccidioides,* etc.

Diagnostic lung puncture to determine specific causative agent as a guide to antibiotic therapy may be indicated in critically ill children.

LIPID PNEUMONIA

Sputum shows fat-containing macrophages that stain with Sudan.

They may be present only intermittently; therefore examine sputum more than once.

DIFFUSE INTERSTITIAL PNEUMONITIS

Serum LDH is increased.

LUNG ABSCESS

Sputum
    Abundant, foul
    Purulent; may be bloody; contains elastic fibers
    Bacterial cultures (including tubercle bacilli)—anaerobic as well as aerobic (*rule out amebas, parasites*)
    Cytologic examination for malignant cells
Blood culture—may be positive in acute stage
Increased WBC in acute stages (15,000—30,000/cu mm)
Increased ESR
Normochromic normocytic anemia in chronic stage
Albuminuria frequent
Findings of underlying disease—especially bronchogenic car-

cinoma; also drug addiction, postabortion state, coccidioidomycosis, amebic abscess, tuberculosis, alcoholism

BRONCHOGENIC CARCINOMA

Cytologic examination of sputum for malignant cells—positive in 40% of patients on first sample, 70% with three samples, 85% with five samples. False positive tests are <1%.

Sputum cytology gives highest positive yield with squamous cell carcinoma (67–85%), intermediate with small cell undifferentiated carcinoma (64–70%), lowest with adenocarcinoma (55%).

Biopsy of scalene lymph nodes for metastases to indicate inoperable status—positive in 15% of patients

Findings of complicating conditions (e.g., pneumonitis, atelectasis, lung abscess)

Findings due to metastases (e.g., Addison's disease, diabetes insipidus, liver metastases with functional hepatic changes, malignant cells in pleural fluid)

Findings due to secretion of active hormone substances (e.g., Cushing's syndrome, hypercalcemia, serotonin production by carcinoid of bronchus) (see p. 423)

Biopsy of bronchus, pleura, lung, metastatic sites in appropriate cases

Transthoracic needle aspiration provides definitive cytologic diagnosis of cancer in 80–90% of cases; useful when other methods (e.g., sputum cytology, bronchoscopy) fail to provide a microscopic diagnosis.

Cancer cells in bone marrow and rarely in peripheral blood

PULMONARY ALVEOLAR PROTEINOSIS

Serum LDH increases when protein accumulates in lungs and drops to normal when infiltrate resolves.

PAS-positive material appears in sputum.

PSP dye injected intravenously is excreted in sputum for long periods of time.

Biopsy of lung for histologic examination is in order.

HYALINE MEMBRANE SYNDROME

Laboratory findings of
    Increased catabolism: increased BUN and serum potassium
    Impaired ventilation: increased pCO_2 and decreased pO_2; decreased blood pH (to $\leqq 7.3$) (Acidosis is first respiratory, later also metabolic.)

PULMONARY INFILTRATIONS ASSOCIATED WITH EOSINOPHILIA

Due To

Allergic conditions (e.g., asthma, serum sickness, drug reaction, farmer's lung)

Collagen disorders (e.g., polyarteritis nodosa, Wegener's granulomatosis, SLE)

Neoplasms (e.g., malignant lymphoma, eosinophilic leukemia)
Infections (e.g., fungus, tuberculosis, brucellosis)
Infestations (e.g., trichinosis, ascariasis, tropical eosinophilia due to *Dirofilaria immitis*)
Idiopathic causes, including Loeffler's syndrome of recurrent transient pulmonary infiltration

PNEUMOCONIOSIS

Biopsy of lung, scalene lymph node—histologic, chemical, spectrographic, and x-ray diffraction studies (e.g., silicosis, berylliosis; also metastatic tumor, sarcoidosis, tuberculosis, fungus infection)
Increased WBC if associated infection
Secondary polycythemia or anemia
Bacterial smears and cultures of sputum (especially for tubercle bacilli)
Cytologic examination of sputum and bronchoscopic secretions for malignant cells

Additional Types of Pneumoconiosis
Asbestosis
  Asbestos bodies sometimes in sputum after exposure to asbestos dust even without clinical disease
  Associated malignancy, especially mesothelioma of pleura and squamous cell carcinoma of bronchus
Acute beryllium disease
  Occasional transient hypergammaglobulinemia
Chronic beryllium disease
  Secondary polycythemia
  Increased serum gamma globulin
  Increased urine calcium
  Increased beryllium in urine long after beryllium exposure has ended
Coal worker's pneumoconiosis
Diatomaceous earth pneumoconiosis
Talcosis
Bauxite fume fibrosis
Siderosis
Byssinosis (dust from carding and spinning of cotton contains fibers, mold, fungi, etc.)
Bagassosis (dust from sugar cane fibers)

FARMER'S LUNG
(bagassosis; thresher's lung; respiratory disease of mushroom workers, etc.)

Due to
Hypersensitivity to inhaled organic dusts (e.g., sugar cane, wheat, corn, oats, straw, hay, barley, tobacco)

Laboratory Findings
Normal WBC; increased in presence of infection
Eosinophilia $\leq 45\%$
Increased ESR

Sputum smear and culture nonspecific
Lung biopsy—acute granulomatous interstitial pneumonitis

IDIOPATHIC PULMONARY HEMOSIDEROSIS
Hemosiderin-laden macrophages in sputum and gastric washings
Hypochromic microcytic anemia due to pulmonary hemorrhages
   with decreased serum iron; sometimes findings of hemolytic type
   of anemia (increased indirect serum bilirubin and urine urobilinogen) (see pp. 305–306)
Eosinophilia in $\leq 20\%$ of patients

GOODPASTURE'S SYNDROME
Malignant hypertension associated with pulmonary hemorrhages
Eosinophilia absent and iron deficiency anemia more marked than
   in idiopathic pulmonary hemosiderosis
Proteinuria and RBCs and RBC casts in urine
Renal function may deteriorate rapidly
Renal biopsy may show characteristic linear immunofluorescent
   deposits or focal or diffuse proliferative glomerulonephritis

IDIOPATHIC PULMONARY FIBROSIS
(HAMMAN-RICH SYNDROME)
May be associated with a collagen-vascular disorder (e.g.,
   rheumatoid arthritis, SLE, polymyositis, Sjögren's syndrome)
   or not associated with any known disorder
Arterial blood oxygen (arterial pO_2) is decreased at rest and falls
   further with exercise
Polycythemia is absent
Serologic changes with associated diseases (see above)

PULMONARY HEMOSIDEROSIS SECONDARY TO MITRAL STENOSIS
Hemosiderin-laden macrophages in sputum

PULMONARY EMBOLISM AND INFARCTION
Pulmonary embolism is unlikely if arterial pO_2 is normal (>90 mm
   Hg).
Serum LDH increased (isoenzymes LDH_2 and LDH_3) (may be
   useful as screening test); rises on first day, peaks on second day,
   normal by tenth day; increased in $<80\%$ of patients
Lung scan (radioactive isotope scans) (see p. 156)
Serum bilirubin increased (as early as fourth day $\cong 5$ mg/100 ml)
   in $\cong 20\%$ of cases
Urine urobilinogen increased
Serum SGOT usually normal or only slightly increased
Serum aldolase slightly increased
Leukocytosis up to 15,000/cu mm in $\cong 50\%$ of patients
ESR increased
"Triad" of increased LDH and bilirubin with normal SGOT found
   in $\cong 15\%$ of cases
Pleural effusion occurs in 50% of patients and shows no character-
   istic diagnostic findings. Bloody pleural effusion in one-third to
   two-thirds of cases. "Typical" pattern of bloody pleural fluid,

predominance of polynuclear leukocytes, and characteristics of exudate is found in only 25% of patients.

See Table 18, p. 170.

These laboratory findings depend on the size and duration of the infarction, and the tests must be performed at the appropriate time to detect abnormalities.

CAVERNOUS HEMANGIOMA (CONGENITAL ARTERIOVENOUS ANEURYSM OR VARIX) OF LUNG
Polycythemia

PULMONARY SEQUESTRATION
The only laboratory findings are due to associated localized chronic bronchitis and bronchiectasis.

TUMORS (PRIMARY OR SECONDARY) OF PLEURA
Examination of pleural fluid (see Table 14, p. 145)
Biopsy of pleura

RHEUMATOID PLEURISY WITH EFFUSION
Decreased glucose level (<30 mg/100 ml in 25% of patients) is the most useful finding clinically. Nonpurulent nonmalignant effusions other than those due to tuberculosis or rheumatoid arthritis almost always have glucose levels >70 mg/100 ml.
Exudate is frequently turbid and may be milky.
Smears and cultures for bacteria, tubercle bacilli, and fungi are negative.
Cytologic examination for malignant cells is negative. RA cells may be found.

Table 19. Endocrine Syndromes That May Be Associated with Pulmonary Disease

Syndrome	Pulmonary Lesion
Hypokalemic alkalosis, edema, Cushing's syndrome	Oat cell carcinoma, adenoma
Hyponatremia (syndrome of inappropriate secretion of antidiuretic hormone)	Oat cell carcinoma, adenoma, tuberculosis, pneumonia, aspergillosis
Hypercalcemia	Squamous cell carcinoma
Gynecomastia (adults), precocious puberty (children)	Anaplastic, "large cell" carcinoma
Hypertrophic osteoarthropathy	Squamous cell carcinoma
"Carcinoid"	Bronchial adenoma, oat cell carcinoma
Hypoglycemia	Mesenchymal cell tumors
Diabetes	Fibrosarcoma
Galactorrhea (or no symptoms)	Anaplastic cell carcinoma
Multiple syndromes	Anaplastic cell carcinoma

Source: Adapted from H.H. Friedman and Solomon Papper, Problem-Oriented Medical Diagnosis. Boston: Little, Brown, 1975.

Table 20. Effect of Respiratory Abnormalities on Arterial Blood Gases[a]

Abnormality	Response To	Arterial pO$_2$	Arterial pCO$_2$	pH
Ventilation-perfusion abnormality	Resting	D	D–I	
	Oxygen[b]	Variably I	N–I	
	Exercise test[c]	Slightly I	D–I	
Generalized alveolar hypoventilation	Resting	D	I	If acute, pH is D; if chronic, pH is near N
	Oxygen	Markedly I	I	
	Exercise test	V	V	
Decreased pulmonary diffusing capacity	Resting	D	Usually D; may be N	
	Oxygen	Markedly I	I	
	Exercise test	Especially D	D	

| Right-to-left shunt or increased venous admixture | Resting | | D | D–N | Oxygen effect measures extent of shunt |
	Oxygen	Exercise test			
	Poorly		D	I	
		Slightly D	D		
Hyperventilation	Resting	Slightly	I	Always D	If acute, pH is I; if chronic, pH is normal

N = normal; V = variable; I = high or increased; D = low or decreased.

[a] See also Hypoxemia; Hypercapnia; Hypocapnia, pp. 45–46, and Respiratory Acidosis; Respiratory Alkalosis, p. 347.

[b] Oxygen = effect of breathing 100% O_2 for 15 minutes.

[c] Exercise test = effect of standard physical exercise test.

Source: Adapted from H. H. Friedman and Solomon Papper, *Problem-Oriented Medical Diagnosis* (Boston: Little, Brown, 1975) and G. L. Baum, *Textbook of Pulmonary Disease* (Boston: Little, Brown, 1974).

Rheumatoid Pleurisy with Effusion *(Continued)*
Protein level is >3 gm/100 ml.
Increased LDH (usually higher than in serum) is commonly found
in other chronic pleural effusions and is not useful in differential
diagnosis.
Rheumatoid factor may be present but may also be found in other
types of pleural effusion (e.g., with carcinoma, tuberculosis,
bacterial pneumonia).
Needle biopsy of pleura usually shows nonspecific chronic inflammation, but characteristic changes of rheumatoid pleuritis may
be found histologically.
Other laboratory findings or rheumatoid arthritis are found (see pp.
276–277).

PNEUMOTHORAX
No abnormal laboratory findings
Laboratory findings *if* underlying disease is present (e.g., tuber-
culosis, sarcoidosis, lung abscess, silicosis, carcinoma)

PNEUMOMEDIASTINUM
Leukocytosis—variable, nonspecific

MEDIASTINAL NEOPLASMS
See
       Thymoma
       Malignant lymphoma
       Ganglioneuroma
       Neuroblastoma
       Pheochromocytoma
       Substernal goiter
       Parathyroid adenoma
       Metastatic tumors
       Sarcoidosis
       Tuberculosis
       Other

DERMOID CYST OF MEDIASTINUM
Hair in sputum may occur with rupture into bronchus.

DIAPHRAGMATIC HERNIA
Microcytic anemia (due to blood loss) may be present.
Stool may be positive for blood.

TIETZE'S SYNDROME
(costochondritis; costochondralgia; rib syndrome, etc.)
No abnormal laboratory findings

LABORATORY FINDINGS IN ORAL MANIFESTATIONS OF SOME SYSTEMIC DISEASES

Infections
- Bacterial (e.g., diphtheria, scarlet fever, syphilis, Vincent's angina)
- Viral (e.g., herpes simplex, herpangina, measles, infectious mononucleosis)
- Fungal (e.g., actinomycosis, histoplasmosis, mucormycosis, moniliasis)

Hematologic diseases
- Pernicious anemia—glossitis
- Iron deficiency anemia—atrophy
- Polycythemia—erosions
- Granulocytopenia—ulceration and inflammation
- Acute leukemia—edema and hemorrhage

Vitamin deficiencies
- Pellagra
- Riboflavin deficiency
- Scurvy

Systemic diseases
- Systemic lupus erythematosus (SLE)
- Primary amyloidosis
- Hereditary hemorrhagic telangiectasia (Osler-Weber-Rendu disease)

GASTROINTESTINAL MANIFESTATIONS OF SOME SYSTEMIC DISEASES

Lymphoma and leukemia
Metastatic carcinoma
Collagen diseases (e.g., scleroderma, polyarteritis nodosa, SLE)
Amyloidosis
Parasitic infestation (schistosomiasis)
Bacterial infection (lymphogranuloma venereum)
Osler-Weber-Rendu disease
Henoch's purpura
Hemolytic crises (e.g., sickle cell disease)
Porphyria
Lead poisoning
Embolic accidents in rheumatic heart disease, bacterial endocarditis
Ischemic vascular disease
Uremia
Allergy
Cystic fibrosis of pancreas
Hirschsprung's disease
Cirrhosis (esophageal varices, hemorrhoids, peptic ulcer)
Zollinger-Ellison syndrome (peptic ulcer)
Peptic ulcer associated with other diseases (in 8–22% of patients

with hyperparathyroidism, 10% of patients with pituitary tumor, etc.)
Other

SYSTEMIC MANIFESTATIONS OCCURRING IN SOME GASTROINTESTINAL DISEASES
Carcinoid syndrome
Anemia (e.g., due to bleeding occult neoplasm)
Arthritis, uveitis, etc., in ulcerative colitis
Vitamin deficiency (e.g., sprue, malabsorption)
Endocrine manifestations due to replacement by metastatic tumors of GI tract

MALLORY-WEISS SYNDROME
(spontaneous cardioesophageal laceration following retching)
Laboratory findings due to hemorrhage from cardioesophageal laceration

SPONTANEOUS PERFORATION OF ESOPHAGUS
Gastric contents in thoracocentesis fluid

PLUMMER-VINSON SYNDROME
Hypochromic anemia associated with dysphagia and cardiospasm in women

CARCINOMA OF ESOPHAGUS
Cytologic examination of esophageal washings is positive for malignant cells in 75% of patients. It is false positive in <2% of patients.

DIAPHRAGMATIC HERNIA
Microcytic anemia (due to blood loss) may be present.
Stool may be positive for blood.

ESOPHAGEAL INVOLVEMENT DUE TO PRIMARY DISEASES ELSEWHERE
Scleroderma (*esophageal involvement in >50% of patients with scleroderma*)
Esophageal varices (see Cirrhosis of Liver, pp. 216–217)
Malignant lymphoma

SOME CONDITIONS OF GASTROINTESTINAL TRACT IN WHICH NO USEFUL ABNORMAL LABORATORY FINDINGS OCCUR
Acute esophagitis
Chronic esophagitis
Diverticula of esophagus and stomach
Esophageal spasm
Prolapse of gastric mucosa
Foreign bodies in stomach

PEPTIC ULCER OF STOMACH
Laboratory findings due to underlying conditions

Administration of ACTH and adrenal steroids
Acute burns (Curling's ulcer)
Cerebrovascular accidents and trauma and inflammation
(Cushing's ulcer)
Various drugs (e.g., salicylates)
Uremia
Cirrhosis
Laboratory findings due to complications
Gastric retention—dehydration, hypokalemic alkalosis
Perforation—increased WBC with shift to the left, dehydration, increased serum amylase, increased amylase in peritoneal fluid
Hemorrhage

Curling's ulcer—hemorrhage 8–10 days and perforation 30 days after burn, causes death in 15% of fatal burn cases

See Chronic Duodenal Ulcer, p. 196.

NONSPECIFIC GASTRITIS
Hypochromic microcytic anemia due to blood loss
Occult blood in stool
Gastric analysis
Hypochlorhydria in early cases
Achlorhydria with complete atrophy
Hypoalbuminemia possible

BENIGN GIANT HYPERTROPHIC GASTRITIS (MENETRIER'S DISEASE)
See Protein-Losing Enteropathy, p. 201.

ADENOMATOUS POLYP OF STOMACH
Gastric analysis—achlorhydria in 85% of patients
Sometimes evidence of bleeding

Polyps occur in 5% of patients with pernicious anemia and 2% of patients with achlorhydria.

CARCINOMA OF STOMACH
Anemia due to chronic blood loss
Occult blood in stool
Gastric analysis
Achlorhydria following histamine or betazole in 50% of patients
Hypochlorhydria in 25% of patients
Normal in 25% of patients
Hyperchlorhydria rare
Exfoliative cytology positive in 80% of patients; false positive in less than 2%
Lymph node biopsy for metastases; needle biopsy of liver, bone marrow, etc.

Carcinoma of the stomach should always be searched for by periodic prophylactic screening in high-risk patients, especially those with pernicious anemia, gastric atrophy, gastric polyps.

LEIOMYOMA, LEIOMYOSARCOMA, MALIGNANT LYMPHOMA OF STOMACH
May show evidence of bleeding

CHRONIC DUODENAL ULCER
Laboratory findings due to associated conditions
> Zollinger-Ellison syndrome (ulcerogenic tumor of pancreas) (see pp. 396–397)
> Chronic pancreatitis
> Mucoviscidosis
> Rheumatoid arthritis
> Chronic pulmonary disease (e.g., pulmonary emphysema)
> Cirrhosis
> Certain drugs (e.g., ACTH)
> Hyperparathyroidism
> Polycythemia vera

Laboratory findings due to treatment
> Milk-alkali (Burnett's) syndrome—alkalosis, hypercalcemia, azotemia, renal calculi or nephrocalcinosis
> Inadequate vagotomy—use insulin test meal (see p. 144)
>> Gastric acidity shows late response of >4.5 mEq total free acid in 30 minutes or any early response.

> *To obtain valid collection, Levin tube must be correctly placed fluoroscopically.*

Dumping syndrome (occurs in $\leqq 70\%$ of post-subtotal gastrectomy patients)—during symptoms may have
> Rapid prolonged alimentary hyperglycemia
> Decreased plasma volume
> Decreased serum potassium
> Increased blood and urine serotonin

Hypoglycemic syndrome (occurs in $<5\%$ of post-subtotal gastrectomy patients)
> Prolonged alimentary hyperglycemia followed after 2 hours by precipitous hypoglycemia
> Late hypoglycemia shown by 6-hour oral GTT

Stomal gastritis—anemia due to chronic bleeding
Postgastrectomy malabsorption
Postgastrectomy anemia (due to chronic blood loss, malabsorption, vitamin B_{12} deficiency, etc.)
Afferent-loop obstruction—marked increase in serum amylase to >1000 units

Laboratory findings due to complications of gastric or duodenal ulcer
> Hemorrhage
> Perforation
> Obstruction
> Other

Gastric analysis
> True achlorhydria following maximum stimulation rules out duodenal ulcer. Normal secretion or hypersecretion does not prove the presence of an ulcer.

Duodenal ulcer is absent in patients with ulcerative colitis (unless under steroid therapy), carcinoma of stomach, pernicious anemia, pregnancy.

REGIONAL ENTERITIS (CROHN'S DISEASE)
Inflammation—increased WBC and ESR
Iron deficiency type of anemia due to blood loss
Malabsorption
Laboratory findings due to complications
    Perforation and peritonitis
    Hemorrhage
    Arthritis
    Secondary amyloidosis

ACUTE APPENDICITIS
Increased WBC (12,000–14,000/cu mm) with shift to the left in acute catarrhal stage; higher and more rapid rise with suppuration or perforation
ESR—may be normal during first 24 hours
Later—laboratory findings due to complications (e.g., dehydration, abscess formation, perforation with peritonitis)

ACUTE DIVERTICULITIS
Increased WBC and ESR
Hypochromic microcytic anemia (some patients)
Occult blood in stool
Cytologic examination of stool—negative for malignant cells
Laboratory findings due to complications
    Hemorrhage
    Perforation
    Obstruction

MOST COMMON AGENTS OF FOODBORNE DISEASE OUTBREAKS (GASTROENTERITIS)

	% of Cases (known etiology)
Viral	5.5
Parasitic	0.8
Chemical (scromboid)	5.1
Bacterial[a]	88.6
Salmonella	31.9
Staphylococcus aureus	16.5
Clostridium botulinum	0.4
Clostridium perfringens	18.5
Shigella	18.0
Vibrio parahaemolyticus	0.03
Bacillus cereus	0.03
Streptococcus, Group A	3.2
Brucella melitensis	0.1

[a]Confirm by culture of food, patient's stool, or food handler's stool.
Source: H. L. Kazal, Laboratory diagnosis of foodborne diseases. *Ann. Clin. Lab. Sci.* 6:381, 1976.

ACUTE MEMBRANOUS ENTEROCOLITIS
Laboratory findings due to antecedent condition
  Disease for which antibiotics are administered
  Myocardial infarction
  Surgical procedure
  Other
Laboratory findings due to shock, dehydration
Culture of staphylococci from stool or rectal swab

WHIPPLE'S DISEASE (INTESTINAL LIPODYSTROPHY)
Characteristic biopsy of intestine and mesenteric lymph nodes
Malabsorption syndrome (see p. 199)
Arthritis

CELIAC DISEASE (GLUTEN-SENSITIVE ENTEROPATHY, NONTROPICAL SPRUE, IDIOPATHIC STEATORRHEA)
Malabsorption syndrome (see p. 199); return to normal on gluten-free diet
Biopsy of small intestine

TUMORS OF SMALL INTESTINE
Laboratory findings due to complications
  Hemorrhage
  Obstruction
  Intussusception
  Malabsorption
Laboratory findings due to underlying condition
  Peutz-Jeghers syndrome
  Malignant lymphoma
  Carcinoid syndrome

MULTIPLE DIVERTICULA OF JEJUNUM
Laboratory findings due to malabsorption syndrome

MECKEL'S DIVERTICULUM
Laboratory findings due only to complications
  Gastrointestinal hemorrhage
  Intestinal obstruction
  Perforation or intussusception ($\cong 20\%$ of patients; the other 80% of patients are asymptomatic)

CLASSIFICATION OF MALABSORPTION
Inadequate mixing of food with bile salts and lipase (e.g., pyloroplasty, subtotal or total gastrectomy, gastrojejunostomy)
Inadequate lipolysis due to lack of lipase (e.g., cystic fibrosis of the pancreas, chronic pancreatitis, cancer of the pancreas or ampulla of Vater, pancreatic fistula, vagotomy)
Inadequate emulsification of fat due to lack of bile salts (e.g., obstructive jaundice, severe liver disease)
Primary absorptive defect in small bowel
  Inadequate absorptive surface due to extensive mucosal disease (e.g., regional enteritis, tumors, amyloid disease, scleroderma, irradiation)

Biochemical dysfunction of mucosal cells (e.g., celiac-sprue syndrome, severe starvation, intestinal infections, infestations, or administration of drugs such as neomycin sulfate, colchicine, or PAS)

Obstruction of mesenteric lymphatics (e.g., by lymphoma, carcinoma, Whipple's disease, intestinal tuberculosis)

Inadequate length of normal absorptive surface (e.g., surgical resection, fistula, shunt)

Miscellaneous (e.g., "blind loops" of intestine, diverticula, Zollinger-Ellison syndrome, agammaglobulinemia, endocrine and metabolic disorders)

LABORATORY DIAGNOSIS OF MALABSORPTION

Direct stool examination
>   Gross—oil droplets, egg particles, buttery materials
>   Sudan III stain—3 globules/microscopic hpf or globules >75 μ
>   Weight—much heavier than normal (normal weight is <200 gm/24 hours or normal fecal solids of 25–30 gm/24 hours)

Chemical analysis of fecal fat
>   Normal—<6 gm of fat/24 hours as average of 3-day collection when diet includes 100 gm of fat/day
>   Chronic pancreatic disease—>10 gm/24 hours

Indirect indices of fat absorption
>   Serum carotene (for screening purposes) is always abnormal in steatorrhea unless therapy is successful.
>>   Normal is 70–290 μg/ml.
>>   30–70 μg/100 ml indicates mild depletion; <30 indicates severe depletion.
>>   May also be low in liver disease and diets low in carotene-containing foods
>   Vitamin A tolerance test (for screening steatorrhea)
>>   Measure plasma vitamin A level 5 hours after ingestion.
>>   Normal rise is 9 times fasting level.
>>   Flat curve in liver disease
>>   Not useful after gastrectomy
>>   With vitamin A as ester of long-chain fatty acid, flat curve occurs in both pancreatic disease and intestinal mucosal abnormalities; when water-soluble forms of vitamin A are used, the curve becomes normal in patients with pancreatic disease but remains flat in intestinal mucosal abnormalities.
>   Triolein ^{131}I absorption with measurement of blood and fecal radioactivity (see p. 153)
>   Oleic acid [131]I (see p. 154)

Carbohydrate absorption indices
>   Oral glucose tolerance test—limited value
>>   Flat curve or delayed peak occurs in celiac disease and nontropical sprue.
>>   Curve is normal in pancreatic insufficiency.
>   D-xylose tolerance test—useful test of carbohydrate absorption
>>   Measure total 5-hour urine excretion; perhaps also measure blood levels at ½, 1, and 2 hours (almost no ab-

sorption from ileum). Accuracy is 90% in distinguishing pancreatic disease from intestinal mucosal disease.

Absorption is normal, but urinary excretion is decreased in renal disease and myxedema; also decreased in the elderly.

Na_2CO_3 and Nile blue dye give blue color to stool proportional to the concentration of oleates.

Protein absorption indices

Normal fecal nitrogen is < 2 gm/day. There is marked increase in sprue and severe pancreatic deficiency.

Measure plasma glycine or urinary excretion of hydroxyproline after gelatin meal. Plasma glycine increases 5 times in 2½ hours in normal persons. In those with cystic fibrosis of the pancreas, the increase is < 2½ times.

Schilling test (using [60]Co- or [57]Co-labeled vitamin B_{12}) shows poor absorption of vitamin B_{12} that is not improved by the addition of intrinsic factor.

PVP-^{131}I test is indicated (see p. 154)

[51]Cr albumin test (IV dose of 30–50 μc) shows increased excretion in 4-day stool collection due to protein-losing enteropathy.

Biopsy of small intestine mucosa is excellent for verification of sprue, celiac disease, and Whipple's disease.

Anemia is due to deficiency of iron, folic acid, vitamin B_{12}, or various combinations, depending on their decreased absorption.

DISACCHARIDE MALABSORPTION

Due to

Primary malabsorption (congenital or acquired) due to absence of specific disaccharidase in brush border of small intestine mucosa

Sucrose-isomaltose malabsorption (inherited recessive defect)

Oral sucrose tolerance curve is flat, but glucose plus fructose tolerance test is normal. Occasionally there is an associated malabsorption with increased stool fat and abnormal D-xylose tolerance test although intestinal biopsy is normal.

Isolated lactase deficiency (most common defect; occurs in > 10% of whites and 60% of blacks; congenital or acquired)

Oral lactose tolerance curve is flat, but glucose plus galactose tolerance test is normal. Intestinal biopsy shows normal histology but decreased lactase activity.

Glucose-galactose malabsorption (inherited autosomal recessive defect that affects kidney and intestine)

Oral glucose or galactose tolerance curve is flat but intravenous tolerance curves are normal. Glucosuria is common. Fructose tolerance test is normal.

Secondary malabsorption

Resection of > 50% of disaccharidase activity

Lactose is most marked, but there may also be sucrose.

Oral disaccharide tolerance (especially lactose) is abnormal, but intestinal histology and enzyme activity are normal.

Diffuse intestinal disease—especially celiac disease in which activity of all disaccharidases may be decreased, with later increase as intestine becomes normal on gluten-free diet; also cystic fibrosis of pancreas, severe malnutrition, ulcerative colitis, severe *Giardia* infestation, blind-loop syndrome, beta-lipoprotein deficiency, effect of drugs (e.g., colchicine, neomycin, birth control pills)

Oral tolerance tests (especially lactose) are frequently abnormal, with later return to normal with gluten-free diet. Tolerance tests with monosaccharides may also be abnormal because of defect in absorption as well as digestion.

Laboratory Findings

Oral carbohydrate (disaccharide) tolerance test is abnormal (blood glucose rises 0–21 mg/100 ml above fasting level).

Oral tolerance test using constituent monosaccharides. Normal result demonstrates normal absorption of monosaccharides.

Examine stool during disaccharide tolerance test.

pH of $\leqq 5$ is abnormal.

Measure disaccharide (Clinitest tablet).

$> 0.5\%$ is abnormal.

0.25–0.5% is suspicious.

$< 0.25\%$ is normal.

Biopsy of small intestine mucosa will reveal activity of specific disaccharidase.

PROTEIN-LOSING ENTEROPATHY

Secondary (i.e., disease states in which clinically significant protein-losing enteropathy may occur as a manifestation)

Giant hypertrophy of gastric rugae

Gastric neoplasms

Regional enteritis

Whipple's disease

Nontropical sprue

Inflammatory and neoplastic diseases of small and large intestine

Ulcerative colitis

Constrictive pericarditis

Primary (i.e., hypoproteinemia is the major clinical feature)

Intestinal lymphangiectasia

Nonspecific inflammatory or granulomatous disease of small intestine

Serum total protein, albumin and gamma globulin decreased

Serum alpha and beta globulins normal

Serum cholesterol usually normal

Mild anemia

Eosinophilia (occasionally)

Serum calcium decreased

Steatorrhea with abnormal tests of lipid absorption

Increased permeability of GI tract to large molecular substances shown by IV PVP-^{131}I test (see p. 154)

Proteinuria absent

PERORAL BIOPSY OF THE PROXIMAL SMALL INTESTINE*
For differential diagnosis of malabsorption, diarrhea, and associated nutritional deficiencies

Biopsy is always useful in
    Celiac sprue
    Whipple's disease
    Agammaglobulinemia
    A-beta-lipoproteinemia (see p. 70: acanthotic RBCs, steatorrhea, failure of beta-lipoprotein manufacture, neurologic findings)

Biopsy may or may not be of specific diagnostic value in
    Amyloidosis
    Intestinal lymphangiectasia
    Malignant lymphoma of small bowel
    Eosinophilic gastroenteritis
    Regional enteritis
    Hypogammaglobulinemia and dysgammaglobulinemia
    Systemic mastocytosis
    Parasitic infestations (giardiasis, coccidiosis, strongyloidiasis, capillariasis)

Biopsy may be abnormal but not diagnostic in
    Tropical sprue
    Folate deficiency
    Vitamin B_{12} deficiency
    Irradiation enteritis
    Zollinger-Ellison syndrome
    Stasis with intraluminal bacterial overgrowth
    Drug-induced lesions (neomycin, antimetabolites)
    Malnutrition

Biopsy is normal in
    Cirrhosis
    Pancreatic exocrine insufficiency
    Postgastrectomy malabsorption without intestinal mucosal disease
    Functional bowel disease (irritable colon, nonspecific diarrhea)

Biopsy taken at duodenojejunal junction by x-ray localization, prompt fixation of tissue, proper orientation of tissue for histologic sectioning, and serial sectioning of specimen are all necessary for proper interpretation.

RECTAL BIOPSY
Rectal biopsy is particularly useful in diagnosis of
    Cancer of rectosigmoid
    Polyps of rectosigmoid
    Secondary amyloidosis
    Amebic ulceration
    Schistosomiasis (even when no lesions are visible)
    Hirschsprung's disease

*J. S. Trier, Diagnostic value of peroral biopsy of the proximal small intestine. *N. Engl. J. Med.* 285: 1470, 1971.

HIRSCHSPRUNG'S DISEASE (AGANGLIONIC MEGACOLON)

Rectal biopsy to include muscle layers shows absence of myenteric plexus ganglia in muscle layers.

CHRONIC NONSPECIFIC ULCERATIVE COLITIS

Laboratory findings parallel severity of the disease
  Anemia due to blood loss (frequently Hb = 6 gm/100 ml)
  WBC usually normal unless complication occurs (e.g., abscess)
  ESR often normal or only slightly increased
Stools
  Positive for blood (gross and/or occult)
  Negative for usual enteric bacterial pathogens and parasites; high total bacterial count
Changes in liver function
  Microscopic changes in needle biopsy of liver
  BSP test sometimes abnormal
  Serum alkaline phosphatase often increased slightly
  Other liver function tests usually normal
Changes in serum electrolytes due to diarrhea or to therapy with adrenal steroids or ACTH
Laboratory changes due to complications or sequelae
  Malabsorption due to involvement of small intestine
  Perforation
  Abscess formation
  Hemorrhage
  Carcinoma
  Arthritis
  Other
Rectal biopsy

GONOCOCCAL PROCTITIS

See pp. 459–460.

HEREDITARY GASTROINTESTINAL POLYPOSIS

Laboratory findings due to intestinal polyps and due to associated lesions
  Familial polyposis of colon
  Occasional discrete polyps of colon and rectum
  Peutz-Jeghers syndrome
  Gardner's syndrome (see next section)
  Turcot sydrome (CNS tumors)
  Oldfield's syndrome (extensive sebaceous cysts)
  Zollinger-Ellison syndrome
  Generalized juvenile polyposis
Laboratory findings due to complications (e.g., bleeding, intussusception, obstruction, malignancy)

GARDNER'S SYNDROME
(multiple osteomas, fibrous and fatty tumors of skin and mesentery, epidermoid inclusion cysts of skin, multiple polyposis)

Polyposis of the colon and rectum may develop before puberty and show great tendency to become malignant.

CARCINOMA OF COLON
Blood in stool (occult or gross)
Evidence of inflammation
  Increased WBC and ESR
Anemia
  May be the only symptom of carcinoma of right side of colon
    (present in >50% of these patients)
  Usually hypochromic
  Stools sometimes negative for occult blood
Evidence of metastases (see Metastatic or Infiltration Disease of
  Liver, p. 222)
Biopsy of colon lesion

Villous tumor of rectum may cause potassium depletion with decreased serum potassium.
Carcinoid tumors may cause increased 5-HIAA in urine.

Laboratory findings due to complications
  Hemorrhage
  Perforation
  Obstruction
Laboratory findings due to underlying condition
  Hereditary polyposis (see above)
  Chronic nonspecific ulcerative colitis
  Granulomatous colitis (Crohn's disease)

VILLOUS ADENOMA OF RECTUM
Stool
  Large amount of mucus tinged with blood; frequent watery
    diarrhea
Serum potassium sometimes decreased
Biopsy of lesion

MESENTERIC VASCULAR OCCLUSION
Chronic (mesenteric arterial insufficiency)
  Laboratory findings due to malabsorption and starvation
Acute
  Marked increase in WBC ($\geq$ 15,000–25,000/cu mm) with shift
    to the left
  Laboratory findings due to intestinal hemorrhage, intestinal
    obstruction, metabolic acidosis, shock
  Infarction of intestine causes increased serum LDH; selective
    increase of intestinal isoenzyme of serum alkaline
    phosphatase is described.

INTESTINAL OBSTRUCTION
WBC is normal early. Later it tends to rise, with increase in
  polynuclear leukocytes; 15,000–25,000/cu mm suggests
  strangulation; >30,000/cu mm suggests mesenteric thrombosis.
Hemoglobin and hematocrit levels are normal early but later increase, with dehydration.
Urine
  Specific gravity increases, with deficit of water and electro-

lytes unless preexisting renal disease is present. Urinalysis helps rule out renal colic, diabetic acidosis, etc.

Gastric contents
Positive guaiac test suggests strangulation; there may be gross blood if strangulated segment is high in jejunum.

Rectal contents
Gross rectal blood suggests carcinoma of colon or intussusception.

Decreased serum sodium, potassium, chloride, and pH, and increased CO_2 are helpful indications for following the course of the patient and to guide therapy.

Increased BUN suggests blood in intestine or renal damage.

Serum amylase may be moderately increased in absence of pancreatitis.

Increased serum LDH may indicate strangulation (infarction) of small intestine.

GALLSTONE ILEUS

Laboratory findings due to preceding chronic cholecystitis and cholelithiasis

Laboratory findings due to acute obstruction of terminal ileum (*accounts for 1–2% of patients*)

GASTROINTESTINAL COMPLICATIONS OF ANTICOAGULANT THERAPY

Hemorrhage into gastrointestinal tract occurs in 3–4% of patients on anticoagulant therapy; may be spontaneous or secondary to unsuspected disease (e.g., peptic ulcer, carcinoma, diverticula, hemorrhoids). Occasionally there is hemorrhage into the wall of the intestine with secondary ileus. Prothrombin time may be in the therapeutic range or, more commonly, is increased. *Coumarin drug action is potentiated by administration of aspirin, antibiotics, phenylbutazone, and thyroxine and T-tube drainage of the common bile duct, especially if pancreatic disease is present.*

Hypersensitivity to phenindione may cause hepatitis or steatorrhea.

GASTROINTESTINAL HEMORRHAGE

Due To

Duodenal ulcer (25% of patients)
Esophageal varices (18% of patients)
Gastric ulcer (12% of patients)
Gastritis (12% of patients)
Esophagitis (6% of patients)
Mallory-Weiss syndrome (5% of patients)
Other (22% of patients)

With previously known GI tract lesions, 40% of patients bled from a different lesion.

In addition to the main cause of bleeding, 50% of patients have an additional lesion that could cause hemorrhage (especially duodenal ulcer, esophageal varices, hiatus hernia).

Table 21. Rectal Bleeding in Children

Cause	Newborn	Ages 1 Week– 2 Years	Ages 2–13 Years
Swallowed blood	3+	–	–
Rectal trauma	1+	1+	–
Milk allergy	1+	1+	–
Bleeding diathesis	2+	1+	1+
Peptic ulcer	2+	2+	1+
Congenital anomalies	1+	2+	1+
Meckel's diverticulum	–	2+	1+
Intussusception	–	2+	1+
Anal fissure	–	4+	4+
Polyps	–	2+	3+
Portal hypertension	–	1+	2+
Ulcerative colitis	–	1+	3+

4+ = most frequent; 1+ = least frequent; – = rare or absent.
Source: Adapted from H. L. Barnett. *Pediatrics.* New York: Appleton-Century-Crofts, 1972.

In newborn, perform alkaline denaturation test on vomited blood to determine if it is of maternal or infant origin.

ACUTE PERITONITIS
Primary. Gram stain of direct smear of peritoneal fluid shows streptococci or pneumococci in absence of *Escherichia coli.*
   Marked increase in WBC ($\leq 50,000$/cu mm) and PMN (80–90%)
Secondary. Laboratory findings due to underlying condition (e.g., appendicitis, perforated ulcer, volvulus)

CHYLOUS ASCITES
Fat content $\leq 5\%$; varies with diet
Protein content 2–3 gm/100 ml

Due To
Filariasis
Inflammation, tumor, or obstruction of small intestine
Trauma to chest or abdomen

HEPATOBILIARY DISEASES AND DISORDERS OF THE PANCREAS

HEPATIC INVOLVEMENT IN SYSTEMIC DISEASES
Infections (e.g., infectious mononucleosis, cytomegalic inclusion disease, Q fever, leptospirosis, lobar pneumonia, typhoid, granulomas, such as those with tuberculosis and brucellosis)

Infestations (e.g., schistosomiasis, echinococciasis, ascariasis, infection with *Toxocara canis,* amebiasis, toxoplasmosis)

Intoxications (e.g., alcohol)

Vascular diseases (e.g., congestive heart failure)

Hematologic diseases (e.g., leukemias, lymphomas, hemolytic anemias, polycythemia)

Endocrine diseases (e.g., hyperthyroidism, diabetes mellitus, pregnancy)

Hereditary and metabolic diseases (e.g., mucopolysaccharidoses, glycogen-storage diseases, sickle cell disease, histiocytoses, Wilson's disease, mucoviscidosis, fatty liver, ulcerative colitis)

Collagen diseases (e.g., systemic lupus erythematosus (SLE), polyarteritis)

ACUTE VIRAL HEPATITIS
Prodromal period

HB_sAg appears in serum (see p. 126).

BSP retention is the earliest abnormality, followed by bilirubinuria before serum bilirubin increases.

Cephalin flocculation becomes positive at the same time that direct serum bilirubin increases.

There is an increase in urinary urobilinogen and total serum bilirubin just before clinical jaundice occurs.

Serum SGOT and SGPT both rise during the preicteric phase and show very high peaks (> 500 units) by the time jaundice appears.

ESR is normal.

Leukopenia (lymphopenia and neutropenia) is noted with onset of fever, followed by relative lymphocytosis and monocytosis; atypical lymphocytes and plasma cells may be found.

Acute icteric period (tests show parenchymal cell damage)

Serum bilirubin is 50–75% direct in the early stage; later, indirect bilirubin is proportionately more.

Serum SGOT and SGPT fall rapidly in the several days after jaundice appears and become normal 2–5 weeks later.

In hepatitis associated with infectious mononucleosis, peak levels are usually <200 units and peak occurs 2–3 weeks after onset, becoming normal by the fifth week. *In toxic hepatitis*, levels depend upon severity; slight elevations may be associated with therapy with anticoagulants, anovulatory drugs, etc.; poisoning (e.g., carbon tetrachloride) may cause levels $\leqq 300$ units. *In severe toxic hepatitis (especially carbon tetrachloride poisoning)*, serum enzymes may be 10–20 times higher than in acute hepatitis and show a different pattern, i.e., increase in LDH is > SGOT is > SGPT. *In acute hepatitis,* SGPT is > SGOT is > LDH.

Serum aldolase is increased in 90% of patients, ≦ 10 times normal. It parallels transaminase with a sharp rise before serum bilirubin and a return to normal 2–3 weeks after jaundice begins.

Serum isocitric dehydrogenase (ICD) is usually elevated in the early stage (5–10 times normal) but returns to normal in 2–3 weeks; increase persists in chronic hepatitis.

Abnormal thymol turbidity and cephalin flocculation occur frequently; changes in toxic hepatitis are less striking.

Other liver function tests are often abnormal, depending on severity of the disease—bilirubinuria, abnormal serum protein electrophoresis, alkaline phosphatase, etc.

Serum cholesterol–ester ratio is usually depressed early; total serum cholesterol is decreased only in severe disease. Serum phospholipids are increased in mild but decreased in severe hepatitis. Plasma vitamin A is decreased in severe hepatitis.

Urine urobilinogen is increased in the early icteric period; at peak of the disease it disappears for days or weeks; urobilinogen simultaneously disappears from stool.

ESR is increased; falls during convalescence.

Serum iron is often increased.

Urine. Cylindruria is common; albuminuria occurs occasionally; concentrating ability is sometimes decreased.

In acute viral hepatitis, very high SGOT and serum bilirubin are not reliable indicators of patient's clinical course, but prolonged prothrombin time, especially > 20 seconds, indicates the likely development of acute hepatic insufficiency; therefore the prothrombin time should be performed when patient is first seen. Triad of prolonged prothrombin time, increased PMN, and nonpalpable liver is omen of massive hepatic necrosis and likely development of coma.

Acute viral hepatitis completely resolves in 90% of patients within 12 weeks. Fulminant hepatitis occurs in 1–2% of patients with Type B hepatitis, and 90% die within 2–4 weeks. Relapse, usually within 1 year, has been recognized in 20% of patients by some elevation of SGOT and changes in liver biopsy.

Defervescent period

Diuresis occurs at onset of convalescence.

Bilirubinuria disappears while serum bilirubin is still increased.

Urine urobilinogen increases.

Serum bilirubin becomes normal after 3–6 weeks.

Later, cephalin flocculation becomes normal. Still later, thymol turbidity is normal.

ESR falls.

Anicteric Hepatitis

Laboratory findings are the same as in the icteric type, but abnormalities are usually less marked and there is slight or no increase of serum bilirubin.

Acute Fulminant Hepatitis with Hepatic Failure
Findings are the same as in acute hepatitis but more severe.
There are findings of hepatic failure.
Serum bilirubin is very high unless death occurs in the prodromal period.
Serum cholesterol and esters are markedly decreased.
Aminoaciduria occurs.
Patient may show anemia, leukocytosis, thrombocytopenia, etc.

Cholangiolitic Hepatitis
Same as acute hepatitis but evidence of obstruction is more prominent (e.g., increased serum alkaline phosphatase and direct serum bilirubin) and tests of parenchymal damage are less marked (e.g., thymol turbidity is frequently normal; SGOT increase may be 3–6 times normal).

Viral Hepatitis Carrier State
Usually liver function tests and needle biopsy are normal.

Comparison of Chronic Active Hepatitis (Patients Who Are Positive or Negative for HB$_s$Ag)

	Positive	*Negative (Lupoid)*
Serum HB$_s$Ag	Present	Absent
Autoimmune diseases	Rare	Frequent
Serum gamma globulin increase	Moderate	Marked
Smooth muscle antibody titer	Low or absent	High (60%)
LE cells	Absent	15%
HB$_s$Ag in liver biopsy	Present in the few ground-glass cells	Absent
Primary liver cancer	Present	Rare
Sex predominance	Male	Female
Response to corticosteroid therapy	Uncertain	Good

SERUM ENZYME DETERMINATIONS IN LIVER DISEASES

Useful In
Diagnosis of asymptomatic, prodromal, or anicteric hepatitis (e.g., in infectious mononucleosis). Occurs earlier than other chemical abnormalities (e.g., thymol turbidity, increased serum bilirubin).
Following the course of hepatitis. Determine return to physical activity (if enzymes increase in response to activity, return to bed rest). Determine prognosis by recurring acute episodes or prolonged course with increased serum enzymes levels.
Differential diagnosis of diseases of liver, biliary tract, etc. (see Tables 24, 25, pp. 212–213, 214–215).

Table 22. Comparison of Infectious Hepatitis and Serum Hepatitis

	Infectious Hepatitis	Serum Hepatitis
Incubation period	15–40 days	50–160 days
Abnormal SGOT	Transient 1–3 weeks	More prolonged 1–8+ months
Thymol turbidity	Usually increased during acute phase	Usually normal
Serum IgM levels	Usually increased to >400 mg/100 ml during acute phase	Usually normal
HB_sAg	Not present	Present during incubation period and acute phase; occasionally may persist

Screening prior to surgery for carcinoma (e.g., sudden rise in SGOT may indicate early liver metastases)

Screening of all blood donors

FATTY LIVER
Laboratory findings are due to underlying conditions (most commonly alcoholism; also diabetes mellitus, poor nutritional state, toxic chemicals, etc.).

Needle biopsy of liver establishes the diagnosis.

Liver function tests are normal in at least 50% of patients; others may show abnormalities of 1 or several tests, including clinical jaundice.

Mild anemia and increased WBC may occur.

Not infrequently, fatty liver is the only postmortem finding in cases of sudden, unexpected death.

ALCOHOLIC HEPATITIS
Occurs in 10–30% of chronic alcoholics; many have normal liver biopsy; others show characteristic alcoholic hyalin.

Anemia in >50% of patients may be macrocytic (folic acid or vitamin B_{12} deficiency), microcytic (iron or pyridoxine deficiency), mixed, or hemolytic.

Increased WBC (usually 10,000–16,000/cu mm); normal WBC indicates folic acid depletion.

Increased SGOT (usually 50–200 units) and SGPT (usually <100 units).

Increased alkaline phosphatase (may be marked).

Increased serum bilirubin.

Decreased serum albumin and increased serum globulin are frequent.

Increased prothrombin time is often found.

Table 23. Increased Serum Enzyme Levels in Liver Diseases

Serum Enzyme	Acute Viral Hepatitis		Obstructive Jaundice		Cirrhosis		Liver Metastases[a]	
	Frequency	Amplitude	Frequency	Amplitude	Frequency	Amplitude	Frequency	Amplitude
SGOT	>95%	14	>95%	3	75%	2	50%	1–2
SGPT	>95%	17	>95%	4	50%	1	25%	1–2
Alkaline phosphatase	60%	1–2	>95%	4–5	55%	1–2	50%	2
LAP	80%	1–2	85%	3	30%	1	70%	2–3
ICD	>95%	6	10%	1	20%	1	40%	2
5'-Nucleotidase	70%	1–2	>95%	6	50%	1–2	65%	3–4
Aldolase	90%	10		N		N	20%	

Frequency = average % frequency of patients with increased serum enzyme level when blood taken at optimal time.

Amplitude = average number of times normal that serum level is increased.

[a] For example, tumor, tuberculosis, sarcoid, amyloid.

Table 24. Serum Enzymes in Differential Diagnosis of Various Liver Diseases

Disease	Alkaline Phosphatase	SGOT	SGPT	ICD
Hepatitis	5–15 BU in > 80% of patients; 15–70 BU in 100% of patients during obstructive phase	Both rise during preicteric phase to peaks (> 500 U) by the time jaundice appears; then rapid fall in several days; become normal 2–5 weeks after onset of jaundice		500–2000 in first week; < 800 after 2 weeks; slightly elevated in third week
Cirrhosis	5–15 BU 40–50% of patients	≦300 U in 65–75% of patients	≦200 U in 50% of patients; wide fluctuation	< 500; poor prognosis if higher
Metastatic disease		≦300 in 50% of patients	40–150 U	250–1000
Metastatic cancer	≦70 BU in 80% of patients			
Tuberculosis	≦50 BU in 50% of patients			
Sarcoidosis	≦18 BU in 40% of patients			
Amyloidosis	≦100 BU frequently			
Biliary obstruction				
Complete	≦70 BU in 100% of patients	≦300 U	20–200 U	100–500
		Both return to normal within 1 week after obstruction is relieved		

Incomplete (occlusion of 1 duct or incomplete occlusion of bile ducts)	Frequently 10–14 BU
Congenital intrahepatic atresia	50–70 BU in 100% of patients
Congenital extrahepatic atresia	Normal unless rickets is present

U = units; BU = Bodansky units.

Table 25. Two Forms of Chronic Hepatitis

	Chronic Active Liver Disease	Benign Persistent Hepatitis
Synonyms	Lupoid hepatitis, subacute hepatitis, plasma cell hepatitis, chronic active hepatitis, chronic liver disease in young women, autoimmune hepatitis, juvenile cirrhosis, chronic aggressive hepatitis, active chronic hepatitis	Chronic persistent hepatitis, chronic lobular hepatitis, chronic portal hepatitis, triaditis, transaminitis, unresolved hepatitis
Criteria for diagnosis	After 12 weeks of hepatitis, tenfold increase in SGOT or fivefold increase in SGOT, with a twofold increase in gamma globulin	

		% of Patients	
Laboratory abnormalities in serum	Increase in SGOT	100	Increase in SGOT may be stable or fluctuate widely
	Increase in gamma globulin	90	Other liver function tests are near normal
	Increase in alkaline phosphatase	90	Twofold increase in alkaline phosphatase
	Increase in bilirubin	90	Increase in bilirubin ≤4 mg/100 ml
	Increase in immunoglobulin G	80	Increase in gamma globulin twofold
	Smooth muscle antibody	80	
	Prolonged prothrombin time	50	
	Increase in immunoglobulin M	50	
	Decrease in albumin	50	
	Increase in immunoglobulin A	33	
	Antinuclear antibody	33	
	Antisalmonella antibody	33	
	Antimitochondrial antibody	20	
	HB$_s$Ag	10–60	HB$_s$Ag ≤ 50%

Laboratory findings of associated diseases (e.g., Hashimoto's thyroiditis, Sjögren's syndrome, primary biliary cirrhosis, pernicious anemia, ITP)	25	No associated autoimmune diseases present
Liver biopsy	Different histologic criteria for diagnosis of each condition	
Laboratory findings of sequelae	Cirrhosis, portal hypertension, or liver failure may occur	Do not occur

Decreased levels of folic acid, thiamine, vitamin B_6, and other vitamins in 20–80% of patients.

Administration of corticosteroids may increase serum albumin and decrease serum bilirubin without prognosis.

CIRRHOSIS OF LIVER

Serum bilirubin is often increased; may be present for years. Fluctuations may reflect liver status due to insults to the liver (e.g., alcoholic debauches). Most bilirubin is of the indirect type unless cirrhosis is of the cholangiolitic type. Higher and more stable levels occur in postnecrotic cirrhosis; lower and more fluctuating levels occur in Laennec's cirrhosis. Terminal icterus may be constant and severe.

Serum SGOT is increased ($\leqq 300$ units) in 65–75% of patients. Serum SGPT is increased ($\leqq 200$ units) in 50% of patients. Transaminases vary widely and reflect activity or progression of the process (i.e., hepatic parenchymal cell necrosis).

Serum ICD is normal or only slightly increased (< 500 units) in 20% of patients. A large increase suggests a poorer prognosis.

Serum 5'-nucleotidase is increased in 50% of patients.

Serum alkaline phosphatase is increased ($\leqq 15$ Bodansky units) in 40–50% of patients. Serum LAP is slightly increased in 30% of patients.

Total serum protein is usually normal or decreased. Serum albumin parallels functional status of parenchymal cells and may be useful for following progress of liver disease; but it may be normal in the presence of considerable liver cell damage. Lowering of serum albumin may reflect development of ascites or hemorrhage. Serum globulin level is usually increased; it reflects inflammation and parallels the severity of the inflammation. Increased serum globulin may cause increased total protein, especially in chronic (viral) hepatitis and posthepatitic cirrhosis. Increased globulin is usually gamma. (See Table 5, p. 65.)

Cephalin flocculation and thymol turbidity are usually abnormal and remain so for long periods. Therefore they are useful for differentiating parenchymal cell disease from obstructive or hemolytic jaundice but are not helpful guides for following the course of cirrhosis.

Total serum cholesterol is normal or decreased. Decreased esters reflect more severe parenchymal cell damage.

BSP retention is a rather sensitive index of liver function and is most useful in the absence of jaundice to follow the course of disease when the other liver function tests are normal.

Urine bilirubin is increased; urobilinogen is normal or increased.

Laboratory findings due to complications or sequelae
  Ascites
  Bleeding esophageal varices
  Hypersplenism
  Hepatoma
  Portal vein thrombosis
  Hepatic coma
  Other

BUN is often decreased (< 10 mg/100 ml); increased with gastrointestinal hemorrhage.

Serum uric acid is often increased.

Electrolytes and acid-base balance are often abnormal and reflect various combinations of circumstances at the time, such as malnutrition, dehydration, hemorrhage, metabolic acidosis, respiratory alkalosis. In cirrhosis with ascites, the kidney retains increased sodium and excessive water causing dilutional hyponatremia.

Anemia reflects increased plasma volume and some increased destruction of RBCs. If more severe, rule out hemorrhage in gastrointestinal tract, folic acid deficiency, excessive hemolysis, etc.

WBC is usually normal with active cirrhosis; increased (≦ 50,000/cu mm) with massive necrosis, hemorrhage, etc.; decreased with hypersplenism.

Blood ammonia level is increased in liver coma and cirrhosis and with portacaval shunting of blood.

Abnormalities of coagulation mechanisms
>Prolonged prothrombin time (does not respond to parenteral vitamin K as frequently as in patients with obstructive jaundice)
>Abnormal TGT reflecting various abnormalities

Biopsy of liver is valuable.

Laboratory findings due to associated diseases or conditions (see appropriate separate sections)
>Alcoholism
>Wilson's disease
>Hemochromatosis
>Mucoviscidosis
>Glycogen-storage diseases
>Galactosemia
>Alpha$_1$ antitrypsin deficiency
>Porphyria
>Fanconi syndrome
>Schistosomiasis
>Gaucher's disease
>Ulcerative colitis
>Osler-Weber-Rendu disease

CHOLANGIOLITIC CIRRHOSIS (HANOT'S HYPERTROPHIC CIRRHOSIS, PRIMARY INTRAHEPATIC BILIARY CIRRHOSIS, ETC.)

Laboratory findings of complete biliary obstruction are of long duration (may last for years) and often of fluctuating intensity.

Direct serum bilirubin is increased in 80% of patients; levels >5 mg/100 ml in only 20% of patients; levels > 10 mg/100 ml in only 6% of patients. Indirect bilirubin is normal or slightly increased.

Serum alkaline phosphatase is markedly increased; in 50% of cases >70 King-Armstrong units (normal is ≦ 13). Be wary of making this diagnosis with values < 40.

Serum IgM is increased in ≅ 75% of patients; levels may be very high.

Table 26. Liver Function Tests in Differential Diagnosis of Jaundice

Disease	Urine Bilirubin	Urine Urobilinogen	Stool Bilirubin	Stool Urobilinogen	Serum Bilirubin Direct	Serum Bilirubin Indirect	Serum Cholesterol Total	Serum Cholesterol Esters	Cephalin Flocculation and Thymol Turbidity
Viral hepatitis	I	N or I	D	D	I early	I predom.	N or D	Mildly to markedly D	I
Hepatitis due to drugs Hepatitic type	I	N or I	D	D	I early	I predom.	N		I
Cholestatic type	I	N or D	D	D	I	Slightly I	I		N or slightly I
Cirrhosis	I	N or I			I < indirect	I > direct	N or D	Mildly to markedly D	I
Extrahepatic biliary obstruction	I	D	Markedly D	Markedly D	I	N or slightly I	Mildly to markedly I		N or slightly I

I = increased; D = decreased; N = normal.

Table 27. Comparison of Three Main Types of Liver Disease Due to Drugs

	Predominantly Cholestatic	Predominantly Hepatitic	Mixed Biochemical Pattern
Laboratory findings	Obstructive type of jaundice (see pp. 209, 223–224). Average duration of jaundice = 2 weeks; may last for years Serum bilirubin may be > 30 mg/100 ml		Some aspects of each type, but one may be more marked
	Alkaline phosphatase and LAP are markedly increased; may remain increased for years after jaundice has disappeared	Less markedly increased	
	SGOT, SGPT, LDH show mild to moderate increase	More markedly increased	
Some causative drugs	Organic arsenicals Anabolic steroids	Cinchophen Monamine oxidase inhibitors (particularly iproniazid)	
	Sulfonyl urea derivatives (including sulfonamides, phenothiazine tranquilizers, antidiabetic drugs, oral diuretics) Chlorpromazine PAS (usually this type but may be mixed) Erythromycin	Isonicotinic acid hydrazide	PAS and other antituberculosis agents
Pathology	Centrilobular bile stasis Low incidence High mortality (20%)	Same as acute viral hepatitis	

The previously mentioned triad should strongly suggest primary biliary cirrhosis. Serum mitochondrial antibody test (M test) is positive in 90% of patients.

Biopsy of liver is often diagnostic or compatible with the diagnosis.

Marked increase in total cholesterol and phospholipids takes place, with normal triglycerides; serum is not lipemic. The increase is associated with xanthomas and xanthelasmas.

Serum globulins (especially beta and alpha$_2$) are increased. Albumin is normal or slightly decreased early; later decreased.

Laboratory findings show relatively little evidence of parenchymal damage.

Thymol turbidity is usually increased; cephalin flocculation is negative or positive.

There are laboratory findings of steatorrhea, but prothrombin time is normal or restored to normal by parenteral vitamin K.

Urine contains urobilinogen and bilirubin.

Laboratory findings due to associated diseases (e.g., rheumatoid arthritis, autoimmune thyroiditis, Sjögren syndrome)

Laboratory findings due to complications (e.g., portal hypertension)

HEMOCHROMATOSIS

Primary (idiopathic) (rare, familial form)

Serum iron is increased (usually 200–300 μg/100 ml).

Serum unsaturated iron-binding capacity (UIBC) is decreased (often approaching zero).

Liver biopsy shows much iron in parenchymal cells and some in reticuloendothelial cells.

No anemia or laboratory changes due to alcoholism.

Laboratory findings due to cirrhosis and diabetes.

Increased stainable iron in bone marrow.

Secondary (more common, not familial)

Serum iron is increased.

Decreased serum UIBC is generally higher than in primary type.

Liver biopsy shows iron deposits predominantly in reticuloendothelial cells, with some iron in parenchymal cells.

Anemia (frequently).

Laboratory changes due to alcoholism, which is usually present.

Laboratory findings due to cirrhosis and diabetes.

Laboratory findings due to underlying disease (see p. 111).

Increased stainable iron in bone marrow.

WILSON'S DISEASE

Serum ceruloplasmin is decreased (<20 mg/100 ml). (*It is normal in 5% of patients with overt Wilson's disease.*)

Total serum copper is decreased.

Nonceruloplasmin copper is increased.

Urinary copper is increased (>100μg/24 hours).

Liver biopsy shows high copper concentration (>250 μg/gm of dry liver).

Liver biopsy may show no abnormalities, moderate to marked fatty changes with or without fibrosis, or active or inactive cirrhosis.

Liver function tests are abnormal, depending on the type and severity of disease (e.g., transaminase).

Aminoaciduria, especially cystine and threonine, may be found.

Decreased serum uric acid may occur.

Decreased serum ceruloplasmin (<20 mg/100) with increased hepatic copper (>250 µg/gm) occurs only in Wilson's disease or normal infants aged <6 months.

Heterozygous gene for Wilson's disease occurs in 1 of 200 in the general population; 10% of these have decreased serum ceruloplasmin.

Homozygous gene (clinical Wilson's disease) occurs in 1 of 200,000 in the general population.

Measure serum ceruloplasmin in any patient under age 30 with hepatitis, hemolysis, or neurologic symptoms to allow early diagnosis and treatment of Wilson's disease.

PORTAL HYPERTENSION (WITH SHUNT FROM PORTAL SYSTEM VIA COLLATERAL CIRCULATION)

Increased blood ammonia

Increased postprandial blood glucose

Increased urine urobilinogen

Laboratory findings due to underlying disease

Posthepatic obstruction (e.g., constrictive pericarditis, obstruction of hepatic veins, obstruction of inferior vena cava, cirrhosis)

Intrahepatic obstruction (e.g., sickle cell disease)

Prehepatic obstruction (e.g., occlusion of portal vein by thrombus or tumor, tumors, scars—as from schistosomiasis)

Shunts (e.g., arteriovenous fistulas, hamartomas of liver)

Laboratory findings due to complications and sequelae

Hypersplenism

Intestinal malabsorption or protein loss

Bleeding from esophageal varices

SURGICAL PORTACAVAL ANASTOMOSIS

In cirrhosis

Operative mortality is <5% if

Serum bilirubin is <3.0 mg/100 ml.

Serum albumin is at least 3.5 gm/100 ml.

Operative mortality is ≅50% if

Serum bilirubin is >8.0 mg/100 ml.

Serum albumin is ≅2.5 gm/100 ml.

Following surgery

Serum indirect bilirubin is slightly increased.

Blood ammonia is increased.

Laboratory findings of hypersplenism decrease.

PORTAL VEIN THROMBOSIS

Laboratory findings due to underlying conditions (e.g., polycythemia, cirrhosis, neoplastic invasion of portal vein)

Laboratory findings due to infarction of intestine

HEPATOMA

Serum alpha-fetoprotein present in 50% of white and 75–90% of nonwhite patients

Laboratory findings associated with metastatic lesions of liver

Laboratory findings associated with underlying disease (>60% occur with preexisting cirrhosis)

> Hemochromatosis ($\leqq$20% of patients die of hepatoma)
> More frequent in postnecrotic than in alcoholic cirrhosis

Sudden progressive worsening of laboratory findings of underlying disease

Hemoperitoneum—ascites in $\cong$50% of patients but tumor cells found irregularly

Laboratory findings due to obstruction of hepatic or portal veins or inferior vena cava

Occasional marked hypoglycemia unresponsive to adrenalin injection

ESR and WBC sometimes increased

Anemia uncommon unless hemorrhage occurs

METASTATIC OR INFILTRATIVE DISEASE OF LIVER

Increased serum alkaline phosphatase is the most useful index of *partial obstruction of the biliary tree* when serum bilirubin is usually normal and urine bilirubin is increased.

> Increased in 80% of patients with metastatic carcinoma ($\leqq$70 Bodansky units)
> Increased in 50% of patients with tuberculosis ($\leqq$50 Bodansky units)
> Increased in 40% of patients with sarcoidosis ($\leqq$18 Bodansky units)
> Increased frequently in patients with amyloidosis ($\leqq$100 Bodansky units)

Increased serum LAP parallels alkaline phosphatase but is not affected by bone disease.

Whenever the alkaline phosphatase is increased, a simultaneous increase of 5'-N establishes biliary disease as the cause of the elevated alkaline phosphatase.

SGOT is increased in 50% of patients ($\leqq$300 units).

SGPT is increased less frequently ($\leqq$150 units).

ICD may show a moderate increase.

Increased serum alkaline phosphatase and increased BSP retention is 65% reliable to establish this diagnosis.

Radioactive scanning of the liver is 80% reliable.

Blind needle biopsy of the liver is positive in 65–75% of patients.

Laboratory findings due to primary disease are noted. See also
> Carcinoid syndrome
> Pyogenic liver abscess
> Other

LIVER FUNCTION ABNORMALITIES IN CONGESTIVE HEART FAILURE

BSP retention is the most frequently abnormal test. It may indicate circulatory stasis as well as cellular damage.

Serum bilirubin is frequently increased (indirect more than direct); usually 1–5 mg/100 ml. It usually represents combined right- and left-sided failure with hepatic engorgement and pulmonary infarcts. Serum bilirubin may suddenly rise rapidly if superimposed myocardial infarction occurs.

Urine urobilinogen is increased. Urine bilirubin is increased in the presence of jaundice.

Thymol turbidity is abnormal in ≅ 30% and cephalin flocculation test is positive in ≅ 20% of patients.

SGOT and SGPT are increased in ≅ 12% of patients.

Serum LDH is increased in ≅ 40% of patients.

Serum alkaline phosphatase shows mild to moderate increase (6–25 Bodansky units) in 45% of cases.

Hypoalbuminemia is common with cardiac fibrosis of liver.

Prothrombin time may be slightly increased, with increased sensitivity to anticoagulant drugs.

Serum cholesterol and esters may be decreased.

These findings may occur with marked liver congestion due to other conditions (e.g., Chiari's syndrome [occlusion of hepatic veins] and constrictive pericarditis).

HEPATIC FAILURE

Serum bilirubin very high
Decreased albumin and also total protein
Previously elevated SGOT and SGPT that fall abruptly with onset of hepatic failure
Decreased blood glucose
Prolonged prothrombin time
Blood ammonia level usually increased
Laboratory findings of hemorrhage, especially in GI tract

COMPLETE BILIARY OBSTRUCTION (INTRAHEPATIC OR EXTRAHEPATIC)

Direct serum bilirubin is increased; indirect serum bilirubin is normal or slightly increased.

Urine bilirubin is increased; urine urobilinogen decreased.

There is decreased stool bilirubin and urobilinogen (clay-colored stools).

Serum alkaline phosphatase is markedly increased (15–70 Bodansky units). In extrahepatic type, the increase is related to the completeness of obstruction.

Serum LAP parallels alkaline phosphatase.

SGOT is increased (≦ 300 units) and SGPT is increased ≦ 200 units); they usually return to normal in 1 week after relief of obstruction.

Thymol turbidity, cephalin flocculation, and BSP test are normal or may later become only slightly increased.

Serum cholesterol is increased (acute, 300–400 mg/100 ml; chronic, ≦ 1000 mg/100 ml).

Serum phospholipids are increased.

Prothrombin time is prolonged, with response to parenteral vitamin K more frequent than in hepatic parenchymal cell disease.

Laboratory findings due to underlying causative disease are noted (e.g., stone, carcinoma of duct, metastatic carcinoma to periductal lymph nodes).

OBSTRUCTION OF ONE HEPATIC BILE DUCT

Serum bilirubin remains normal in the presence of serum alkaline phosphatase that is markedly increased.

CONGENITAL EXTRAHEPATIC BILIARY ATRESIA

Direct serum bilirubin increased in early days of life in some infants but not until second week in others. Level is often < 12 mg/100 ml during first months, with subsequent rise later in life.

Laboratory findings as in Complete Biliary Obstruction (see p. 223 and above).

Liver biopsy to differentiate from neonatal hepatitis.

Laboratory findings due to sequelae (e.g., biliary cirrhosis, portal hypertension, frequent infections, rickets, hepatic failure)
[131]I-rose bengal excretion test (see next section)

Most important to differentiate this condition from neonatal hepatitis, for which surgery may be harmful.

>90% of cases of extrahepatic biliary obstruction in newborns are due to biliary atresia; occasional cases may be due to choledochal cyst (causes intermittent jaundice in infancy), bile plug syndrome, or bile ascites (associated with spontaneous perforation of the common bile duct).

NEONATAL HEPATITIS*

Due To
Unknown agent
Toxoplasmosis
Syphilis
Listeria
Cytomegalovirus
Rubella
Herpes
Varicella
Coxsackie
Hepatitis A and B viruses (?)

Clinical and Laboratory Findings
Jaundice at birth, or days or weeks later. Both direct and indirect bilirubin levels are increased in variable proportions.

Mild hemolytic anemia is usual.

Increased SGOT, SGPT, etc., may be marked and usually greater

---

*J. D. Johnson, Current concepts. Neonatal nonhemolytic jaundice. *N. Engl. J. Med.* 292:194, 1975.

than in biliary atresia, but increases are not reliable for differentiating the two conditions.

Laboratory findings as in acute viral hepatitis, (p. 207).

Liver biopsy to differentiate from biliary atresia and to avoid unnecessary surgery is useful in ≅65% of patients but it may be misleading.

[131]I-rose bengal excretion test indicates complete biliary obstruction if <10% of the radioactivity is excreted in stools during 48–72 hours and incomplete obstruction if excretion is >10%. Complete obstruction is found in all infants with biliary atresia and in ≅20% with neonatal hepatitis and severe cholestasis. Administration of phenobarbital and cholestyramine increases the ^{131}I-rose bengal excretion in neonatal hepatitis but not in extrahepatic atresia. Some authors have suggested a repeat test in 3–4 weeks prior to exploratory surgery if rose bengal test indicates complete obstruction.

Laboratory tests for various etiologic agents

Laboratory findings of chronic liver disease, which develops in 30–50% of these infants.

DUBIN-JOHNSON SYNDROME (SPRINZ-NELSON DISEASE)

Inherited familial disease may resemble mild viral hepatitis. It is characterized by mild recurrent jaundice with hepatomegaly and right upper quadrant abdominal pain. It is due to inability to transport bilirubin-glucuronide through the parenchymal hepatic cell into the canaliculi; however, conjugation of bilirubin-glucuronide is normal. Usually it is compensated, except in periods of stress. Jaundice (innocuous and reversible) may be produced by estrogens, last trimester of pregnancy, or birth control pills.

Serum direct bilirubin is increased (3–10 mg/100 ml).

Urine contains bile and urobilinogen.

BSP excretion is impaired with late (1½- and 2-hour) rise.

Other liver function tests are normal (thymol turbidity and cephalin flocculation may be somewhat abnormal).

Serum alkaline phosphatase is normal.

Liver biopsy shows large amounts of yellow-brown or slate-black pigment in hepatic cells in centrilobular location; small amounts of Kupffer's cells.

ROTOR SYNDROME

Inherited condition of defective transfer of bilirubin from liver to bile; usually detected in adolescents or adults. Jaundice may be produced or accentuated by pregnancy, birth control pills, alcohol, infection, surgery.

Mild chronic conjugated hyperbilirubinemia

BSP excretion impaired, with late rise

Other liver function tests normal

GILBERT'S DISEASE (UNCONJUGATED HYPERBILIRUBINEMIA WITHOUT OVERT HEMOLYSIS)

Mild symptomatic benign condition with an evanescent increase of indirect serum bilirubin, which is usually discovered on routine laboratory examinations. The disease may be due to inadequacy of glucuronyl-transferase or bilirubin transfer from plasma to liver and probably represents a heterogeneous group (e.g., late infectious hepatitis, mild familial congenital disease), or it may be an inherited defect that is aggravated by other medical conditions. Jaundice is usually accentuated by pregnancy, fever, exercise, and various drugs, including alcohol and birth control pills.

Indirect serum bilirubin is increased. It may rise to 18 mg/100 ml but usually is <4 mg/100 ml. Fasting (<400 calories/day) for 72 hours causes elevated indirect bilirubin to increase >100% in Gilbert's disease but not in normal persons or those with liver disease or hemolytic anemia.

Fecal urobilinogen may be decreased.

Urine shows no increased bilirubin.

BSP retention may be slightly increased.

Liver function tests are usually normal.

HEREDITARY GLUCURONYL-TRANSFERASE DEFICIENCY, GROUP I (CRIGLER-NAJJAR SYNDROME)

This rare familial autosomal recessive disease is due to marked congenital deficiency or absence of glucuronyl-transferase that conjugates bilirubin to bilirubin-glucuronide in hepatic cells (counterpart is the homozygous Gunn rat).

Indirect serum bilirubin is increased; it appears on first or second day of life, rises to 12–45 mg/100 ml, and persists for life.

Fecal urobilinogen is very low.

Liver function tests are normal.

Liver biopsy is normal.

There is no evidence of hemolysis.

Nonjaundiced parents have diminished capacity to form glucuronide conjugates with menthol, salicylates, and tetrahydrocortisone.

This syndrome has been divided into two groups:

	Group I	Group II
Transmission	Autosomal recessive	Autosomal dominant
Hyperbilirubinemia	More severe	Less severe and more variable (normal ≅ 22 mg/100 ml)
Kernicterus	Frequent	Absent
Bile	Essentially colorless	Normal color
	Only traces of unconjugated bilirubin	Contains bilirubin-glucuronide
Phenobarbital administration	Hyperbilirubinemia unaffected	Jaundice disappears

BREAST-MILK JAUNDICE

Severe unconjugated hyperbilirubinemia that develops in 1% of breast-fed infants by the fourth to seventh day. Reaches peak of 15–25 mg/100 ml by the second to third week; then gradually disappears by 3–10 weeks in all cases. If nursing is interrupted

Table 28. Differential Diagnosis of Adult Jaundice When Other Liver Chemistries Are Normal and There Are No Signs or Symptoms of Liver Disease

	When Increased Bilirubin Is Conjugated (direct)		When Increased Bilirubin Is Unconjugated (indirect)		
	Dubin-Johnson Syndrome	Rotor Syndrome	Gilbert's Disease	Crigler-Najjar Syndrome	Hemolytic Jaundice
Serum Bilirubin					
Direct	I	I			
Indirect	I		I	I	I
Urine					
Bilirubin	I	N or I	N	N	Absent
Urobilinogen	I	N or I	N or D	N or D	I
Stool					
Bilirubin			D	D	I
Urobilinogen			N or D	N or D	I
Impaired excretion of dyes (e.g., BSP) requiring conjugation	Present	Present	May be slightly impaired		
Liver biopsy	Characteristic pigment	No pigment	N	N	N

N = normal; D = decreased; I = increased.

227

for 3–4 days, serum bilirubin falls rapidly; if interrupted for 6–9 days, serum bilirubin becomes normal.

No other abnormalities are present.

Kernicterus does not occur.

This syndrome occurs in 75% of the infants of such mothers. Is due to the presence in mother's milk of pregnane-3(α),20(β)-diol, which inhibits glucuronyl-transferase activity.

TRANSIENT FAMILIAL NEONATAL HYPERBILIRUBINEMIA (LUCEY-DRISCOLL SYNDROME)

Newborn infants have severe nonhemolytic unconjugated hyperbilirubinemia and a high risk of kernicterus.

Syndrome is due to unidentified substance in mother's serum only during last trimester of pregnancy that inhibits glucuronyltransferase activity.

NEONATAL PHYSIOLOGIC HYPERBILIRUBINEMIA

This is a transient unconjugated hyperbilirubinemia ("physiologic jaundice") that occurs in most newborns. Diagnosis by exclusion of other known causes of jaundice in this age group.

In normal full-term infants, average maximum serum bilirubin is 6 mg/100 ml and occurs during the second to fourth day. In premature infants, average maximum serum bilirubin is 10–12 mg/100 ml and occurs during the fifth to seventh day.

In newborns clinical icterus is not apparent until serum bilirubin is >5 mg/100 ml, but in older children it is apparent clinically when serum bilirubin is >2 mg/100 ml.

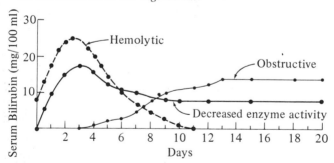

Fig. 6. Comparison of progressive changes in serum bilirubin levels during prolonged jaundice in infancy due to hemolytic jaundice, obstruction (e.g., biliary atresia, cystic fibrosis, "inspissated bile syndrome," neonatal hepatitis, galactosemia), or decreased liver enzyme activity (e.g., prematurity, Gilbert's disease, Crigler-Najjar syndrome, breast-feeding, infections such as cytomegalic inclusion disease and toxoplasmosis, "physiologic" disorders).

SOME CAUSES OF HYPERBILIRUBINEMIA IN THE NEWBORN

Unconjugated

Excessive destruction of RBCs (see Hemolytic Disease of the

Newborn, p. 307, Hereditary Spherocytosis, p. 303, G-6-PD Deficiency, p. 304)
Neonatal physiologic hyperbilirubinema (see p. 228)
Transient familial neonatal hyperbilirubinemia (see p. 228)
Hereditary glucuronyl-transferase deficiency (see p. 226)
 Group I (Crigler-Najjar syndrome)
 Group II
Breast-milk jaundice (see pp. 226, 228)
Associated with other conditions (e.g., high intestinal obstruction, maternal diabetes, hypothyroidism, neonatal respiratory distress, neonatal administration of drugs, such as vitamin K_3 and novobiocin)

Conjugated
Biliary obstruction—usually due to extrahepatic biliary atresia (see p. 224) but may be due to choledochal cyst, obstructive inspissated bile plugs, or bile ascites
Neonatal hepatitis (see p. 224)
Sepsis, especially *Escherichia coli* pyelonephritis (moderate azotemia, acidosis, increased serum bilirubin, slight hemolysis, normal or slightly increased SGOT)
Hereditary diseases (e.g., galactosemia, alpha$_1$ antitrypsin deficiency, cystic fibrosis, hereditary fructose intolerance, tyrosinemia, infantile Gaucher's disease, familial intrahepatic cholestasis [Byler disease])
In the course of hemolytic disease of the newborn—due to liver damage the cause of which is unknown.

SOME CAUSES OF HYPERBILIRUBINEMIA IN OLDER CHILDREN

All cases of conjugated hyperbilirubinemia also show some increase of unconjugated serum bilirubin.

Unconjugated
Gilbert's disease (see pp. 225–226)
Administration of drugs (e.g., novobiocin)
Occasionally in other conditions (e.g., thyrotoxicosis, following portacaval shunt in cirrhosis)

Conjugated
Dubin-Johnson syndrome (see p. 225)
Rotor syndrome (see p. 225)
Acute viral hepatitis causes most cases in children
Cholestasis due to chemicals and drugs (see Table 27, p. 219) or associated with other diseases (e.g., Hodgkin's disease, sickle cell disease)

HEPATIC CHOLESTEROL ESTER STORAGE DISEASE
In this inherited familial disorder, an enlarged liver contains excessive deposition of cholesterol esters and serum bile acid levels are increased.

Liver chemical function tests are normal.

Other blood chemistries are normal (including carotene, vitamin A, ceruloplasmin).

Serum lipid profiles may show a moderate increase in esterified cholesterol, phospholipid, triglyceride.

Lipoprotein electrophoresis may show a slight decrease in alpha-lipoproteins or a slight increase in beta- and pre-beta-lipoproteins.

Biopsy of liver reveals brilliant orange-yellow color. Polarized light shows crystalline material in parenchymal cells. There is chemical and histochemical confirmation of cholesterol esters. Septate cirrhosis may be present histologically.

RECURRENT FAMILIAL CHOLESTASIS

Rare familial condition with early onset of multiple episodes of conjugated hyperbilirubinemia with spontaneous complete remissions and exacerbations.

LIVER TRAUMA

Serum LDH is frequently increased ($>$1400 units) 8–12 hours after major injury. *Shock due to any injury may also increase LDH.*

Other serum enzymes and liver function tests are not generally helpful.

Findings of abdominal paracentesis

    Bloody fluid (in $\cong$ 75% of patients) confirming traumatic hemoperitoneum and indicating exploratory laparotomy

    Nonbloody fluid (especially if injury occurred $>$24 hours earlier)

        Microscopic—some red and white blood cells

        Determine amylase, protein, pH, presence of bile.

SUPPURATIVE CHOLANGITIS

Marked increase in WBC ($\leqq$ 30,000/cu mm) with increase in granulocytes

Blood culture often positive

Laboratory findings of incomplete duct obstruction due to inflammation or of preceding complete duct obstruction that caused the cholangitis (e.g., stone, tumor, scar)

Laboratory findings of parenchymal cell necrosis and malfunction

    Increased serum SGOT, SGPT, etc.

    Increased urine urobilinogen

SEPTIC PYLEPHLEBITIS

Polynuclear leukocytosis in $>$90% of patients; usually $>$20,000/cu mm

Anemia of varying severity

Moderate increase in serum bilirubin in $\cong$33% of patients

Other liver function tests positive in $\cong$25% of patients

Needle biopsy of liver not helpful; contraindicated

Blood culture sometimes positive

Laboratory findings due to preceding disease (e.g., acute appendicitis, diverticulitis, ulcerative colitus)

Laboratory findings due to complications (e.g., portal vein occlusion)

PYOGENIC LIVER ABSCESS
Increase in WBC due to increase in granulocytes
Abnormalities of liver function tests.
>   BSP retention
>   Decreased serum albumin, increased serum globulin
>   Positive cephalin flocculation
>   Increased serum alkaline phosphatase
>   Increased serum bilirubin (>10 mg/100 ml usually indicates pyogenic rather than amebic and suggests poorer prognosis because of more tissue destruction)
>   Other laboratory findings (see Metastatic or Infiltrative Disease of Liver, p. 222)

Anemia frequent
Laboratory findings due to complications (e.g., subphrenic abscess, pneumonia, empyema, bronchopleural fistula)

Patients with amebic abscess of liver due to *Entamoeba histolytica* also show positive serologic tests for ameba (see p. 505).
>   Stools may be negative for cysts and trophozoites.
>   Needle aspiration of abscess may show *Entamoeba histolytica* in 50% of patients. (*Characteristic brown or anchovy-sauce color may be absent; secondary bacterial infection may be superimposed.*)

ACUTE CHOLECYSTITIS
Increased ESR, WBC (average 12,000/cu mm; if >15,000 suspect empyema or perforation) and other evidence of acute inflammatory process
Increased serum bilirubin in 20% of patients (usually <4 mg/100 ml; if higher, suspect associated choledocholithiasis)
Increased BSP retention (some patients) even if serum bilirubin is normal
Increased serum alkaline phosphatase (some patients) even if serum bilirubin is normal
Increased serum amylase and lipase in some patients
Laboratory findings of associated biliary obstruction if such obstruction is present
Laboratory findings of preexisting cholelithiasis (some patients)
Laboratory findings of complications (e.g., empyema of gallbladder, perforation, cholangitis, liver abscess, pylephlebitis, pancreatitis, gallstone ileus)

Serum SGOT is increased in 75% of patients.

CHRONIC CHOLECYSTITIS
May be mild laboratory findings of acute cholecystitis or no abnormal laboratory findings
May be laboratory findings of associated cholelithiasis

CHOLELITHIASIS
Laboratory findings of underlying conditions causing hypercholesterolemia (e.g., diabetes mellitus)
Laboratory findings of causative chronic hemolytic disease (e.g., hereditary spherocytosis)

Laboratory findings of resultant cholecystitis or choledocholithiasis, etc.

CHOLEDOCHOLITHIASIS
During or soon after an attack of biliary colic
    Increased WBC
    Increased serum bilirubin in $\cong$ one-third of patients
    Increased urine bilirubin in $\cong$ one-third of patients
    Increased serum and urine amylase
Fluctuating laboratory evidence of biliary obstruction (see p. 223)
Laboratory findings due to secondary cholangitis
In duodenal drainage, crystals of both calcium bilirubinate and cholesterin (some patients); 50% accurate (only useful in nonicteric patients)

BILIARY DYSKINESIA
Normal laboratory tests of biliary, hepatic, and pancreatic function
Normal WBC

CANCER OF GALLBLADDER AND BILE DUCTS
Laboratory findings reflect varying location and extent of tumor infiltration that may cause partial intrahepatic duct obstruction or obstruction of hepatic or common bile duct, metastases in liver or associated cholangitis (see pp. 223, 224, 222, 230); 50% of patients have jaundice at the time of hospitalization.
Laboratory findings of duct obstruction are of progressively increasing severity in contrast to the intermittent or fluctuating changes due to duct obstruction caused by stones. A papillary intraluminal duct carcinoma may undergo periods of sloughing, producing the findings of intermittent duct obstruction.
Stool is frequently positive for occult blood.
Anemia is present.
Cytologic examination of aspirated duodenal fluid may demonstrate malignant cells.
Laboratory findings of the preceding cholelithiasis are present (gallbladder cancer occurs in $\cong$ 3% of patients with gallstones).

PARASITIC INFESTATION OF BILIARY SYSTEM
Laboratory findings due to biliary obstruction and to cholangitis
Infestation due to *Echinococcus, Ascaris,* liver flukes

POSTOPERATIVE JAUNDICE
This is usually due to a combination of factors.

Overproduction of bilirubin
    Resorption of blood (e.g., hematoma, hemoperitoneum)
    G-6-PD deficiency (see p. 304)
    Sickle cell disease (see p. 297)
    Hemolysis of transfused RBCs. The amount of hemoglobin produced is insufficient to cause jaundice unless other conditions (e.g., sepsis, hypoxemia, anesthesia) are present.
Impaired hepatocellular function:

Halothane toxicity. Occurs 1:10,000 cases. WBC is increased in 2 days. Jaundice may not appear for several weeks but may occur earlier if there has been previous exposure. Laboratory findings of severe liver necrosis are present (e.g., marked increase of SGOT, prolonged prothrombin time), and there is 20% fatality.

Shock. Severe jaundice in 2% of patients is due to trauma. (*Multiple factors are usually present, e.g., drugs, infection, transfusions.*) Serum bilirubin reaches 5–20 mg/100 ml 2–10 days after surgery; SGOT is 100–500 units; serum alkaline phosphatase is 2–3 times normal. *Clinical jaundice is found in only 20% of patients with massive liver necrosis.*

Syndrome of benign postoperative intrahepatic cholestasis. Occurs in patients with difficult prolonged surgery, multiple transfusions, postoperative complications (e.g., hemorrhage, sepsis, kidney failure, heart failure). Serum bilirubin reaches 15–40 mg/100 ml 2–10 days after surgery; SGOT is usually <200 units; serum alkaline phosphatase shows marked but variable increase. Liver biopsy reveals dilated bile canaliculi with bile casts, and minimal necrosis or infiltration of lymphocytes.

Bacterial infections, especially gram-negative septicemia and pneumococcal pneumonia. Occurs 5–12 days after onset of infection. Increased serum bilirubin is mild; there is variable increase in SGOT and serum alkaline phosphatase. Liver biopsy reveals intrahepatic cholestasis with mild periportal infiltration of leukocytes; there is little or no hepatic cell necrosis.

Preexisting anicteric hepatitis or cirrhosis

Drugs (see Table 27, p. 219)

Extrahepatic bile duct obstruction

Injury to bile duct. Jaundice usually occurs within 1 week. See also Cholangitis, p. 230.

See also Cholecystitis, p. 231; Choledocholithiasis, p. 232.

ACUTE PANCREATITIS

Serum amylase increase begins in 3–6 hours, rises to >250 Somogyi units within 8 hours in 75% of patients, reaches maximum in 20–30 hours, and may persist for 48–72 hours. The increase may be ≦40 times normal, but the height of the increase does not correlate with the severity of the disease. The level should be ≧ 500 Somogyi units/100 ml to be significant of acute pancreatitis. *Similar high values may occur in obstruction of pancreatic duct; they tend to fall after several days. >10% of patients with acute pancreatitis may have normal values, even when dying of acute pancreatitis.*

Serum lipase increases in 50% of patients and may remain elevated for as long as 14 days after amylase returns to normal. *(Lipase should always be determined whenever amylase is determined since the amylase may have already returned to normal values.)* Urinary lipase is not clinically useful.

Serum calcium is decreased in severe cases 1–9 days after onset (due to binding to soaps in fat necrosis). The decrease usually occurs after amylase and lipase levels have become normal. Tetany may occur. (*Rule out hyperparathyroidism if serum calcium is high or fails to fall in hyperamylasemia of acute pancreatitis.*)

Increased urinary amylase tends to reflect serum changes by a time lag of 6–10 hours, but sometimes increased urine levels are higher and of longer duration than serum levels. The 24-hour level may be normal even when some of the 1-hour specimens show increased values. Amylase levels in hourly samples of urine may be useful (>40 Somogyi units/hour). Ratio of amylase clearance to creatinine clearance is increased (>5%) and avoids the problem of timed urine specimens. Simplest and most useful is increased ratio of urinary amylase to urinary creatinine (on random specimen).

Serum bilirubin may be increased when pancreatitis is of biliary tract origin but is usually normal in alcoholic pancreatitis.

Other nonspecific serum enzymes may also be increased (e.g., LDH, MDH, LSP, ALD, SGOT). Serum SGOT may correlate with serum bilirubin rather than with amylase, lipase, or calcium levels. Serum alkaline phosphatase is increased when serum bilirubin is elevated and parallels serum bilirubin.

Serum trypsin is increased.

WBC is slightly to moderately increased (10,000–20,000/cu mm).

Hemoconcentration occurs (increased hematocrit). Hematocrit may be decreased in severe hemorrhagic pancreatitis.

Mild increase of blood sugar is common.

Glycosuria appears in 25% of patients.

Ascites may develop, cloudy or bloody or "prune juice" fluid, ½–2 L in volume, containing increased amylase with a level higher than that of serum amylase. No bile is evident (unlike the situation in perforated ulcer). Gram stain shows no bacteria (unlike the situation in infarct of intestine).

Poorer prognosis is indicated when ≧ 3 of the following laboratory findings are present:

> Initial WBC >16,000/cu mm
> Initial blood glucose >200 mg/100 ml
> Initial serum LDH >700 IU/L
> Initial serum SGOT >250 IU/L
> Decreased serum calcium
> Fall in hematocrit >10%
> Rise in BUN >5 mg/100 ml
> Arterial pO_2 <60 mm Hg
> Metabolic acidosis with base deficit >4 mEq/L

CHRONIC PANCREATIC DISEASE (CHRONIC PANCREATITIS; CARCINOMA OF PANCREAS)

Examine duodenal contents (volume, bicarbonate concentration, amylase output) after IV administration of pancreozymin and secretin. Some abnormality occurs in >85% of patients with chronic pancreatitis. Amylase output is the most frequent abnormality. When all three are abnormal, there is a greater frequency of abnormality in the tests listed below.

Serum amylase and lipase increase after administration of pancreozymin and secretin in $\cong 20\%$ of patients with chronic pancreatitis. They are more often abnormal when duodenal contents are normal.

Fasting serum amylase and lipase increase in 10% of patients with chronic pancreatitis.

There will be a diabetic oral glucose tolerance test (GTT) in 65% of patients with chronic pancreatitis and frank diabetes in >10% of patients with chronic relapsing pancreatitis. When GTT is normal in the presence of steatorrhea, the cause should be sought elsewhere than in the pancreas.

Chemical determination of fecal fat demonstrates steatorrhea. It is more sensitive than tests using triolein [131]I.

Triolein ^{131}I is abnormal in one-third of patients with chronic pancreatitis.

Starch tolerance test is abnormal in 25% of patients with chronic pancreatitis.

Radioactive scanning of pancreas (selenium) yields variable findings in different clinics.

See Laboratory Diagnosis of Malabsorption, p. 199.

Laboratory findings due to underlying conditions are noted (e.g., alcoholism, trauma, duodenal ulcer, cholelithiasis).

PSEUDOCYST OF PANCREAS

Serum direct bilirubin is increased (>2 mg/100 ml) in 10% of patients.

Serum alkaline phosphatase is increased (>5 Bodansky units) in 10% of patients.

Fasting blood sugar is increased in < 10% of patients.

Laboratory findings of preceding acute pancreatitis are present (this is mild and unrecognized in one-third of patients). Persistent increase of serum amylase and lipase after an acute episode may indicate formation of a pseudocyst.

Duodenal contents after secretin-pancreozymin stimulation usually show decreased bicarbonate content (<70 mEq/L) but normal volume and normal content of amylase, lipase, and trypsin.

Laboratory findings due to conditions preceding acute pancreatitis are noted (e.g., alcoholism, trauma, duodenal ulcer, cholelithiasis).

CYSTIC FIBROSIS OF PANCREAS (MUCOVISCIDOSIS)

Striking increase in sweat sodium and chloride (>60 mEq/L) and, to a lesser extent, potassium is present in virtually all homozygous patients. It is present throughout life from time of birth and is not related to severity of disease or organ involvement. There is a broad range of values in this disease and in normal but minimal overlap (see Sweat Electrolytes, p. 146). *(Sweat chloride is somewhat more reliable than sodium for diagnostic purposes.)* Sweat sodium and chloride increase is not useful for determination of heterozygosity or genetic counseling.

Serum chloride, sodium, potassium, calcium, and phosphorus are normal unless complications occur (e.g., chronic pulmonary disease with accumulation of CO_2, massive salt loss due to sweating).

Urine electrolytes are normal.

Submaxillary saliva has slightly increased chloride and sodium but not potassium; however, considerable overlap with normal persons prevents diagnostic use. Submaxillary saliva also is more turbid, with increased calcium, total protein, and amylase. These changes are not generally found in parotid saliva.

Serum protein electrophoresis shows increasing gamma globulin with progressive pulmonary disease, mainly due to immunoglobulins G and A; M and D are not appreciably increased.

Serum albumin is often decreased (because of hemodilution due to cor pulmonale; may be found before cardiac involvement is clinically apparent). In late stages of chronic lung disease, decreased serum electrolytes, hemoglobin, hematocrit level, etc., may also reflect hemodilution.

Bacteriology. Hemolytic *Staphylococcus aureus* is the most frequent and important organism in the respiratory tract; *Pseudomonas aeruginosa* has recently been found increasingly often.

Adrenal and pituitary function tests are normal.

Laboratory changes secondary to complications (e.g., pancreatic deficiency, chronic pulmonary disease, excessive loss of electrolytes in sweat, cirrhosis of liver, intestinal obstruction)

> Pancreas (see Laboratory Diagnosis of Malabsorption, p. 199
> > 80% of patients show loss of all pancreatic enzyme activity.
> > 10% of patients show decrease of pancreatic enzyme activity.
> > 10% of patients show normal pancreatic enzyme activity.
> Cirrhosis (in >25% of patients at autopsy)
> Chronic lung disease (especially upper lobes) with laboratory changes due to accumulation of CO_2, severe recurrent infection, secondary cor pulmonale, etc.
> Meconium ileus during early infancy

Stool shows lack of trypsin digestion of x-ray film gelatin; this is a useful screening test up to age 4.

CARCINOMA OF BODY OR TAIL OF PANCREAS

Laboratory tests are often normal.

Serum amylase and lipase may be slightly increased in early stages (<10% of cases); with later destruction of pancreas, they are normal or decreased. They may increase following secretin-pancreozymin stimulation before destruction is extensive; therefore, the increase is less marked with a diabetic glucose tolerance curve. Serum amylase response is less reliable.

Glucose tolerance curve is of the diabetic type in 50% of patients. Flat blood sugar curve with IV tolbutamide tolerance test indicates destruction of islet cell tissue. Unstable, insulin-sensitive diabetes that develops in an older man should arouse suspicion of carcinoma of the pancreas.

Secretin-pancreozymin stimulation evidences duct obstruction when duodenal intubation shows decreased volume of duodenal contents (<10 ml/10-minute collection period) with usually normal bicarbonate and enzyme levels in duodenal contents. Acinar destruction (as in pancreatitis) shows normal volume (20-30 ml/10-minute collection period), but bicarbonate and enzyme levels may be decreased. In carcinoma, the test result depends on the relative extent and combination of acinar destruction and of duct obstruction. Cytologic examination of duodenal contents shows malignant cells in 40% of patients.

Serum leucine aminopeptidase (LAP) is increased (>300 units) in 60% of patients with carcinoma of pancreas due to liver metastases or biliary tract obstruction. *It may also be increased in chronic liver disease.*

Triolein ^{131}I test demonstrates pancreatic duct obstruction with absence of lipase in the intestine causing flat blood curves and increased stool excretion.

Radioisotope scanning of pancreas may be done (^{75}Se) for lesions >2 cm.

CARCINOMA OF HEAD OF PANCREAS

The abnormal pancreatic function tests that occur with carcinoma of the body of the pancreas (see above) may be evident.

Laboratory findings due to complete obstruction of common bile duct

> Serum bilirubin increased (12–25 mg/100 ml), mostly direct (increase persistent and nonfluctuating)
>
> Serum alkaline phosphatase increased (usually 12–30 Bodansky units)
>
> Urine and stool urobilinogen absent
>
> Increased prothrombin time; normal after IV vitamin K administration
>
> Increased serum cholesterol (usually >300 mg/100 ml) with esters not decreased
>
> Other liver function tests (e.g., thymol turbidity, cephalin flocculation) usually normal

See tests listed in sections on other diseases of pancreas, pp. 233–237.

MACROAMYLASEMIA

Serum amylase persistently increased

Urine amylase normal or low

28

DISEASES OF THE CENTRAL AND PERIPHERAL NERVOUS SYSTEM

METABOLIC CAUSES OF COMA

Hypoglycemia (due to insulin, liver diseases, etc.)

Metabolic deficiencies (e.g., vitamin B_{12}, thiamine, niacin, pyridoxine)

Diseases of other organs
  Hepatic coma
  Uremia
  Lung (CO_2 narcosis)
  Pancreas (diabetic coma, hypoglycemia)
  Thyroid (myxedema, thyrotoxicosis)
  Parathyroid (hypoparathyroidism, hyperparathyroidism)
  Adrenal (Addison's disease, pheochromocytoma, Cushing's disease)
  Pituitary
  Porphyria
  Aminoacidurias
  Also leukodystrophies, lipid storage diseases, Bassen-Kornzweig syndrome, etc.

Abnormalities of electrolytes and acid-base balance
  Acidosis (metabolic, respiratory)
  Alkalosis (metabolic, respiratory)
  Water and sodium (hypernatremia, hyponatremia)
  Serum potassium (increased, decreased)
  Serum calcium (increased, decreased)
  Serum magnesium (increased, decreased)

Poisons
  Sedatives (especially alcolhol, barbiturates)
  Enzyme inhibitors (especially salicylates, heavy metals, organic phosphates, cyanide)
  Other (e.g., methyl alcohol, paraldehyde, ethylene glycol)

Cerebral hypoxia
  Decreased blood O_2 content with normal tension (e.g., anemia, carbon monoxide poisoning, methemoglobinemia)
  Decreased blood O_2 content and tension (e.g., decreased atmospheric pO_2 [high altitude] lung disease, alveolar hypoventilation)

Cerebral ischemia
  Decreased cardiac output (e.g., cardiac arrhythmias and Adams-Stokes disease, congestive heart failure, myocardial infarction, aortic stenosis)
  Decreased peripheral resistance in systemic circulation (e.g., low blood volume, syncope, carotid sinus hypersensitivity)
  Increased cerebral vascular resistance (e.g., increased blood viscosity as in polycythemia, hypertensive encephalopathy, hyperventilation syndrome)

SOME CONDITIONS ASSOCIATED WITH EPILEPSY THAT MAY HAVE ASSOCIATED LABORATORY ABNORMALITIES

Metabolic

Carbohydrate (e.g., glycogen storage disease, hypoglycemia)
Protein (e.g., phenylketonuria, maple syrup urine disease)
Fat (e.g., leukodystrophies, lipidoses)
Electrolytes (e.g., hypocalcemia, hypomagnesemia, hyponatremia, hypernatremia)
Other (e.g., porphyria)
Malformations (e.g., vascular malformations and shunts)
Infections
Fetal (e.g., rubella, cytomegalic inclusion disease, toxoplasmosis)
Encephalitis, meningitis
Postinfectious encephalitis (e.g., measles, mumps)
Allergic (e.g., postvaccinal encephalitis, drug reaction)
Circulatory (e.g., thrombosis, embolism, hemorrhage, hypertensive encephalopathy)
Neoplasms
Degenerative diseases of the brain
Hematologic (e.g., sickle cell anemia, leukemia)
Normal CSF
Found in
Korsakoff's syndrome
Wernicke's encephalopathy
Alzheimer's disease (diffuse cerebral atrophy)
Jakob-Creutzfeld disease
Tuberous sclerosis (protein rarely increased)
Idiopathic epilepsy (*If protein is increased, rule out neoplasms; if cell count is increased, rule out neoplasm or inflammation.*)
Narcolepsy, cataplexy, etc.
Parkinson's disease
Hereditary cerebellar degenerations
Migraine
Ménière's syndrome
Psychiatric conditions (e.g., neurocirculatory asthenia, hysteria, depression, anxiety, schizophrenia) (*Rule out psychiatric condition as a manifestation of primary disease, e.g., drugs, porphyria, primary endocrine diseases.*)
Transient cerebral ischemia
Amyotropic lateral sclerosis
Muscular dystrophy
Progressive muscular atrophy
Syringomyelia
Vitamin B_{12} deficiency with subacute combined degeneration of spinal cord
Pellagra
Beriberi
Subacute myelo-optico-neuropathy (SMON)
Minimal brain dysfunction of childhood
Cerebral palsies
Febrile convulsions of childhood

See Chapter 31 for metabolic and hereditary diseases that affect the nervous system (e.g., gangliosidosis, mucopolysaccharidoses, glycogen storage disease).

Table 29. Cerebrospinal Fluid Findings in Various Diseases

Disease	Appearance	Initial Pressure (mm of water)	Protein (mg/100 ml)	Fasting Sugar (mg/100 ml)	WBC/cu mm
Normal Ventricular	Clear, colorless, no clot	70–180	5–15	45–80	0–10
Cisternal			10–25		
Lumbar			15–45		
Tuberculous meningitis	O, slightly yellow, delicate clot	Usually I	45–500	10–45	25–1000, chiefly L
Acute pyogenic meningitis	O–Pu, slightly yellow, coarse clot	Usually I	50–1500	0–45	25–10,000 chiefly P
Aseptic meningeal reaction	C or T or X	Often N	20–200+	N	≦ 500, occasionally 2000
Syphilis Tabes dorsalis	N	N	25–100	N	10–80
General paresis	N	N	50–300	N	10–150
Meningovascular syphilis	N	N	45–150, N in 30% of patients	N	10–100, N in 45%

Acute anterior poliomyelitis	C or slightly O, may be slightly yellow, may be delicate clot	Usually N, may be I	20–350	N	10–500+, L P
Other virus Mumps	N or O	N or slightly I	20–125	N	0–2000+
Measles	N or O	N or slightly I	Slightly I	N	≦500
Herpes zoster	N		20–110	N	≦300, 40% of patients
Equine, St. Louis, choriomeningitis	N or slightly T	N or I	20–200+	N	10–200, occasionally to 3000
Postinfectious encephalitis	N	May be slightly I	15–75	N	5–200, rarely to 1000
Toxoplasmosis (congenital)	X	I	≦2000		50–500, chiefly monocytes
Cryptococcal meningitis	N		≦ 500 mg/100 ml in 90%	Moderately decreased in 55%	≦ 800 (L > P)
Coccidioidomycosis			I	Frequently D	≦ 200

See Footnotes on page 244.

(*Continued*)

Table 29 (Continued)

Disease	Appearance	Initial Pressure (mm of water)	Protein (mg/100 ml)	Fasting Sugar (mg/100 ml)	WBC/cu mm
Primary amebic meningoencephalitis (due to free-living *Naegleria*)	Sanguino-purulent, may be T or Pu	I	I	Usually D	400–21,000 (predominantly P). Usually RBCs are also found. Amebas seen on Wright's stain
Tumor Cord	C, occasionally X	N or D	≦ 3500 in 85%, N in 15%	N	≦ 100, chiefly L; N in 60%
Brain	C, occasionally X	I	≦ 500	N	≦ 150, N in 75%
Pseudotumor cerebri	N	I	N	N	N
Cerebral thrombosis	N	25% I, 75% N	≦ 100+, N in 60%	N	≦ 50, N in 75%
Cerebral hemorrhage	N in 15%, X in 10%, B in 75%	80% I, 20% N	≦ 2000, usually I	N	Same as in blood, N in 10%
Subarachnoid hemorrhage (ruptured berry aneurysm)	B, X in 24 hours, no clot	Usually I	≦ 1000+, usually I	N	Same as in blood
Bloody tap (traumatic)	B	N or D	I by blood	N	Same as in blood

Head trauma	N, B, or X	Often I	I if bloody	N	Same as in blood
Subdural hematoma	N, B only with contusion	80% I, 20% N	N or slightly I	N	Same as in blood
Multiple sclerosis	N	N	≦130, N in 75%; IgG I in 75%	N	≦40, N in 70%
Polyneuritis Polyarteritis	N; X if protein is very I	N	Usually N	N	N, but albuminocytologic dissociation in Guillain-Barré syndrome that may occur in heavy metal poisoning, infection, etc.
Porphyria		N	Usually N	N	
Beriberi		N	Usually N	N	
Alcohol		N	Usually N	N	
Arsenic		N	Usually N	N	
Diabetes mellitus		N	Often ≦300	N	
Acute infections		N	≦1500	N	
Lead encephalopathy	N or slightly yellow	I	≦100	N	0–100
Alcoholism	N	May be I	N	N	Usually N

(Continued)

243

Table 29 (Continued)

Disease	Appearance	Initial Pressure (mm of water)	Protein (mg/100 ml)	Fasting Sugar (mg/100 ml)	WBCs/cu mm
Diabetic coma	N	D	N	I	Usually N
Uremia	N	Usually I	N or I	N or I	Usually N
Epilepsy	N	N	N	N	N

C = clear; O = opalescent; T = turbid; N = normal; X = xanthochromic; B = bloody; Pu = purulent; I = increased; D = decreased; P = polymorphonuclear neutrophilic leukocyte; L = lymphocyte.

General comments:

1. Spinal fluid sugar decreased by utilization by bacteria (pyogens or tubercle bacilli) or occasionally cancer cells in spinal fluid. Normally is about 20 mg/100 ml less than blood sugar (80% of blood sugar level), a determination of which should be performed simultaneously. In pyogenic meningitis is usually <50% of blood sugar level; may rapidly become N after antibiotic therapy. May be decreased in 10–20% of cases of lymphocytic choriomeningitis, encephalitis due to mumps, or herpes simplex.

2. Blood and spinal fluid serology positive in case of CNS syphilis; positive in 7–10% of active cases of infectious mononucleosis.

3. Must routinely make smears for gram stain and acid-fast stain since the other findings may be normal in these diseases. Occasionally animal inoculations may be required.

4. Cytology smears may be useful in finding cancer cells in occasional cases.

5. Spinal fluid chloride reflects only blood chloride level although in tuberculous meningitis a decrease of 25% may exceed the decrease of serum chlorides on account of dehydration and electrolyte loss.

6. Colloidal gold test is usually not of diagnostic value. Paretic or luetic colloidal gold curve is strongly suggestive of active multiple sclerosis in the absence of syphilis.

7. Cell counts refer to lymphocytes except for monocytes in toxoplasmosis and polynuclear neutrophils in pyogenic meningitis. *Beware of misinterpreting RBCs as leukocytes.*

8. Toxicology examination for drugs (e.g., alcohol, barbiturates), heavy metals (e.g., lead, arsenic).

9. SGOT and LDH are normal in primary brain tumor but may be increased in malignant tumor (carcinoma, leukemia, lymphoma), meningitis, and subarachnoid hemorrhage.

10. Viral isolation and serologic studies.

244

DIFFERENTIATION OF BLOODY CSF DUE TO SUBARACHNOID HEMORRHAGE AND TRAUMATIC LUMBAR PUNCTURE

CSF Findings	Subarachnoid Hemorrhage	Traumatic Lumbar Puncture
CSF pressure	Often increased	Low
Blood in tubes for collecting CSF	Mixture with blood is uniform in all tubes	Earlier tubes more bloody than later tubes
CSF clotting	Does not clot	Often clots
Xanthochromia	Present if more than 8–12 hours since cerebral hemorrhage	Absent unless patient is icteric
Immediate repeat of lumbar puncture at higher level	CSF same as initial puncture	CSF clear

TRANSAMINASE (GOT) IN CEREBROSPINAL FLUID

Normal CSF is not permeable to serum enzymes. Changes in GOT are irregular and generally of limited diagnostic value.

Increased In
Large infarcts of brain during first 10 days. (In severe cases, serum GOT may also be increased; occurs in $\cong$40% of patients.)
$\cong$ 40% of CNS tumors (various benign, malignant, and metastatic), depending on location, growth rate, etc.; chiefly useful as indicator of organic neurologic disease
Some other conditions (e.g., head injury, subarachnoid hemorrhage)

LACTIC DEHYDROGENASE (LDH) IN CEREBROSPINAL FLUID

Changes are of limited diagnostic value.

Increased In
Cerebrovascular accidents. Increase occurs frequently, reaches maximum level in 1–3 days, and is apparently not related to xanthochromia, RBC, WBC, protein, sugar, or chloride levels.
CNS tumors (primary and metastatic), depending on location, growth rate, etc.
Meningitis—mild increase in viral meningitis due to LDH_1 and LDH_2; more marked increase in bacterial meningitis due to LDH_4 and LDH_5

CREATINE PHOSPHOKINASE (CPK) IN SPINAL FLUID
Test not useful because
> It does not consistently increase in various CNS diseases
> No relationship to CSF protein, WBC, or RBC values
> No pattern of relationship of LDH and GOT in CSF
> No correlation of serum CPK and cerebrospinal fluid CPK

See Serum Creatine Phosphokinase, p. 61.

HEAD TRAUMA
Laboratory findings due to single or various combinations of brain injuries
> Contusion
> Laceration
> Subdural hemorrhage
> Extradural hemorrhage
> Subarachnoid hemorrhage

Laboratory findings due to complications (e.g., pneumonia, meningitis)

In possible skull fractures, nasal secretions may be differentiated from CSF by absence of glucose in nasal secretions (test tapes or tablets can be used)

ACUTE EPIDURAL HEMORRHAGE
CSF is usually under increased pressure; clear unless there is associated cerebral contusion, laceration, or subarachnoid hemorrhage.

SUBDURAL HEMATOMA
CSF findings are variable: clear, bloody, or xanthochromic, depending on recent or old associated injuries (e.g., contusion, laceration).
Chronic subdural hematoma fluid is usually xanthochromic; protein content is 300–2000 mg/100 ml.
Anemia is often present in infants.

CEREBROVASCULAR ACCIDENT (NONTRAUMATIC)

Due to
Occlusion (thrombosis, embolism, etc.) in 80% of patients
Hemorrhage
> Ruptured berry aneurysm (45% of patients)
> Hypertension (15% of patients)
> Angiomatous malformations (8% of patients)
> Miscellaneous (e.g., brain tumor, blood dyscrasia)— infrequent
> Undetermined (rest of patients)

CSF
> *In early subarachnoid hemorrhage* (<8 hours after onset of symptoms) the test for occult blood may be positive before xanthochromia develops. After bloody spinal fluid occurs, WBC/RBC ratio may be higher in CSF than in peripheral blood.

Bloody CSF clears by tenth day in 40% of patients. CSF is persistently abnormal after 21 days in 15% of patients. ≅5% of cerebrovascular episodes due to hemorrhage are wholly within the parenchyma with normal CSF.

See Serum Creatine Phosphokinase, p. 61.
See Serum Transaminase, p. 57–58.

CEREBRAL THROMBOSIS
Laboratory findings due to some diseases which may be causative
Hematologic (e.g., polycythemia, sickle cell disease, thrombotic thrombopenia, macroglobulinemia)
Arterial (e.g., polyarteritis nodosa, Takayasu's syndrome, dissecting aneurysm of aorta, syphilis, meningitis)
Hypotension (e.g., myocardial infarction, shock)
CSF
Protein normal or may be increased ≦ 100 mg/100 ml
Cell count normal or ≧ 10 leukocytes/cu mm during first 48 hours and rarely ≧ 2000 leukocytes/cu mm transiently on third day
See Serum Creatine Phosphokinase, p. 61.
See Serum Transaminase, p. 57–58, and Table 29, p. 242.

CEREBRAL EMBOLISM
Laboratory findings due to underlying causative disease
Bacterial endocarditis
Nonbacterial thrombotic vegetations on heart valves
Chronic rheumatic mitral stenosis (*Rule out underlying hypothyroidism*)
Mural thrombus due to underlying myocardial infarctions
Myxoma of left atrium
Myocardial infarction
Fracture of long bones in fat embolism
Neck, chest, or cardiac surgery in air embolism
CSF
Usually findings are the same as in cerebral thrombosis. One-third of patients develop hemorrhagic infarction, usually producing slight xanthochromia several days later; some of these patients may have grossly bloody CSF (10,000 RBC/cu mm). Septic embolism (e.g., bacterial endocarditis) may cause increased WBC (≦ 200/cu mm with variable lymphocytes and polynuclear leukocytes), increased RBC (≦ 1000/cu mm), slight xanthochromia, increased protein, normal sugar, negative culture.

INTRACEREBRAL HEMORRHAGE
Increased WBC (15,000–20,000/cu mm) (*higher than in cerebral occlusion, e.g., embolism, thrombosis*)
Increased ESR
Urine
Transient glycosuria
Laboratory findings of concomitant renal disease
Laboratory findings due to other causes of intracerebral hemor-

rhage (e.g., leukemia, aplastic anemia, purpuras, hemophilias, anticoagulant therapy, SLE, polyarteritis nodosa)

CSF
See Table 29, pp. 240–244.

See Differentiation of Bloody CSF, p. 245.
See Cerebrovascular Accident (Nontraumatic), p. 246.

Especially if blood pressure is normal, always rule out ruptured berry aneurysm, hemorrhage into tumor, angioma.

Laboratory findings due to other diseases that occur with increased frequency in association with berry aneurysm
Coarctation of the aorta
Polycystic kidneys
Hypertension

RUPTURED BERRY ANEURYSM OF CEREBRAL VESSELS
See preceding section and Cerebrovascular Accident (Nontraumatic), p. 246.

CEPHALOHEMATOMA OF INFANCY
If the cephalohematoma is large, it may cause anemia and jaundice.

HYPERTENSIVE ENCEPHALOPATHY
Laboratory findings due to changes in other organ systems
Cardiac
Renal
Endocrine
Toxemia of pregnancy
Laboratory findings due to progressive changes that may occur (e.g., focal intracerebral hemorrhage)
CSF frequently shows increased pressure and protein $\leqq 100$ mg/100 ml.

PSEUDOTUMOR CEREBRI
CSF normal except for increased pressure
Laboratory findings due to underlying causative condition
Corticosteroid administration, usually after reduction of dosage or change to different preparation
Sex hormone administration
Addison's disease
Lateral sinus thrombosis (most commonly after otitis media)
Acute hypocalcemia

BRAIN TUMOR
CSF findings
CSF is clear, occasionally xanthochromic or bloody if there is hemorrhage into the tumor.
WBC may be increased $\leqq 150$ cells/cu mm in 75% of patients; normal in others.

Protein is usually increased.

Tumor cells may be demonstrable.

Glucose may be decreased if cells are present.

CSF protein is particularly increased with meningioma of the olfactory groove and with acoustic neurinoma.

Brain stem gliomas, which are characteristically found in childhood, usually show normal CSF.

"Diencephalic syndrome" of infants due to glioma of hypothalamus usually show normal CSF.

Laboratory findings due to underlying causative disease

Primary brain tumors

Metastatic tumors, especially of bronchus, breast, kidney, GI tract (*hemorrhagic tumor particularly with choriocarcinoma and some bronchogenic carcinomas*)

Leukemias and lymphoma

Infections (e.g., tuberculoma, schistosomiasis, torulosis, hydatid cyst, cysticercosis)

Pituitary adenomas—CSF protein and pressure usually normal

See Brain Scanning, p. 157.

ANGIOMAS OF BRAIN (ARTERIAL-VENOUS COMMUNICATIONS)

Laboratory findings due to complications

Subarachnoid hemorrhage (20% of patients)

Intracerebral hemorrhage (20% of patients)

Convulsion (50% of patients)

Oxygen tension in jugular venous blood may be increased.

LEUKEMIC INVOLVEMENT OF CNS

Intracranial hemorrhage—principal cause of death in leukemia (may be intracerebral, subarachnoid, subdural)

More frequent when WBC is > 100,000/cu mm and with rapid increase in WBC, especially in blastic crises

Platelet count frequently decreased

Evidence of bleeding elsewhere

Cerebrospinal fluid findings of intracranial hemorrhage (see pp. 246–248)

Meningeal infiltration of leukemic cells

CSF may show

Increased pressure

Increased cells that are not usually recognized as blast cells because of poor preservation

Increased protein

Glucose decreased to < 50% of blood level

Complicating meningeal infection (see next two sections)

Various bacteria

Opportunistic fungi (see pp. 493–494, 498, 499, 502, 512)

Table 30. Etiology of Bacterial Meningitis by Age

	Newborns	Less Than Age 1	Ages 1–5	Ages 5–14	More Than Age 15
Most frequent	*Escherichia coli*	*Haemophilus influenzae*	*Haemophilus influenzae*	*Neisseria meningitidis*	Pneumococcus
Common	*Klebsiella-Aerobacter* Beta-hemolytic streptococcus *Staphylococcus aureus*	*Neisseria meningitidis* Pneumococcus	*Neisseria meningitidis*	*Haemophilus influenzae* Pneumococcus	*Neisseria meningitidis* *Staphylococcus aureus*
Uncommon	Paracolon bacilli *Pseudomonas* species *Haemophilus influenzae*	*Pseudomonas* species *Staphylococcus aureus* Beta-hemolytic streptococcus *Escherichia coli*	Beta-hemolytic streptococcus		Beta-hemolytic streptococcus *Escherichia coli* *Pseudomonas* species
Rare	*Neisseria meningitidis*	*Klebsiella-Aerobacter,* paracolons, various other gram-negative organisms			*Haemophilus influenzae*

The frequency of different organisms may vary from year to year, in presence of epidemics, or by geographic location. Occasionally more than one organism is recovered.

Haemophilus influenzae (almost always Type B) causes most cases between age 6 months and age 3 but is unusual before age 2 months. Enteric bacteria are so rarely found in older children that in their presence immunologic defect or congenital dermal sinus should be ruled out. If surgery has not been performed, congenital dermal sinus should be ruled out if *Staphylococcus aureus* is present.

A gram stain of CSF should always be done in addition to a culture because it provides a more immediate clue to the causative agent and the proper therapy and because the culture may be negative if the patient received antibiotics soon before the lumbar puncture. Cultures should also be obtained from blood and petechial skin lesions if present. Gram stain of buffy coat of blood is often useful.

CSF glucose is very useful in differentiating bacterial and viral meningitis and is a good index to the severity of the infection, with a lower level in more severe infections. *Newborns with overwhelming pneumococcal infections may have no decrease in glucose or increase of cells.*

CSF should be reexamined in 24 hours as a guide to therapeutic response; a good response shows negative gram-stained smear and culture, increased glucose level, and a changing cell count from predominance of polymorphonuclear cells to predominance of mononuclear cells; total cell count and protein may show an initial rise. CSF should be reexamined when therapy is to be stopped; treatment should not be stopped unless CSF is normal except for slight increase of cells ($\leqq$ about 20 lymphocytes).

BACTERIAL MENINGITIS
CSF
See Table 29, pp. 240–244.

75% of cases are due to *Neisseria meningitidis*, pneumococcus, *Haemophilus influenzae*. *Bacteria can be identified in only 90% of cases; culture is more reliable than gram stain although the stain offers a more immediate guide to therapy.*

Laboratory findings due to preceding diseases
    Pneumonia, otitis media, sinusitis, skull fracture prior to pneumococcal meningitis
    Neisseria epidemics prior to this meningitis
    Bacterial endocarditis, septicemia, etc.

Laboratory findings due to complications (e.g., Waterhouse-Friderichsen syndrome, subdural effusion

ASEPTIC MENINGITIS
CSF
    Protein is normal or slightly increased.
    Increased cell count shows predominantly leukocytes at first, mononuclear cells later.
    Glucose is normal.
    Bacterial cultures are negative.

    If glucose levels are decreased, rule out tuberculosis, cryptococcosis, leukemia, lymphoma, metastatic carcinoma, sarcoidosis.

Due To (clinically most important types)
Viral infections (especially poliomyelitis, Coxsackie, ECHO, lymphocytic choriomeningitis, infectious mononucleosis, and many others)
Leptospirosis, syphilis
Tuberculosis, cryptococcosis (*CSF glucose levels may not be decreased until later stages.*)
Brain abscess, incompletely treated bacterial meningitis
Neoplasm (leukemia, carcinoma)

RECURRENT MENINGITIS
May Be Associated with
Bacterial Infections
    Anatomic defects (traumatic or congenital)
    Adjacent foci of infection (e.g., paranasal sinusitis, mastoiditis, brain abscess, epidural abscess, subdural empyema)
    Immunologic deficiencies (e.g., sickle cell anemia, lymphoma, decreased immunoglobulins)
    Various infections (brucellosis, leptospirosis, tuberculosis, idiopathic)
Fungal infections
    Cryptococcosis
    Treatment failure in cases of blastomycosis, coccidioidomycosis, and histoplasmosis

Other infections
    Viral
    Cerebral hydatid cyst
Neoplasms of brain and spinal cord (e.g., hemangioma of third
    ventricle, ependymoma, craniopharyngioma)
Unknown etiology
    Sarcoidosis
    Mollaret's meningitis
    Behçet's syndrome
    Vogt-Koyanagi syndrome
    Harada's syndrome

PRIMARY AMEBIC MENINGOENCEPHALITIS
(due to free-living amebas—*Naegleria*)
Increased WBC, predominantly neutrophils
CSF findings (see Table 29, p. 242)
    Fluid may be cloudy, purulent, or sanguinopurulent.
    Protein is increased.
    Glucose is usually decreased; may be normal.
    Increased WBCs are chiefly polynuclear neutrophilic leuko-
        cytes. RBCs are frequently present also. Motile amebas are
        seen in hemocytometer chamber.
    Amebas are seen on Wright's stain. Gram's stain and cultures
        are negative for bacteria and fungi.

VON ECONOMO'S ENCEPHALITIS LETHARGICA
CSF changes appear in 50% of patients: increase in lymphocytes
and variable increase in protein.

ACUTE ENCEPHALOMYELITIS
(postvaccinal, postexanthematous, postinfectious)
CSF shows increased protein and lymphocytes.
Laboratory findings due to preceding condition (e.g., measles) are
    noted.

REYE'S SYNDROME
Childhood syndrome of pernicious vomiting without clinical jaun-
    dice, beginning one week after an infection, with acute altera-
    tions of consciousness or coma, not due to CNS infection, intox-
    ication (e.g., salicylates, lead), or brain trauma.
SGOT and SGPT are increased to >100 units.
Blood ammonia is increased (often > 200 $\mu g/100$ ml).
Prothrombin time is prolonged by 2 seconds or more.
Blood amino acids are increased (alanine, glutamine, lysine,
    alpha-amino-n-butyrate), which distinguishes condition from se-
    vere salicylism.
Liver biopsy shows marked fatty changes.
Serum LDH and CPK (isoenzyme MM) may be increased due to
    muscle damage.
Plasma free fatty acids are increased with pyruvic and lactic
    acidosis (severe metabolic acidosis).
Hypoglycemia is often present.
Serum bilirubin and GGT are usually normal.

Serum uric acid and BUN may be increased.

CSF shows normal cell count; glucose is decreased proportional to decreased serum level.

MOLLARET'S MENINGITIS

Numerous recurrent episodes (2–7 days each) of aseptic meningitis occur over a period of several years with symptom-free intervals showing mild leukopenia and eosinophilia. Other organ systems are not involved. There is frequently a history of previous severe trauma with fractures and concussions.

CSF during first 12–24 hours may contain $\leqq$ several thousand cells/cu mm, predominantly polynuclear neutrophils and 66% of a large type of mononuclear cell. The mononuclear cells (sometimes called "endothelial" cells) are of unknown origin and significance and are characterized by vague nuclear and cytoplasmic outline with rapid lysis even while being counted in the hemocytometer chamber; they may be seen only as "ghosts" and are usually not detectable after the first day of illness. After the first 24 hours, the polynuclear neutrophils disappear and are replaced by lymphocytes, which, in turn, rapidly disappear when the attack subsides.

CSF protein may be increased $\leqq$ 100 mg/100 ml. CSF glucose is normal or may be slightly decreased.

GUILLAIN-BARRÉ SYNDROME

CSF shows albuminocytologic dissociation with normal cell count and increased protein (average 50–100 mg/100 ml). Protein increase parallels increasing clinical severity; increase may be prolonged.

Laboratory findings due to underlying disease are noted (e.g., infectious mononucleosis, Refsum's disease).

MENTAL RETARDATION

Laboratory findings due to underlying causative condition (see appropriate separate sections)

Prenatal

Infections (e.g., syphilis, rubella, toxoplasmosis, cytomegalic inclusion disease)

Metabolic (e.g., diabetes mellitus, toxemia, placental dysfunction)

Chromosomal (e.g., Down's syndrome, E_{18} trisomy, cri du chat syndrome, Klinefelter's syndrome)

Metabolic abnormalities

    Amino acid metabolism (e.g., phenylketonuria, maple syrup urine disease, homocystinuria, cystathioninuria, hyperglycinemia, arginosuccinicaciduria, citrullinemia, histidinemia, hyperprolinemia, oasthouse urine disease, Hartnup disease, Joseph's syndrome, familial iminoglycinuria)

    Lipid metabolism (e.g., Batten's disease, Tay-Sachs disease, Niemann-Pick disease, a-beta-lipoproteinemia, Refsum's disease, metachromatic leucodystrophy)

Carbohydrate metabolism (e.g., galactosemia, mucopolysaccharidoses)

Purine metabolism (e.g., Lesch-Nyhan syndrome, hereditary orotic aciduria)

Mineral metabolism (e.g., idiopathic hypercalcemia, pseudo- and pseudopseudohypoparathyroidism)

Other syndromes (e.g., tuberous sclerosis, Louis-Bar syndrome)

Perinatal
Kernicterus
Prematurity
Anoxia
Trauma

Postnatal
Poisoning (e.g., lead, arsenic, carbon monoxide)
Infections (e.g., meningitis, encephalitis)
Metabolic (e.g., hypoglycemia)
Postvaccinal encephalitis
Cerebrovascular accidents
Trauma

SENILE DEMENTIA (ALZHEIMER-PICK DISEASE; CEREBRAL ATROPHY)
There are no abnormal laboratory findings, but laboratory findings are useful to rule out other diseases that may resemble these syndromes but are amenable to therapy
Neurosyphilis
Bromism
Myxedema
Vitamin B_{12} deficiency
Brain tumors
Other (see conditions listed under Metabolic Causes of Coma, p. 238)

REFSUM'S DISEASE
This is a rare hereditary recessive lipidosis of the nervous system with retinitis pigmentosa, peripheral neuropathy, cerebellar ataxia, nerve deafness, and ichthyosis.
CSF shows albuminocytologic dissociation.

METACHROMATIC LEUKODYSTROPHY
Urine sediment may contain metachromatic lipids (from breakdown of myelin products).
CSF protein may be normal or elevated ≤ 200 mg/100 ml.
Biopsy of dental or sural nerve with demonstration of accumulated metachromatic sulfatide is diagnostic.

PROGRESSIVE CEREBELLAR ATAXIA WITH SKIN TELANGIECTASIAS (LOUIS-BAR SYNDROME)
This is an autosomal recessive multisystem disease with cerebellar ataxia and oculocutaneous telangiectasia.

Some patients have
Glucose intolerance
Abnormal liver function tests
Decreased or absent serum IgA and IgE causing recurrent
pulmonary infections; IgM present
Increased serum alpha-fetoprotein

See also Table 44, pp. 326–327.

TUBEROUS SCLEROSIS
This is a hereditary, familial, congenital anomaly of adenoma
sebaceum, epilepsy, and mental retardation associated with
sclerotic areas in the brain.
There are no abnormal laboratory findings.
Rarely, CSF protein is increased.

BASSEN-KORNZWEIG SYNDROME
Abnormal RBCs (acanthocytes) are present in the peripheral blood
smear.
There may be
Marked deficiency of serum beta-lipoprotein and cholesterol
Abnormal pattern of RBC phospholipids
Marked impairment of GI fat absorption

LINDAU-VON HIPPEL DISEASE (HEMANGIOBLASTOMAS OF RETINA AND CEREBELLUM)
Laboratory findings due to associated conditions
Polycythemia
Pheochromocytomas
Various tumors (e.g., kidney)

MULTIPLE SCLEROSIS
CSF shows a slight increase in mononuclear cells and normal or
slightly increased protein (50% of patients). (*Diagnosis is probably multiple sclerosis if >20% is gamma globulin and not at-
tributable to an elevation in the blood*.) The protein increase
causes abnormal colloidal gold curves.

CRANIAL ARTERITIS
ESR is markedly increased.

CAVERNOUS SINUS THROMBOPHLEBITIS
CSF is usually normal unless there is associated subdural empyema or meningitis, or it may show increased protein and WBC
with normal glucose, or it may be hemorrhagic. *In the diabetic
patient, mucormycosis may cause this clinical appearance.*
Laboratory findings due to preceding infections of paranasal
sinuses, mastoid, etc., are noted.
Laboratory findings due to complications (e.g., meningitis, brain
abscess) are noted.
Laboratory findings due to other causes of venous thromboses
(e.g., sickle cell disease, polycythemia, dehydration) in patients
with sinus thrombosis rather than thrombophlebitis.

INTRACRANIAL EXTRADURAL ABSCESS
CSF shows a slight increase in neutrophils and lymphocytes (20–100/cu mm) and a slight increase in protein.
Laboratory findings due to underlying osteomyelitis of middle ear or paranasal sinus are noted.

ACUTE SUBDURAL EMPYEMA
CSF
> Cell count is increased to a few hundred, with predominance of either mononuclear or polynuclear leukocytes.
> Protein is increased.
> Glucose is normal or slightly decreased.
> Bacterial cultures are negative.

WBC is usually increased ($\leqq$ 25,000/cu mm).

Laboratory findings due to preceding diseases
> ENT infections, especially acute sinusitis
> Intracranial surgery

Streptococci are the most common organisms when preceding condition is sinusitis. Staphylococcus aureus *or gram-negative organisms are the most common organisms following trauma or surgery.*

BRAIN ABSCESS
CSF shows increased neutrophils, lymphocytes, RBCs, and WBC $\cong$ 25–300/cu mm. There may be increased protein level (75–300 mg/100 ml). The sugar level is normal. Bacterial cultures are negative.
Associated primary disease
> Ear, nose, and throat diseases (e.g., frontal sinusitis, middle ear infections, mastoiditis)
> Primary septic lung disease (e.g., lung abscess, bronchiectasis, empyema)
> Congenital heart disease with septal defects and pulmonary arteriovenous shunts

Due To
Usually mixed anaerobic (e.g., streptococci or *Bacteroides*) and aerobic organisms (e.g., streptococci, staphylococci, or pneumococci).
May be caused by almost any organism, including fungi, *Nocardia*.

TUBERCULOMA OF BRAIN
CSF shows increased protein with small number of cells. The tuberculoma may be transformed into tuberculous meningitis with increased protein and cells (50–300/cu mm), decreased sugar and chloride.
Laboratory findings due to tuberculosis elsewhere are noted.

SPINAL CORD TUMOR
CSF protein is increased. It may be very high and associated with xanthochromia when there is a block of the subarachnoid space. See Table 29, pp. 240–244.

EPIDURAL ABSCESS OF SPINAL CORD
CSF protein is increased (usually 100–400 mg/100 ml), and WBCs (lymphocytes and neutrophils) are relatively few in number.
Most common organism is *Staphylococcus aureus,* followed by streptococci and gram-negative bacilli.
Laboratory findings due to preceding condition
    Vertebral osteomyelitis
    Bacteremia due to dental, respiratory, or skin infections
    Postoperative state

MYELITIS
CSF may be normal or may show increased protein and cells (20–1000/cu mm—lymphocytes and mononuclear cells).
See primary disease
    Poliomyelitis
    Herpes zoster
    Tuberculosis, syphilis, parasites, abscess
    Postvaccinal myelitis
    Multiple sclerosis
    Other

INFARCTION OF SPINAL CORD
CSF changes same as in cerebral hemorrhage or infarction
Laboratory findings due to causative condition
    Polyarteritis nodosa
    Dissecting aneurysm of aorta
    Arteriosclerosis of aorta with thrombus formation
    Iatrogenic (e.g., aortic arteriography, clamping of aorta during cardiac surgery)

CHRONIC ADHESIVE ARACHNOIDITIS
(due to spinal anesthesia, syphilis, etc.)
CSF protein may be normal or increased.

CERVICAL SPONDYLOSIS
CSF shows increased protein in some cases.

POLYNEURITIS OR POLYNEUROPATHY
Due To
Infectious mononucleosis—CSF shows increased protein and ≦ several hundred mononuclear cells
Diphtheria—CSF protein is 50–200 mg/100 ml
Leprosy
Metabolic condition (e.g., pellagra, beriberi, combined system disease, pregnancy, porphyria)—CSF usually normal

Uremia—CSF protein is 50–200 mg/100 ml; occurs in a few chronic cases of uremia

Neoplasm (leukemia, multiple myeloma, carcinoma)—CSF protein often increased; may be associated with an occult primary neoplastic lesion outside CNS

Amyloidosis—CSF protein often increased

Sarcoidosis

Polyarteritis nodosa—CSF usually normal; nerve involvement in 10% of patients

Systemic lupus erythematosus

Toxic condition caused by drugs and chemicals (especially lead, arsenic, etc.)

Alcoholism—CSF usually normal

Bassen-Kornzweig syndrome

Refsum's disease

Chédiak-Higashi syndrome

DISEASES CAUSING NEURITIS OF ONE NERVE OR PLEXUS

Due To

Diphtheria

Herpes zoster

Sarcoidosis

Leprosy

Tumor (leukemias, lymphomas, carcinomas)—may find tumor cells in spinal fluid

Serum sickness

Bell's palsy

Idiopathic cause

MULTIPLE CRANIAL NERVE PALSIES

Laboratory findings due to causative condition

    Trauma

    Aneurysms

    Tumors (e.g., meningioma, neurofibroma, carcinoma, cholesteatoma, chordoma)

    Herpes zoster

Benign polyneuritis associated with cervical lymph node tuberculosis or sarcoidosis

FACIAL PALSY

Laboratory findings due to causative disease

    Bell's palsy—occasional slight increase in cells in CSF

    Herpes zoster

    Pontine lesions (tumor or vascular)

    Tumors invading the temporal bone

    Acoustic neuromas

    Sarcoidosis (uveoparotid fever or Heerfordt's syndrome)

    Leprosy

    Acute infectious polyneuritis

TRIGEMINAL NEURALGIA (TIC DOULOUREUX)

Laboratory findings due to causative disease

Usually idiopathic
May also stem from multiple sclerosis, herpes zoster

OPHTHALMOPLEGIA
Laboratory findings due to causative disease
Diabetes mellitus
Myasthenia gravis
Hyperthyroid exophthalmos

VON RECKLINGHAUSEN'S DISEASE (MULTIPLE NEUROFIBROMAS)
CSF findings of brain tumor if acoustic neurinoma occurs

BITEMPORAL HEMIANOPSIA
Laboratory findings due to causative disease
Usually pituitary adenoma
Also metastatic tumor, sarcoidosis, Hand-Schüller-Christian disease, meningioma of sella, aneurysm of circle of Willis

RETROBULBAR NEUROPATHY
CSF is normal or may show increased protein and ≤ 200 lymphocytes.

75% of these patients ultimately develop multiple sclerosis.

GLOMUS JUGULARE TUMOR
CSF protein may be increased.

MUSCULOSKELETAL DISEASES

MYASTHENIA GRAVIS

Serum enzymes are normal.

Complete blood count and ESR are normal (occasional cases of associated macrocytic anemia).

Serum electrolytes are normal.

Thyroid function tests are normal (disease may be associated with, but independent of, hyperthyroidism or hypothyroidism).

Fluorescent antibodies to skeletal muscle cross-striations have been reported in 30–40% of patients.

High frequency of associated diabetes mellitus is seen, especially in older patients; therefore GTT should be performed with or without cortisone.

Always rule out cancer of lung.

Thymic tumor is present in up to 10% of patients; 70% of patients have thymic hyperplasia with germinal centers in medulla.

POLYMYOSITIS

Total eosinophil count is frequently increased. WBC may be increased in fulminant disease.

Mild anemia may occur.

ESR is moderately to markedly increased; may be normal; not clinically useful.

Thyroid function tests are normal.

Serum enzymes are increased; occasionally they remain normal. The degree of increase reflects the activity of the disease; usually decrease occurs 3–4 weeks before improvement in muscle strength and increase 5–6 weeks before clinical relapse; the level frequently becomes normal with steroid therapy or in chronic myositis.

Serum CPK is increased in two-thirds of patients. Levels may vary greatly. In childhood very high levels may occur.

Serum aldolase is increased in 75% of patients.

Serum LDH is increased in 25% of patients.

Serum SGOT is increased in $\cong 25\%$ of the patients.

Serum alpha-hydroxybutyric dehydrogenase (α-HBD) may be increased, paralleling the increased LDH.

Serum MDH may be increased but offers no additional diagnostic value.

Urine shows a moderate increase in creatine and a decrease in creatinine. Myoglobinuria occurs occasionally in severe cases.

LE tests are usually negative. Latex fixation rheumatoid factor— (RA) tests may be positive in 50% of patients.

Serum gamma globulins may be increased.

Muscle biopsy shows necrosis of muscle, with phagocytosis of muscle fibers and infiltration of inflammatory cells.

Associated carcinoma is present in $\leqq 20\%$ of the patients and in $\leqq 5\%$ of patients over age 40 (especially cancer of lung and cancer

Table 31. Laboratory Findings in the Differential Diagnosis of Some Muscle Diseases

Disease	Complete Blood Count	ESR	Thyroid Function Tests	Percent of Patients with Increase in Various Serum Enzyme Levels	Muscle Biopsy	Comment
Myasthenia gravis	N	N	N	N	Lymphorrhages	Cancer of lung should always be ruled out; high frequency of associated diabetes mellitus, especially in older patients Serum electrolytes N
Polymyositis	Total eosinophil count frequently I	Moderately to markedly I; occasionally N	N	CPK in 65%; levels may vary greatly and become N with steroid therapy; markedly I may occur in children ALD in 75%, LDH in 25%, SGOT in 25%; α-HBD parallels LDH; MDH offers no additional diagnostic value	Necrosis of muscle with phagocytosis of muscle fibers, infiltration of inflammatory cells	Associated cancer in ≦ 17% of cases (especially lung; also breast) LE preparation and latex fixations occasionally positive; serum alpha₂ and gamma globulin may be increased.
Muscular dystrophy	N	N	N	In active phase: CPK in 50%, ALD in 20%, LDH in 10%, SGOT in 15%	Various degenerative changes in muscle; late muscle atrophy; no cellular infiltration	

N = normal; I = increased.

261

of breast). The polymyositis may antedate the neoplasm by up to age 2.

MUSCULAR DYSTROPHY
ESR is usually normal.
Thyroid function tests are normal.
Serum enzymes are increased, especially in
> Young patients. Highest levels ($\leqq 50$ times normal) are found at onset in infancy and childhood, with gradual return to normal.
>
> The more rapidly progressive dystrophies (such as the Duchenne type) and may be slightly or inconsistently increased in the limb-girdle and facioscapulohumeral types
>
> The active early phase. Increased levels are not constant and are affected by patient's age and duration of disease. Enzymes may be increased before disease is clinically evident.

> Serum CPK is increased in $\cong 50\%$ of patients.
> Serum aldolase is increased in $\cong 20\%$ of patients.
> Serum LDH is increased in $\cong 10\%$ of patients.
> Serum SGOT is increased in $\cong 15\%$ of patients.
> Serum CPK is increased in $\cong 75\%$ of female *carriers*. It is thus possible to identify carrier state and detect clinically unaffected male infants with Duchenne type.
> Elevated serum enzyme levels are not affected by steroid therapy.

Muscle biopsy shows muscle atrophy but no cellular infiltration.
Urine creatine is increased; urine creatinine is decreased. These changes are less marked in limb-girdle and facioscapulohumeral types than in the Duchenne type.

MYOTONIC DYSTROPHY
Increased creatine in urine may occur irregularly.
Findings due to atrophy of testicle and androgenic deficiency are noted.
Urine 17-ketosteroids are decreased.
Thyroid function may be decreased.
Serum enzyme increases are slight and inconsistent. Female carriers may have higher levels of ALD and CPK than control females.

SERUM ENZYMES IN SOME DISEASES OF THE MUSCULOSKELETAL SYSTEM
CPK is the measurement of choice. It is more specific and sensitive than SGOT and LDH and more discriminating than ALD.

Increased In
Dermatomyositis
Progressive muscular dystrophy (see Muscular Dystrophy, above)
Myotonic dystrophy (see above)

Normal In
Rheumatoid arthritis
Scleroderma
Acrosclerosis
Discoid lupus erythematosus
Muscle atrophy of neurologic origin (e.g., old poliomyelitis, polyneuritis)
Hyperthyroid myopathy

CREATINE AND CREATININE
Decreased creatinine excretion
Increased creatine excretion
Increased blood creatinine

Occurs In
Progressive muscular dystrophy
Decreased muscle mass in
    Neurogenic atrophy
    Polymyositis
    Addison's disease
    Hyperthyroidism
    Male eunuchoidism

MYALGIAS—DIFFERENTIAL DIAGNOSIS
Rheumatoid arthritis
Rheumatic fever
Hyperparathyroidism
Hyperthyroidism and hypothyroidism
Hypoglycemia
Renal tubular acidosis
Myoglobinuria
McArdle syndrome
Brucellosis
Other infections (bacterial, viral, rickettsial, etc.)

METABOLIC DISEASES OF MUSCLE
Hyperthyroidism
    Increased urine creatine
    Decreased creatine tolerance
    Normal serum enzyme levels
    Normal muscle biopsy

    causes some cases of hypokalemic periodic paralysis.

Hypothyroidism (rarely associated with myotonia)
    Decreased urine creatine
    Increased creatine tolerance
    Increased serum CPK, especially when PBI is < 2.5 μg/100 ml
Other serum enzyme levels normal
Associated with administration of adrenal corticosteroids and with Cushing's syndrome
    Increased urine creatine

Table 32. Increased Serum Enzyme Levels in Muscle Diseases

| Enzyme | Muscular Dystrophy | | | | | | | Myotonic Dystrophy | Polymyositis |
| | Duchenne | | Limb-Girdle | | Facioscapulohumeral | | | | |
	Frequency	Amplitude	Frequency	Amplitude	Frequency	Amplitude		Frequency	Frequency
CPK	>95%	65	75%	25	80%	5		50%	70%
ALD	90%	9	25%	3	30%	2		20%	75%
SGOT	90%	4	25%	2	25%	1½		15%	25%
LDH	90%	4	15%	1½	10%	1		10%	25%

Frequency = average % frequency of patients with increased serum enzyme level when blood is taken at optimal time.
Amplitude = average number of times normal that serum level is increased.

Increased serum enzymes (SGOT, aldolase)—uncommon, and may be due to the primary disease

Muscle biopsy—degenerative and regenerative changes in scattered muscle fibers; no inflammatory cell infiltration.

CONGENITAL MYOTONIA (THOMSEN'S DISEASE)
Mild creatine intolerance is found.
Urine creatine may be increased in some patients.
Muscle biopsy shows few changes that are not specific.
Serum enzymes are normal.

STIFF-MAN SYNDROME
BMR is often increased ($\leqq 75$).
Other laboratory examinations are normal.
CSF is normal.
Biopsy of muscle is normal or shows minimal nonspecific changes (e.g., slight atrophy).
Occasionally other alterations are present (e.g., persistent leukopenia with eosinophilia).

MYOTUBULAR MYOPATHY
Routine laboratory studies including measurement of serum enzymes are normal; occasionally serum CPK is slightly increased.
Biopsy of muscle establishes the diagnosis.

MITOCHONDRIAL MYOPATHY
Routine laboratory studies including measurement of serum enzymes are normal.
Biopsy of muscle with histochemical staining reaction demonstrates hyperactivity of certain mitochondrial enzymes (e.g., DPNH diaphorase, succinate dehydrogenase, cytochrome oxidase).

NEMALINE (ROD) MYOPATHY
Routine laboratory tests are normal.
Serum enzymes are normal; occasionally serum CPK is slightly increased.
Endocrine studies (including measurements of urine 17-ketosteroids and 11-oxysteroids) are normal.
Biopsy of muscle with appropriate special stains establishes the diagnosis.

MYOPATHY ASSOCIATED WITH ALCOHOLISM
Acute
> Increased serum CPK, SGOT, and other enzymes. Serum CPK increases in 1–2 days; reaches peak in 4–5 days. CPK in CSF is normal, even when serum level is elevated.
> Gross myoglobinuria
> Acute renal failure (some patients)

Chronic—may show some or all of the following changes
> Increased urine creatine
> Increased serum CPK and SGOT

Diminished ability to increase blood lactic acid with ischemic exercise

Abnormalities on muscle biopsy (support the diagnosis)

Myoglobinuria

FAMILIAL PERIODIC PARALYSIS

Serum potassium is decreased during the attack.

Urine potassium excretion decreases at the same time.

Serum enzymes are normal.

ADYNAMIA EPISODICA HEREDITARIA (GAMSTORP'S DISEASE)

Transient increase in serum potassium occurs during the attack; attack is induced by administration of potassium.

Urine potassium excretion is unchanged during or before the attack.

Table 33.   Types of Periodic Paralysis

	Hypokalemic (familial, sporadic, associated with hyperthyroidism)	Hyperkalemic (adynamia episodica hereditaria)	Normokalemic
Induced by	Glucose and insulin, ACTH, DOCA, epinephrine	KCl	KCl
Serum potassium during attack	Decreased	Increased	Normal or slightly decreased
Urine potassium excretion	Decreased	Normal	Decreased

MALIGNANT HYPERTHERMIA
(autosomal dominant syndrome triggered by potent inhalational anesthetic agents)

Early Changes

Respiratory and metabolic acidosis

Hypoxemia

Increased serum potassium and magnesium

Increased serum glucose, lactate, and pyruvate

Later Changes

Decreased serum potassium and calcium

Increased serum phosphorus

Increased serum CPK and other enzymes

Possibly, consumption coagulopathy

Possibly, acute renal shutdown

NORMAL LABORATORY FINDINGS IN DISEASES OF BONE

Polyostotic fibrous dysplasia (Albright's syndrome) (occasionally increased serum alkaline phosphatase)

Giant-cell tumor of bone
Achondroplasia
Dyschondroplasias
Tietze's syndrome
Osteitis pubis
Osteogenesis imperfecta

OSTEOMYELITIS

WBC may be increased, especially in acute case.
ESR is increased in <50% of patients but may be important clue in occult cases (e.g., intervertebral disk space infection).
Bacteriology
> *Staphylococcus aureus* causes almost all infections of hip and two-thirds of infections of skull, vertebrae, and long bones. Other bacteria may simultaneously be present and contribute to infection.
> Gram-negative bacteria cause most infections of mandible, pelvis, and small bones.
> *Salmonella* is more commonly found in patients with sickle hemoglobinopathy.

Laboratory findings due to underlying conditions
> Postoperative status
> Irradiation therapy
> Foreign body, tissue gangrene, contiguous infection, etc.

SKELETAL INVOLVEMENT ASSOCIATED WITH SOME METABOLIC ABNORMALITIES

Primary hypophosphatemia
Hypophosphatasia
Rickets
Gaucher's disease
Gargoylism (mucopolysaccharides in urine; sometimes Riley bodies in white cells)
Gout
Alkaptonuria
Phenylketonuria
Familial hyperparathyroidism
Idiopathic hypercalcemia
Osteogenesis imperfecta
Marfan's syndrome
Other

SKELETAL INVOLVEMENT ASSOCIATED WITH SOME HEMATOLOGIC DISEASES

Anemia
> Hereditary hemolytic (e.g., sickle cell disease, thalassemia, hereditary spherocytosis)
> Iron deficiency anemia of childhood
> Congenital aplastic anemia (Fanconi syndrome)

Coagulation defects (e.g., deficiency of AHG, PTC, or PTA)
Malignant lymphoma (e.g., leukemia, lymphosarcoma, Hodgkin's disease, multiple myeloma)
Primary reticulum cell sarcoma of bone
Reticuloendothelioses (e.g., Niemann-Pick disease, Gaucher's disease, Hand-Schüller-Christian disease; Letterer-Siwe disease, eosinophilic granuloma)
Myelosclerosis
Osteopetrosis (marble bone disease)
Other

OSTEOPOROSIS

Urine calcium may be increased, normal, or decreased but is not influenced by intake; calcium restriction does not produce the normal fall.

Laboratory tests (including serum calcium, phosphorus, and alkaline phosphatase) are normal.

In secondary osteoporosis, see primary condition for laboratory findings.

Administration of steroids	Neoplasms
Cushing's syndrome	Immobilization
Acromegaly	Hypophosphatasia
Hyperthyroidism	Uremia
Gonadal insufficiency	Sprue
Hyperparathyroidism	Other

RICKETS

Serum alkaline phosphatase is increased. This is the earliest and most reliable biochemical abnormality; parallels severity of the rickets. It may remain elevated until bone healing is complete.

Serum calcium is usually normal or slightly decreased.

Serum phosphorus is usually decreased. In some persons, serum calcium and phosphorus may be normal.

Generalized renal aminoaciduria is present; it disappears when adequate vitamin D is given.

Serum calcium and phosphorus rapidly become normal after institution of vitamin D therapy.

OSTEOMALACIA

Serum calcium and phosphorus may be normal or decreased, but the calcium × phosphorus product is decreased.

Serum alkaline phosphatase is increased in active cases, except in hypophosphatasia. This is the earliest biochemical alteration.

Blood chemistries may be normal.

IV infusion of a standard dose of calcium results in 24-hour retention of >60%.

Biopsy of bone. Undercalcified sections show an increased number of osteoid seams which are wider than normal. Biopsy can show a decreased rate of mineralization by oral tetracycline labeling prior to biopsy and examination of bone under fluorescent light.

Due To

Primary vitamin D deficiency

Gastrointestinal malabsorption

    Partial gastrectomy

    Diseases of the small intestine (e.g., regional enteritis)

    Pancreatic disease (e.g., chronic pancreatitis)

    Hepatobiliary disease (e.g., chronic biliary obstruction)

Primary hypophosphatemia

Renal disease

    Renal tubular diseases (e.g., renal tubular acidosis)

    Chronic renal insufficiency

Hypophosphatasia

Axial osteomalacia (see next section)
Other (e.g., hypoparathyroidism, hyperthyroidism, Paget's disease, osteoporosis, osteopetrosis, fluoride ingestion, ureterosigmoidostomy)

AXIAL OSTEOMALACIA
Axial skeleton shows x-ray changes resembling those in Paget's disease and metastatic tumor.
Bone biopsy is characteristic of osteomalacia.
Blood chemistries are normal.
There is no recognizable cause for axial osteomalacia.

RENAL TUBULAR HYPOPHOSPHATEMIA WITH ASSOCIATED RICKETS

Due To
Toxic injury or intrinsic metabolic defect of renal tubule cell

PRIMARY HYPOPHOSPHATEMIA (FAMILIAL VITAMIN D–RESISTANT RICKETS)
(hereditary metabolic defect in phosphate transport in renal tubules and possibly intestine)
See discussion of vitamin D–resistant rickets, p. 364.

Serum phosphorus is markedly decreased.
Serum calcium is relatively normal.
Serum alkaline phosphatase is moderately increased.
Stool calcium is increased, and urine calcium is decreased.
Administration of vitamin D does not cause serum phosphorus to rise (in contrast to ordinary rickets), but urine and serum calcium may be increased with sufficiently large dose.
Renal aminoaciduria is absent, in contrast to ordinary rickets.
Treatment is monitored by choosing dose of vitamin D that will not increase serum calcium > 11 mg/100 ml or urine calcium > 200 mg/day. Serum phosphorus usually remains low; increase > 4 mg/100 ml may indicate renal injury due to vitamin D toxicity.

RENAL TUBULAR ACIDOSIS WITH RICKETS AND OSTEOMALACIA
(inborn error of renal tubular metabolism)

FANCONI SYNDROME
See pp. 363–364.

VITAMIN D–DEPENDENT RICKETS
Serum calcium is frequently decreased, sometimes causing tetany.
Serum phosphorus is decreased but not as markedly or as consistently as in hypophosphatemic rickets.
Serum alkaline phosphatase is increased.
Urine calcium is decreased.
Generalized renal aminoaciduria is present; it disappears when adequate vitamin D is given.
Serum chemistries return to normal after adequate vitamin D is given (may require very large doses).
May be due to familial genetic pattern.

METAPHYSEAL DYSOSTOSIS
Rare congenital disorder with progressive long bone deformities that mimic chronic rickets.
Serum calcium, phosphorus, and alkaline phosphatase are normal.

VITAMIN D INTOXICATION
Serum calcium may be increased.
Serum phosphorus is usually also increased but sometimes is decreased, with increased urinary phosphorus.

FAMILIAL OSTEOECTASIA
(uncommon inherited disorder of membranous bone showing painful swelling of the periosteal soft tissue and spontaneous fractures)
Serum alkaline phosphatase is increased.
Serum acid phosphatase and aminopeptidase are also increased.

INFANTILE CORTICAL HYPEROSTOSIS (CAFFEY'S DISEASE)
ESR is increased.
WBC may be increased.

A similar picture may occur in children over age 1 because of hypervitaminosis A.

OSTEOSCLEROSIS

Due To
Osteopetrosis (see next section)
Heavy-metal poisoning (e.g., lead, bismuth)
Hypoparathyroidism
Hypothyroidism

OSTEOPETROSIS (ALBERS-SCHÖNBERG DISEASE; MARBLE BONE DISEASE)
Normal serum calcium, phosphorus, alkaline phosphatase
Serum acid phosphatase increased (some patients)
Myelophthisic anemia (some patients)
Laboratory findings due to complications
    Osteomyelitis
    Other infections

PAGET'S DISEASE OF BONE (OSTEITIS DEFORMANS)
Marked increase in serum alkaline phosphatase directly related to severity and extent of disease; sudden additional increase with development of osteogenic sarcoma
Normal serum calcium increased during immobilization (e.g., due to intercurrent illness or fracture)
Normal or slightly increased serum phosphorus
Frequently increased urine calcium; renal calculi common
Increase in hydroxyproline in urine may be marked.

OSTEOGENIC SARCOMA
Marked increase in serum alkaline phosphatase ($\leqq 40$ times nor-

mal); reflects new bone formation and parallels clinical course (development of metastases, response to therapy, etc.)

OSTEOLYTIC TUMORS OF BONE
(e.g., Ewing's sarcoma)
Usually normal serum calcium, phosphorus, alkaline phosphatase

METASTATIC CARCINOMA OF BONE
Osteolytic metastases (especially from primary tumor of bronchus, breast, kidney, thyroid)

Urine calcium is often increased; marked increase may reflect increased rate of tumor growth.

Serum calcium and phosphorus may be normal or increased.

Serum alkaline phosphatase is usually normal or slightly to moderately increased.

Serum acid phosphatase is often slightly increased, especially in prostatic metastases.

Osteoblastic metastases (especially from primary tumor in prostate)

Serum calcium is normal; it is rarely increased.

Urine calcium is low.

Serum alkaline phosphatase is usually increased.

Serum acid phosphatase is increased in prostatic carcinoma.

Serum phosphorus is variable.

FAT EMBOLISM
This occurs after trauma (e.g., fractures, insertion of femoral head prosthesis).

Unexplained fall in hemoglobin

Decreased platelet count

Free fat in urine in 50% of patients

Fat globules in sputum (some patients)

Decreased arterial pO_2 with normal or decreased pCO_2

Increased serum lipase in 30–50% of patients. Increased free fatty acids. Not of diagnostic value.

Increased serum triglycerides

Fat globulinemia in 42–67% of patients and in 17–33% of controls

Normal cerebrospinal fluid

Labaratory findings alone are inadequate for diagnosis.

CONDITIONS ASSOCIATED WITH THE DEVELOPMENT OF AVASCULAR (ASEPTIC) NECROSIS OF THE HEAD OF THE FEMUR
Due To
Traumatic interruption of blood supply

> 25% of patients with fracture of neck of femur

Dislocation of hip

Slipped femoral capital epiphysis

Nontraumatic interference with blood supply

Caisson disease

Sickle cell disease and trait and sickle cell-C hemoglobin disease

Infection

Gout
Rheumatoid arthritis
Systemic lupus erythematosus (SLE)
Fabry's disease
Scleroderma
Gaucher's disease
Cushing's syndrome
Corticosteroid treatment
Alcoholism
Pancreatitis
X-ray irradiation
Idiopathic (Chandler's disease)

CLASSIFICATION OF ARTHRITIS*

Polyarthritis of unknown etiology
    Rheumatoid arthritis
    Juvenile rheumatoid arthritis (Still's disease)
    Ankylosing spondylitis (Marie-Strümpell disease)
    Psoriatic arthritis
    Reiter's syndrome
    Other
Collagen diseases (acquired connective tissue disorders)
    SLE
    Scleroderma (progressive systemic sclerosis)
    Polymyositis and dermatomyositis
    Necrotizing arteritis and other forms of vasculitis (e.g.,
        polyarteritis nodosa, hypersensitivity angiitis, Wegener's
        granulomatosis, Takayasu's disease, Cogan's syndrome,
        giant cell arteritis)
    Amyloidosis
    Other
Rheumatic fever
Degenerative joint disease (osteoarthritis)
    Primary
    Secondary
Diseases with frequently associated arthritis
    Sarcoidosis
    Relapsing polychondritis
    Schönlein-Henoch purpura
    Ulcerative colitis
    Regional ileitis
    Whipple's disease
    Sjögren's syndrome
    Familial Mediterranean fever
    Psoriatic arthritis
    Other
Associated with infectious agents
    Bacterial (e.g., *Brucella,* gonococcus, tubercle bacillus, *Sal-
        monella,* pneumococcus, *Staphylococcus, Streptococcus
        moniliformis,* syphilis, yaws)

---

* Adapted from American Rheumatism Association, Primer on the
Rheumatic Diseases, *J.A.M.A.* 224:662, 1973.

Rickettsial
Viral (especially rubella; also mumps, viral hepatitis)
Fungal (especially coccidioidomycosis; also histoplasmosis, blastomycosis, cryptococcosis, sporotrichosis)
Parasitic
Traumatic and/or neurogenic causes
Direct trauma
Tertiary syphilis (tabes dorsalis)
Diabetes mellitus with neurologic complications
Syringomyelia
Shoulder-hand syndrome
Mechanical derangement of joints
Endocrine diseases
Hyperparathyroidism
Acromegaly
Hypothyroidism
Biochemical and metabolic diseases
Gout
Pseudogout (chondrocalcinosis articularis)
Ochronosis
Hemophilias
Hemoglobinopathies
Agammaglobulinemia
Scurvy
Gaucher's disease
Hemochromatosis
Hyperlipoproteinemia Type II (xanthoma tuberosum and tendinosum)
Other
Inherited and congenital diseases
Mucopolysaccharidoses (e.g., Hurler's syndrome, Morquio's disease)
Homocystinuria
Ehlers-Danlos syndrome
Marfan's syndrome
Osteogenesis imperfecta
Congenital hip dysplasia
Tumors
Multiple myeloma
Leukemia
Metastatic tumors
Primary juxta-articular bone
Synovioma
Other
Allergy and drug reactions (e.g., serum sickness)
Miscellaneous
Aseptic necrosis of bone
Stevens-Johnson syndrome
Erythema nodosum
Hypertrophic osteoarthropathy
Juvenile osteochondritis
Osteochondritis dissecans
Pigmented villonodular synovitis

Table 34. Synovial Fluid Findings in Various Diseases of Joints

Property	Normal	Noninflammatory[a]	Hemorrhagic[b]		Acute Inflammatory[c]			Septic		
					Acute Gouty Arthritis	Rheumatic Fever	Rheumatoid Arthritis	Tuberculous Arthritis	Gonorrheal Arthritis	Septic Arthritis[d]
Volume	3.5 ml	I	I		I			I		
Appearance	Clear, colorless	Clear, straw	Bloody or xanthochromic		Turbid yellow			Turbid yellow		
Viscosity	High	High	V		D			D		
Fibrin clot	0	Usually 0	V		+			+		
Mucin clot	Good	Good	V		Fair to poor			Poor		
WBC (no./cu mm)[e]	<200	<5000	<10,000	Range	750–45,000	300–98,000	300–75,000	2500–105,000	1500–108,000	15,600–213,000
				average	13,500	17,800	15,500	23,500	14,000	65,400
Neutrophils (%)	<25	<25	<50	Range	48–94	8–98	5–96	29–96	2–96	75–100
				average	83	46	65	67	64	95
Blood-synovia glucose difference (mg/100 ml)[f]	<10	<10	<25	Range	0–41		0–88	0–108	0–97	40–122
				average	12	6	31	57	26	71
Culture[g]	0	0	0		0	0	0	See pp. 282–283.		

I = increased; D = decreased; 0 = absent; + = positive; V = variable.

[a] For example, degenerative joint disease, traumatic arthritis, some cases of pigmented villonodular synovitis.

[b] For example, tumor, hemophilia, neuroarthropathy, trauma, some cases of pigmented villonodular synovitis.

[c] For example, rheumatoid arthritis, Reiter's syndrome, acute gouty arthritis, acute pseudogout, systemic lupus erythematosus, etc.

[d] For example, pneumococcal.

[e] Use saline instead of acetic acid, which clumps the joint fluid.

[f] Joint tap should be performed preferably after patient has been fasting for > 4 hours, and a blood glucose determination should be performed simultaneously.

[g] Material should be cultured aerobically and anaerobically. Culture for tubercle bacilli and guinea pig inoculation should be performed.

Tietze's syndrome
Other
Nonarticular rheumatism
Intervertebral disk and low back syndromes
Fibrositis, myositis, tendinitis, bursitis, tenosynovitis, fasciitis
Carpal tunnel syndrome
Neuritis
Panniculitis

NEEDLE BIOPSY OF JOINT (HISTOLOGIC EXAMINATION OF SYNOVIA)

May Be Useful In
Gout
Pseudogout
Ochronosis
Tuberculosis
Coccidioidomycosis
Pyogenic arthritis
Rheumatoid arthritis
Osteoarthritis
Reiter's syndrome
SLE

Provides major diagnostic assistance in about one-third of patients with early or difficult diagnosis.

OSTEOARTHRITIS
ESR may be slightly increased (possibly because of soft-tissue changes secondary to mechanical alterations in joints).
Complete blood count, ESR, serum protein electrophoresis, rheumatoid factor, serum uric acid, calcium, phosphorus, alkaline phosphatase, VDRL tests, etc., are normal.

RHEUMATOID ARTHRITIS
Serologic tests for rheumatoid factor (e.g., using latex, bentonite, or sheep or human RBCs). Tests become positive after disease active for 6 months. Positive in 75% of "typical" cases; positive in 95% of patients with subcutaneous nodules; high titers in patients with splenomegaly, vasculitis, or neuropathy. Positive in only 10–20% of patients with juvenile rheumatoid arthritis. May diminish or disappear during remission. Positive in 5% of normal population. False positive in other diseases (e.g., SLE, sarcoidosis, liver diseases, subacute bacterial endocarditis, syphilis, leprosy, tuberculosis). Negative in osteoarthritis, gout, ankylosing spondylitis, rheumatic fever, suppurative arthritis, arthritis associated with ulcerative colitis (see p. 281).
Anemia is moderate in degree, of the normocytic hypochromic type, and not responsive to administration of iron, folic acid, or vitamin B_{12} or to splenectomy.
Serum iron is decreased.
WBC is usually normal; there may be a slight increase early in the active disease.

Increased ESR and positive C-reactive protein (CRP) test are rough guides to activity and to therapy.

Serum protein electrophoresis shows increase in globulins, especially in gamma and alpha$_2$ globulins, and decreased albumin.

Positive LE test in $\leqq$20% of patients is usually weakly reactive.
Antinuclear factors are present in $\leqq$65% of patients, depending on sensitivity of test.

Serum calcium, phosphorus, alkaline phosphatase, uric acid, and ASOT are normal.

Synovial biopsy is especially useful in monarticular form to rule out tuberculosis, gout, etc.

For synovial fluid examination see Table 34, pp. 274–275.
See Amyloidosis, p. 520.

Table 35. Comparison of Rheumatoid Arthritis and Osteoarthritis

Rheumatoid Arthritis	Osteoarthritis
Synovial fluid has high WBC and low viscosity	Effusions infrequent
	Synovial fluid has low WBC and high viscosity
ESR more markedly increased	ESR may be mildly to moderately increased
Rheumatoid factor usually present	RF usually absent
Positive biopsy of subcutaneous rheumatoid nodule and synovia	Rheumatoid changes in tissue absent

JUVENILE RHEUMATOID ARTHRITIS (STILL'S DISEASE)

Serologic tests for rheumatoid factor RA are positive in only 10–20% of patients.

WBC may be normal or increased, $\leqq$50,000/cu mm.

Hypochromic anemia is frequent; varies from mild to severe.

Other findings are similar to those in adult rheumatoid arthritis.
Increased ESR and CRP parallels degree of inflammation.
Serum protein electrophoresis shows increased globulins, especially gamma.
Secondary amyloidosis appears in long-standing active disease (see Amyloidosis, p. 520).

Table 36. ESR in Differential Diagnosis of Juvenile Rheumatoid Arthritis

Disease	ESR Falls to Normal
Untreated acute rheumatic fever	9–12 weeks
Salicylate-treated acute rheumatic fever	5 weeks
Steroid-treated acute rheumatic fever	2 weeks
Chronic rheumatic fever	Occasionally shows persistent elevation
Juvenile rheumatoid arthritis	May remain elevated for months or years despite therapy

Table 37. Synovial Fluid Findings in Acute Inflammatory Arthritis of Various Etiologies

Disease	WBC	Complement Activity	Rheumatoid Factor (RF)	Crystals[a]	Other Findings
Acute gouty arthritis	I	I	0	Monosodium urate; within PMNs during acute stage	
Acute chondrocalcinosis (pseudogout)	I	I	0	Calcium pyrophosphate	
Reiter's syndrome	Markedly I	Markedly I	0		Macrophages with ingested leukocytes
Rheumatoid arthritis	I	Low	Usually +		
Juvenile rheumatoid arthritis	I	Low	0		Abundant lymphocytes (sometimes > 50%); immature lymphocytes and monocytes present

	Usually very low	Low or 0	V	0	LE cells may be present
Systemic lupus erythematosus	I			0	LE cells may be present
Arthritis associated with psoriasis, ulcerative colitis, ankylosing spondylitis		I			

I = increased; 0 = absent; V = variable; PMN = polynuclear leukocyte; + = positive.

[a] Crystals should be identified using polarized light microscopy. Finding of characteristic crystals is diagnostic of gout and of chondrocalcinosis.

FELTY'S SYNDROME

The syndrome occurs in 5–10% of patients with rheumatoid arthritis associated with splenomegaly and leukopenia.
Rheumatoid arthritis is far advanced.
Serologic tests for rheumatoid factor are positive; RF may be present in high titers.
Positive LE test is more frequent than in rheumatoid arthritis.
Leukopenia is present. Anemia and thrombocytopenia may occur; they respond to splenectomy.

SJÖGREN'S SYNDROME

This immunologic abnormality is associated with decreased secretion of exocrine glands.
50% of patients have rheumatoid arthritis.
Mild anemia and leukopenia occur in one-third of patients.
ESR is usually increased.
Serologic tests for rheumatoid factor are positive even in patients without arthritis.
LE test is positive in 10% of patients, all of whom have arthritis.
Serum protein electrophoresis shows increased globulins, largely due to 7S gamma globulin.
Occasionally nonthrombocytopenic purpura occurs.
The syndrome may be associated with Waldenström's macroglobulinemia, collagen diseases (SLE, polyarteritis nodosa, etc.), and Felty's syndrome.
Rule out other causes of Mikulicz's syndrome (e.g., sarcoidosis, tuberculosis, cirrhosis, leukemia).

ANKYLOSING RHEUMATOID SPONDYLITIS (MARIE-STRÜMPELL DISEASE)

ESR is increased in $\leq 80\%$ of cases.
Mild to moderate hypochromic anemia appears in $\leq 30\%$ of cases.
Serologic tests for rheumatoid factor are positive in $< 15\%$ of patients with arthritis of only the vertebral region.
CSF protein is moderately increased in $\leq 50\%$ of patients.
Secondary amyloidosis appears in 6% of patients.
Laboratory findings of carditis and aortitis with aortic insufficiency, which occur in 1–4% of patients, are noted.
Laboratory findings of frequently associated diseases
    Chronic ulcerative colitis
    Regional ileitis
    Psoriasis

ARTHRITIS ASSOCIATED WITH PSORIASIS

Arthritis occurs in 2% of patients with psoriasis. There is no correlation between activity of skin and of joint manifestations; either one may precede the other.
Increased serum uric acid is due to increased turnover of skin cells in psoriasis.
Serologic tests for rheumatoid factor are negative.

ARTHRITIS ASSOCIATED WITH ULCERATIVE COLITIS OR REGIONAL ENTERITIS

There may be rheumatoid arthritis, ankylosing spondylitis, or acute synovitis (monarticular or polyarticular—absent rheumatoid factor).

Joint fluid is sterile bacteriologically and microscopically. It is similar to fluid of rheumatoid arthritis and Whipple's disease (cell count, differential count, specific gravity, viscosity, protein, sugar, poor mucin clot formation). Joint fluid examination is principally useful in monarticular involvement to rule out suppurative arthritis.

Synovial biopsy is similar to rheumatoid arthritis biopsy.

ARTHRITIS ASSOCIATED WITH WHIPPLE'S DISEASE

This is a nonspecific synovitis.

HEMOCHROMATOSIS-ASSOCIATED ARTHRITIS

Laboratory findings of hemochromatosis

Negative RA factor

No subcutaneous nodules

Biopsy of synovia—iron deposits in synovia lining but not in cartilage, little iron in deep macrophages

    Hemarthrosis—iron diffusely distributed in macrophages (e.g., in hemophilia, trauma, and pigmented villonodular synovitis)

    Osteoarthritis—small amount of iron that is limited to deep macrophages

    Rheumatoid arthritis—iron in both deep macrophages and lining cells

Chondrocalcinosis frequently associated

REITER'S SYNDROME

This triad of arthritis, urethritis, and conjunctivitis has additional features: dermatitis, buccal ulcerations, circinate balanitis, and keratosis blennorrhagica.

Increased ESR parallels the clinical course.

WBC is increased (10,000–20,000/cu mm), as are granulocytes.

Serum globulins are increased in long-standing disease.

Nonbacterial cystitis, prostatitis, or seminal vesiculitis is found (significance of culturing pleuropneumonia-like organisms is not determined).

GOUT

Serum uric acid is increased. Several determinations may be required to establish elevated values; beware of serum levels reduced to normal range by recent aspirin ingestion.

Serum uric acid levels are increased in $\cong 25\%$ of asymptomatic relatives.

Moderate leukocytosis and increased ESR occur during acute attacks; normal at other times.

Presence of crystals of monosodium urate from tophi and joint fluid (viewed microscopically under polarized light) establishes the diagnosis.

See Tables 34, pp. 274–275, and 37, p. 278.
Uric acid crystals and amorphous urates are normal findings in urinary sediment.
Uric acid stones are found in the urinary system in 15% of patients.
Low-grade proteinuria occurs in 20–80% of gouty persons for many years before further evidence of renal disease appears.
Histologic examination of gouty nodule should be made.
Diabetes mellitus develops with increased frequency.

See also sections on renal diseases.

DISEASES ASSOCIATED WITH GOUT
Hypertension in one-third of patients with gout
Diabetes mellitus
Familial hypercholesterolemia
Acute intermittent porphyria
von Gierke's disease
Sarcoidosis
Other

SECONDARY GOUT

Occurs In
Lead intoxication
Hematologic diseases (e.g., leukemia, polycythemia vera, secondary polycythemia, malignant lymphomas). *Blood dyscrasias are found in* $\cong 10\%$ *of patients with clinical gout.*
Psoriasis

CHONDROCALCINOSIS ("PSEUDOGOUT")
Joint fluid contains crystals of calcium pyrophosphate dihydrate, inside and outside of WBCs; differentiated from urate crystals under polarized light.
Blood and urine findings are normal.
See Tables 34, pp. 274–275, and 37, p. 278.

CONDITIONS THAT MAY PRESENT AS ACUTE ARTHRITIS
Beware of conditions that may present as acute arthritis
    Acute leukemia in children
    Hypertrophic pulmonary osteoarthropathy (clubbing) in lung tumors—may have acute onset and be painful
    Drug reaction causing lupus erythematosus-like syndrome (e.g., procaine amide)
    Aortic insufficiency starting with back pain and symptoms of spondylitis

SEPTIC ARTHRITIS (SUPPURATIVE OR PURULENT ARTHRITIS)
Laboratory findings due to preexisting infections (e.g., subacute bacterial endocarditis, meningococcic meningitis, pneumococcal pneumonia, typhoid, gonorrhea, tuberculosis) are noted.

See Table 34, 274–275.

Joint fluid
> In purulent arthritis
>> Gram stain is particularly useful for establishing diagnosis promptly and in cases in which cultures are negative.
>> Culture may be negative because of prior administration of antibiotics.
> In tuberculous arthritis
>> Gram stain and bacterial cultures are negative, but acid-fast stain, culture for tubercle bacilli, guinea pig inoculation, and biopsy of synovia confirm the diagnosis.

PIGMENTED VILLONODULAR SYNOVITIS
Complete blood count, ESR, blood cholesterol, and urinalysis are normal.

See Table 34, pp. 274–275.

POLYMYALGIA RHEUMATICA
ESR is usually markedly increased.
Mild hypochromic or normochromic anemia is commonly found.
WBC count is usually normal.
Abnormalities of serum proteins are frequent although there is no consistent or diagnostic pattern. Most frequently the albumin is decreased with an increase in alpha$_1$ and alpha$_2$ globulins and fibrinogen. Cryoglobulins are sometimes present.
Rheumatoid factor is present in serum in 7.5% of patients.
LE test is negative.
Serum enzymes (e.g., SGOT, CPK, aldolase) are normal.
Muscle biopsy is usually normal or may show mild nonspecific changes.
Temporal artery biopsy is often positive because of the high incidence of associated cranial arteritis.

HYPERTROPHIC OSTEOARTHROPATHY (CLUBBING; HYPERTROPHIC "PULMONARY" OSTEOARTHROPATHY)
Due To
Pulmonary diseases (especially bronchogenic carcinoma, bronchiectasis, lung abscess)
Pleural disease (especially tumors, empyema)
Mediastinal lesions (e.g., malignant lymphoma, aortic aneurysm)
Cardiac diseases (especially subacute bacterial endocarditis, cyanotic congenital heart disease)
Hepatic disease (especially cholangiolitic cirrhosis)
Intestinal diseases (especially tuberculosis, amebic infection, regional enteritis, ulcerative colitis, neoplasms)
Rare hereditary and idiopathic causes

CARPAL TUNNEL SYNDROME
Rule out underlying conditions
> Amyloidosis
> Pregnancy
> Acromegaly

Rheumatoid inflammation
Many others (e.g., fibrosis, trauma)

NORMAL LABORATORY FINDINGS IN DISEASES OF JOINTS
Slipped femoral epiphysis
Aseptic (avascular) necrosis of bone
Juvenile osteochondritis
Osteochondritis dissecans
Hypertrophic osteoarthropathy
Congenital dysplasia of hip
Joint mice
Intervertebral disk syndrome

NORMAL LABORATORY FINDINGS IN DISEASES OF MUSCULOSKELETAL SYSTEM
Fibrositis
Fasciitis
Bursitis
Capsulitis
Tenosynovitis
Tendinitis
Dupuytren's contracture

HEMATOLOGIC DISEASES

CLASSIFICATION OF ANEMIAS ACCORDING TO PATHOGENESIS
Marrow hypofunction with decreased RBC production
    Marrow replacement (myelophthisic anemias due to tumor or granulomas [e.g., tuberculosis])

In absence of severe anemia or leukemoid reaction, nucleated RBCs in blood smear suggest miliary tuberculosis or marrow metastases.

    Marrow injury (hypoplastic and aplastic anemias)
    Nutritional deficiency (e.g., megaloblastic anemias due to lack of vitamin B_{12} or folic acid)
    Endocrine hypofunction (e.g., pituitary, adrenal, thyroid)
Marrow hypofunction due to decreased hemoglobin production (hypochromic microcytic anemias)
    Deficient heme synthesis (iron deficiency anemia, pyridoxine-responsive anemias)
    Deficient globin synthesis (thalassemias, hemoglobinopathies)
Excessive loss of RBCs (hemolytic anemias due to genetically defective RBCs)
    Abnormal shape (hereditary spherocytosis, hereditary elliptocytosis)
    Abnormal hemoglobins (sickle cell anemia, thalassemias, hemoglobin C disease)
    Abnormal RBC enzymes (G-6-PD deficiency, congenital nonspherocytic hemolytic anemias)
Excessive loss of RBCs
    Hemolytic anemias with acquired defects of RBC and positive Coombs' test (autoantibodies, as in systemic lupus erythematosus [SLE], malignant lymphoma; or exogenous allergens, as in penicillin allergy)
Excessive loss of normal RBCs
    Hemorrhage
    Hypersplenism
    Chemical agents (e.g., lead)
    Infectious agents (e.g., *Clostridium welchii, Bartonella,* malaria)
    Miscellaneous diseases (e.g., uremia, liver disease, cancers)
    Physical agents (e.g., burns)
    Mechanical trauma (e.g., artificial heart valves, tumor microemboli)

Blood smear shows fragmented bizarre-shaped RBCs in patients with artificial heart valves.

RED BLOOD CELL INDICES IN VARIOUS ANEMIAS
Macrocytic (MCV >95 cu μ; MCHC >30 gm/100 ml)
    Megaloblastic anemia
        Pernicious anemia

Table 38. Red Blood Cell Indices

Type of Anemia	Mean Corpuscular Volume (MCV)[a] (cu μ)	Mean Corpuscular Hemoglobin (MCH)[b] ($\mu\mu$g)	Mean Corpuscular Hemoglobin Concentration (MCHC)[c] (gm/100 ml)
Normal	82–92	27–31	32–36
Normocytic anemias	82–92	25–30	32–36
Macrocytic anemias	95–150	30–50	32–36
Microcytic (usually hypochromic) anemias	50–80	12–25	25–30

[a]Mean corpuscular volume (MCV) (cu μ) = $\dfrac{\text{hematocrit}}{\text{RBC}}$

[b]Mean corpuscular hemoglobin (MCH) ($\mu\mu$g) = $\dfrac{\text{hemoglobin}}{\text{RBC}}$; represents weight of hemoglobin in average RBC. Not as useful as MCHC.

[c]Mean corpuscular hemoglobin concentration (MCHC) (gm/100 ml) = $\dfrac{\text{hemoglobin}}{\text{hematocrit}}$; represents concentration of hemoglobin in average RBC.

MCHC is increased only in hereditary spherocytosis. MCHC is not increased in pernicious anemia.

          Sprue (e.g., steatorrhea, celiac disease, intestinal resection or fistula)
          Macrocytic anemia of pregnancy
          Megaloblastic anemia of infancy
          Fish tapeworm infestation
          Carcinoma of stomach, following total gastrectomy
          Antimetabolite therapy
          Orotic aciduria
          Di Guglielmo's disease
          Other
     Miscellaneous macrocytic nonmegaloblastic anemias that are usually normocytic
          Anemia of hypothyroidism
          Chronic liver disaease
          Other
Normocytic (MCV = 80–94; MCHC >30)
     Following acute hemorrhage
     Hemolytic anemias
     Anemias due to inadequate blood formation
          Myelophthisic
          Hypoplastic
          Aplastic
          Associated with various chronic infections, neoplasms, uremia, etc.
Microcytic (usually hypochromic) (MCV <80; MCHC <30)
     Iron deficiency
          Inadequate intake

Poor absorption
Excessive iron requirements
Chronic blood loss
Other
Pyridoxine-responsive anemia
Thalassemia (major or combined with hemoglobinopathy)

MYELOPHTHISIC ANEMIA
Anemia is present.
Increased nucleated RBCs and normoblasts in peripheral smear are out of proportion to the degree of anemia and may be found even in the absence of anemia. Polychromatophilia, basophilic stippling, and increased reticulocyte count may also occur.
WBC may be normal or decreased; occasionally it is increased up to a leukemoid picture; immature WBC may be found in peripheral smear.
Platelets may be normal or decreased, and abnormal forms may occur. Abnormalities may occur even when WBC is normal.
Bone marrow demonstrates primary disease.
Metastatic carcinoma of bone marrow (especially breast, lung, prostate, thyroid)
Hodgkin's disease
Multiple myeloma (5% of patients)
Gaucher's, Niemann-Pick, and Hand-Schüller-Christian diseases
Osteopetrosis
Myelofibrosis

IDIOPATHIC MYELOFIBROSIS (AGNOGENIC MYELOID METAPLASIA)
Normocytic anemia is usual.
Peripheral smear shows anisocytosis; teardrop poikilocytosis is striking; polychromatophilia and occasional nucleated RBCs are found.
Reticulocyte count is increased ($\leq 10\%$)
WBC may be normal (50% of patients), increased or decreased, and abnormal forms may occur. Immature cells ($\leq 15\%$) are usual. Basophils and eosinophils may be increased.
Platelets may be normal or decreased, and abnormal forms may occur.
Repeated bone marrow aspiration often produces no marrow elements. Surgical biopsy of bone for histologic examination shows fibrosis of marrow which is usually hypocellular.
Needle puncture of spleen and a lymph node shows extramedullary hematopoiesis.
Hypersplenism causes thrombocytopenia in 30%, and leukopenia in 15% of these patients.
Leukocyte alkaline phosphatase is increased; may be marked.
Serum uric acid is often increased.
Prolonged prothrombin time is found in 75% of patients.
Laboratory findings due to complications
Hemorrhage
Hemolytic anemia

Infection
DIC occurs in 20% of patients.

Rule out other myeloproliferative diseases, underlying poisoning (e.g., phosphorus, fluorine, estrogens).

PURE RED CELL ANEMIA (AREGENERATIVE ANEMIA; IDIOPATHIC HYPOPLASTIC ANEMIA; PRIMARY RED CELL APLASIA, ETC.)

Normochromic normocytic anemia is present that is refractory to all treatment except transfusion and sometimes ACTH or corticosteroids.

Reticulocytes are decreased or absent.

WBC and differential blood count are normal.

Platelet count is normal.

There is no evidence of hemolysis.

Bone marrow usually shows marked decrease in erythroid series but sometimes is normal. Myeloid cells and megakaryocytes are normal.

Plasma iron (^{59}Fe) clearance is markedly reduced.

RBC uptake of ^{59}Fe is markedly decreased.

The disease may be related to thymus tumors (see p. 290), leukemia, which develops in 10% of patients, chemicals, bronchogenic carcinoma (rarely), kwashiorkor, etc.

PANCYTOPENIA

Anemia

Leukopenia—absolute myeloid decrease may be associated with relative lymphocytosis or with lymphocytopenia

Thrombocytopenia

Laboratory findings due to causative disease

Due To

Hypersplenism
  Congestive splenomegaly
  Malignant lymphomas
  Histiocytoses
  Infectious diseases (tuberculosis, kala-azar, sarcoidosis)
  Primary splenic pancytopenia
Diseases of marrow
  Metastatic carcinoma
  Multiple myeloma
  Aleukemic leukemia
  Osteopetrosis
  Myelosclerosis, myelofibrosis, etc.
Aplastic anemias
  Physical and chemical causes (e.g., ionizing irradiation, benzol compounds)
  Idiopathic causes (familial or isolated. *"Isolated" accounts for 50% of all cases of pancytopenia.*)
Megaloblastic macrocytic anemias (e.g., pernicious anemia)
Paroxysmal nocturnal hemoglobinuria (rare)

APLASTIC ANEMIA
Laboratory findings represent the whole spectrum from the most severe condition of the classic type, with marked leukopenia, thrombocytopenia, anemia, and acellular bone marrow, to cases with involvement only of erythroid elements. In some cases the marrow may be cellular or hyperplastic.

Due To
Ionizing irradiation (x-ray, radioisotopes)
Benzene family chemicals
Cytotoxic drugs (e.g., nitrogen mustards, busulfan)
Antimetabolite drugs (e.g., 6-mercaptopurine, antifolates)
Other (e.g., arsenic)
Various agents that are less frequently responsible (especially chloramphenicol, phenylbutazone, Atabrine, gold compounds, anticonvulsant drugs, antibiotics)

HEMATOLOGIC EFFECTS OF CHEMICALS THAT INJURE BONE MARROW
(especially benzene; also trinitrotoluene and others)
In order of decreasing frequency
    Anemia
    Macrocytosis
    Thrombocytopenia
    Leukopenia
    Other (e.g., decreased lymphocytes, increased reticulocytes, increased eosinophils)
Varying degrees of severity up to aplastic anemia
Hemolytic anemia is sometimes produced.

HEMATOLOGIC EFFECTS OF IRRADIATION
(depends on amount of irradiation received)
Severe
    Severe leukopenia with infection
    Thrombocytopenia and increased vascular fragility, causing hemorrhage; begins in 4–7 days, peak severity in 16–22 days
    Aplastic anemia if patient survives 3–6 weeks; laboratory findings due to complications, such as hemorrhage, infection, dehydration
Mild (<300 R)
    Increased neutrophils within a few hours with onset of irradiation sickness
    Decreased lymphocytes after 24 hours, causing decrease in total WBC
    No anemia unless dose of radiation is greater; may appear in 4–8 weeks (*Early appearance of anemia with greater irradiation is due to hemorrhage and changes in fluid homeostasis rather than marrow injury.*)
    Platelets slightly decreased (some patients)
Chronic (occupational)
    Decreased granulocytes

Increased lymphocytes, relative or absolute
Varying degrees of leukocytosis and leukemoid reactions
Varying degrees of anemia, normocytic or macrocytic; erythrocytosis
Thrombocytopenia
Late
Increased incidence of leukemia (e.g., in survivors of atomic bomb explosions)
Increased incidence of visceral malignancy (e.g., liver cancer due to Thorotrast, bone cancer due to radium)

TUMORS OF THYMUS

Associated With
Cushing's syndrome associated with malignant thymoma
Congenital hypogammaglobulinemia
Combinations of lymphopenia with dysgammaglobulinemia or normogammaglobulinemia or agammaglobulinemia and histologic abnormality of thymus associated with marked increase in susceptibility to infection (e.g., widespread moniliasis, death following BCG vaccination)
Acquired hypogammaglobulinemia. 10% of adults with this condition have an associated thymoma. The condition does not respond to thymectomy.
Myasthenia gravis. In 10–20% of patients there is associated thymoma, malignant in 25% of patients. 75% of myasthenia patients show thymic hyperplasia. Response to thymectomy is usually unpredictable and varies from marked improvement to worsening.
Aregenerative anemia of unknown cause (not autoimmune), usually of the normocytic normochromic type, occasionally macrocytic. Tumor may be present for many years before onset of anemia. Anemia may not be prevented or corrected by thymectomy (thymectomy causes remission in 30% of patients) or steroid therapy.

Laboratory Findings
WBC is usually normal. Lymphocytes may be increased. In 15% of patients there is also associated leukopenia or thrombocytopenia or both. Occasionally pancytopenia occurs.
Bone marrow shows selective erythroid hypoplasia with normal myeloid and megakaryocytic elements.

PERNICIOUS ANEMIA
Anemia sometimes shows RBC as low as 500,000/cu mm.
MCV is increased (95–110 cu μ).
MCH is increased.
MCHC is normal.
Poikilocytosis is moderate to marked; it is always present in relapse.
Anisocytosis is moderate to marked; it is always present in relapse.
Reticulocyte count is decreased or normal.
Blood smear may show polychromatophilia, stippled RBCs, Howell-Jolly bodies, Cabot's rings, etc. Large hypersegmented

leukocytes (shift to the right) are usually present and may precede RBC abnormalities. Occasionally there is moderate eosinophilia.

Thrombocytopenia is present; abnormal and giant forms may be seen.

Leukopenia is usual (4000–5000/cu mm).

RBC survival is decreased.

Marrow shows megaloblastic and erythroid hyperplasia and abnormalities of myeloid and megakaryocytic elements.

Achlorhydria occurs even after administration of histamine—this is virtually essential for diagnosis. Decreased volume of gastric juice, high pH, and decreased or absent pepsin and rennin are also shown. Achlorhydria and gastric changes are rarely found in children.

Schilling test is diagnostic.

Serum vitamin B_{12} is decreased.

Serum iron is almost always increased during relapse unless there is complicating iron deficiency. Total iron-binding capacity (TIBC) is normal or slightly decreased.

Serum indirect bilirubin is increased (<4 mg/100 ml).

Urine urobilinogen and coproporphyrin I are increased.

Stool urobilinogen is increased.

Serum LDH is markedly increased.

Serum alkaline phosphatase is decreased; increases after treatment.

Serum cholesterol is moderately decreased.

Cholinesterase activity in RBC, plasma, and whole blood is decreased.

There is a characteristic therapeutic response to vitamin B_{12} administration.

RESPONSE OF LABORATORY TESTS TO SPECIFIC TREATMENT OF PERNICIOUS ANEMIA

Increased urinary urobilinogen and coproporphyrin I immediately revert to normal, preceding reticulocyte response.

Serum folate decreases at the same time reticulocytosis takes place.

Serum iron decreases to normal or less than normal at the same time reticulocytosis takes place.

Serum uric acid increases; peak precedes maximum reticulocyte count by about 24 hours; remains increased as long as rapid RBC regeneration goes on.

Serum LDH falls but is not yet normal by eighth day.

Serum cholesterol rises to greater than normal levels; most marked at peak of reticulocyte response.

RBC count reaches normal between eighth and 12th week regardless of severity of anemia; hemoglobin concentration may rise at a slower rate, producing hypochromia with microcytosis.

Reticulocyte response is proportional to severity of anemia. This response is characteristic: reticulocyte count begins to rise by fourth day after treatment and reaches maximum on eighth to ninth day; returns to normal by 14th day.

Megaloblasts disappear from marrow in 24–48 hours.

Achlorhydria persists.
RBC cholinesterase activity increases.
Serum alkaline phosphatase increases to normal.

MACROCYTIC ANEMIA OF SPRUE, CELIAC DISEASE, STEATORRHEA
See p. 198.

MEGALOBLASTIC ANEMIA OF PREGNANCY AND PUERPERIUM
Anemia may have been present during previous pregnancy with spontaneous remission after delivery.
Hematologic abnormalities are less marked than in pernicious anemia (see p. 290).
If achlorhydria is present, it often disappears after delivery.
Therapeutic response to folic acid but usually not to vitamin B_{12}.
Urinary excretion of formiminoglutamic acid (FIGLU) is increased.

MEGALOBLASTIC ANEMIA OF INFANCY
(Age 6–12 months)
Morphologic findings in peripheral blood smear are similar to, but less severe than, those of pernicious anemia.
Bone marrow shows megaloblastic dysplasia that varies from mild to marked.
Urine FIGLU is increased; disappears after folic acid treatment.

HEREDITARY OROTIC ACIDURIA
This disorder of pyrimidine metabolism is due to a defect in the conversion of orotic acid to uridylic acid.
The severe megaloblastic anemia is refractory to vitamin B_{12} and folic acid but responsive to oral prednisone and yeast extract containing uridylic and cytidylic acids.
Anemia is hypochromic or normocytic; there is marked anisocytosis.

Table 39. Laboratory Tests in Differential Diagnosis of Causes of Vitamin B_{12} Deficiencies

	Gastric Juice		Schilling Test	
Condition	HCl	Intrinsic Factor Assay	Without Intrinsic Factor	With Intrinsic Factor
Lack of intrinsic factor (usually pernicious anemia)	O	O	D	N
Intestinal lesion	P or O	P	D	D
Nutritional	P or O	P	N	N

O = absent; P = present; N = normal; D = decreased.
Presence of free HCl in gastric juice always rules out pernicious anemia (except for very rare cases); absence of HCl is not helpful.

Table 40. Laboratory Tests in Differential Diagnosis of Vitamin B_{12} and Folic Acid Deficiencies

Deficiency	Macrocytosis	Leukopenia and Thrombocytopenia	Serum B_{12}	Serum Folate	Urinary Excretion of	
					FIGLU[a]	MMA[b]
Vitamin B_{12}	More marked	More constant	Markedly D	N	I or N	I
Folic acid	Less marked	Inconstant	N or slightly D	D	I	N

D = decreased; I = increased; N = normal.

[a]Formiminoglutamic acid after histidine load; not a reliable test (since B_{12} is needed for normal folic acid metabolism).

[b]Methylmalonic acid.

293

Table 41. Laboratory Tests in Differential Diagnosis of Microcytic (MCV <80) and Hypochromic (MCHC <30) Anemias

1. Determine serum iron and TIBC (and also perhaps do iron stain on bone marrow smear—the most reliable index of iron deficiency).
2. If serum iron and TIBC are both normal, hemoglobin electrophoresis will establish the diagnosis of thalassemia.
   If serum iron is abnormal, the cause may be iron deficiency (e.g., blood loss, dietary deficiency) or normochromic microcytic anemia of chronic disease.

Type of Anemia	Serum Iron	TIBC	Transferrin Saturation	Marrow Hemosiderin	Sideroblasts	Type of Hemoglobin	Anemia
Normal values	80–160 µg/100 ml in men 50–150 µg/100 ml in women	250–410 µg/100 ml	20–55%		30–50%	AA	
Iron deficiency	D	I	D	O	D	AA	Hypochromic, normocytic, or microcytic
Normochromic, normocytic or microcytic, of chronic disease	D	D or N	D or N	N or I	D	AA	Normochromic, normocytic, or microcytic
Thalassemia Major	I	D	I	I	I	20–90% F	Hypochromic
Minor	N or I	N	N or I	N or I	I	2–8% F, A_2 is I	Microcytic
Sideroblastic	N	D or N	I	I	I	AA	Hypochromic microcytic, or normochromic normocytic

O = absent; D = decreased; I = increased; N = normal.

Iron depletion: Early—serum iron is normal; TIBC may be increased. Later—serum iron decreases; anemia is often normocytic when mild or of rapid onset; anemia first becomes microcytic, then hypochromic.

Iron deficiency may occur without anemia (transferrin saturation < 15%; decreased marrow iron and sideroblasts).

Leukopenia is present with increased susceptibility to infection.
Orotic acid in urine is increased; crystals precipitate when urine stands at room temperature.
RBC orotidylic decarboxylase activity is decreased (<5.5 units).
Iatrogenic orotic aciduria occurs during cancer chemotherapy with 6-azauridine.

ANEMIA IN HYPOTHYROIDISM
Occurs in one-third to two-thirds of patients with hypothyroidism; usually mild (hematocrit reading >35)
Macrocytic or normocytic (*If hypochromic, rule out associated iron deficiency.*)
No anisocytosis or poikilocytosis
Decreased total blood volume and plasma volume
Normal RBC survival
Responds to treatment of hypothyroidism

IRON DEFICIENCY ANEMIA

Due To (usually a combination of these factors)
Chronic blood loss (e.g., menometrorrhagia, bleeding from gastrointestinal tract, especially from carcinoma of colon, hiatus hernia, peptic ulcer, parasites in intestine)
Decreased food intake (e.g., poverty, emotional factors)
Decreased absorption (e.g., steatorrhea, gastrectomy, achlorhydria)
Increased requirements (e.g., pregnancy, lactation)

Laboratory Findings
Hemoglobin is decreased (usually 6–10 gm/100 ml) out of proportion to decrease in RBC (3.5–5.0 million/cu mm); thus MCV is decreased (<80 cu μ), MCHC is decreased (25–30 gm/100 ml), and MCH is decreased (<25 $\mu\mu$g). Hypochromia and microcytosis parallel severity of anemia. Polychromatophilia and nucleated RBCs are less common than in pernicious anemia. Diagnosis from peripheral blood smear is difficult and unreliable.
Serum iron is decreased (usually <40 μg/100 ml), total ironbinding capacity increased (usually 350–460 μg/100 ml) and transferrin saturation decreased (<15%).
Bone marrow shows normoblastic hyperplasia with decreased hemosiderin, later absent, and decreased percentage of sideroblasts.
Reticulocytes are normal or decreased unless there is recent hemorrhage.
WBC is normal or may be slightly decreased; may be increased with fresh hemorrhage.
Serum bilirubin is not increased
Platelet count is normal or may be slightly increased.
Coagulation studies are normal.
RBC fragility is normal or (often) increased to 0.21%.
RBC life span is normal.
Laboratory findings may disclose causative factors (e.g., GI bleeding).

ATRANSFERRINEMIA
(isolated absence of transferrin)
Iron deficiency anemia is unresponsive to therapy.

Hemosiderosis follows transfusions with involvement of adrenals, heart, etc.

Serum protein electrophoresis shows marked decrease in beta globulins.

Absence of transferrin is demonstrated with immunoelectrophoresis.

ANEMIAS OF CHRONIC DISEASES
Due To
Subacute or chronic infections (especially tuberculosis, bronchiectasis, lung abscess, empyema, bacterial endocarditis, brucellosis)

Neoplasms

Chronic liver diseases

Rheumatoid arthritis (*anemia parallels activity of arthritis*)

Rheumatic fever, SLE

Uremia (BUN >70 mg/100 ml)

Laboratory Findings
Anemia is usually mild (hemoglobin >9 gm/100 ml).

Anemia is usually normocytic, normochromic. If hypochromic or microcytic, it is always less marked than in iron deficiency anemia.

Moderate anisocytosis and slight poikilocytosis are present.

Reticulocytosis, polychromatophilia, and nucleated RBCs are absent (*may be present with severe anemia or uremia*).

Serum iron is decreased. TIBC and transferrin saturation are decreased or normal.

Marrow hemosiderin is increased or normal; sideroblasts are decreased.

RBC survival is slightly decreased in patient but not in normal recipient.

See Table 41, p. 294.

SIDEROBLASTIC (SIDEROACHRESTIC) ANEMIAS
This miscellaneous group of diseases is characterized by increased sideroblasts (erythroblasts containing iron inclusions) in marrow.

See Table 41, p. 294.

Due To
Hereditary factors

Certain drugs (e.g., isoniazid and PAS in treatment of tuberculosis)

Preleukemia

Unknown cause

PYRIDOXINE-RESPONSIVE ANEMIA
Severe hypochromic microcytic anemia is present.

Blood smear shows anisocytosis, poikilocytosis with many bizarre

forms, target cells, hypochromia. Polychromatophilia and reticulocytosis are not increased.
Serum iron is increased; TIBC is somewhat decreased; transferrin saturation is markedly increased. Marrow sideroblasts and blood siderocytes are increased. Marrow and liver biopsy show increased hemosiderin.
Bone marrow usually shows normoblastic hyperplasia; occasionally it is megaloblastic.
Response to pyridoxine is always incomplete. Even when hemoglobin becomes normal, morphologic changes in RBCs persist.

LABORATORY SCREENING FOR HEMOGLOBINOPATHIES
Normocytic normochromic RBC except in
    Thalassemia syndromes—microcytic hypochromic
    Hemoglobin (Hb) C, D, E diseases—microcytic normochromic
Osmotic fragility—normal or decreased (especially in thalassemia)
    Symmetric shift in hemoglobin C, D, E diseases
    Asymmetric shift in other hemoglobin diseases
Target cells—in many of hemolytic diseases due to hemoglobinopathies; 50% of RBCs in hemoglobin C, D, E diseases
Sickle cell test—proves presence of hemoglobin S
Inclusion bodies—in hemoglobin H and C disorders
Hemoglobin electrophoresis
Alkali denaturation for hemoglobin F

SICKLE CELL DISEASE
Sickle cell trait (heterozygous sickle cell or hemoglobin AS disease—occurs in $\cong 10\%$ of American blacks)
    Hemoglobin electrophoresis: Hemoglobin S is 20–40% and hemoglobin A is 60–80%, small amount of hemoglobin F ($\leqq 2\%$) may be present.
    Sickle cell preparation is positive.
    Blood smear shows only a few target cells.
    No anemia or hemolysis or jaundice is present.
    Anoxia may cause systemic sickling (see below, Sickle cell anemia).
        Beware anesthesia, airplane flights, etc.
    Hematuria without any other demonstrable cause may be found.
    Hyposthenuria may occur.
Sickle cell anemia (homozygous hemoglobin SS disease); (occurs in 1:625 American blacks)
    Hemoglobin electrophoresis: Hemoglobin S is 80–100% and hemoglobin F comprises the rest (see Fetal Hemoglobin, p. 114); hemoglobin A is absent.
    The anemia is normocytic normochromic (hemoglobin 5–10 gm/100 ml).
    Sickle cell preparation is positive.
    Blood smear shows a variable number of RBCs with abnormal shapes, nucleated RBCs, Howell-Jolly bodies, target cells, spherical cells.
    Reticulocyte count is increased (5–30%).

Table 42. Some Laboratory Findings in Hemoglobinopathies and Thalassemia

Condition	Hb Type	Hb F (Fetal Hemoglobin) % of Total	Sickling (stained blood smear)	% Target Cells	Micro-cytosis	Hypo-chromia	Severity of Anemia	Splenomegaly
Normal adult	AA	0–2	0	0	0	0	0	0
Normal newborn	AF	60–90	0	0	0	0	0	0
Sickle cell trait	AS	0–2	+	4	0	0	0	0
Sickle cell anemia	SS	2–30	++	5–30	0	0–1+	4+	0
Sickle cell–thalassemia	SF	2–20	+	20–40	3+	3+	3–4+	2+
Sickle cell–Hb C	SC	2–8	+	20–85	0	1–2+	2–3+	2+
Sickle cell–Hb D	SD	0–2	+	1+	0–1+	1–2+	3–4+	2+
Sickle cell–Hb G	SG	0–2	+	0	0	0	0	0
Sickle cell–hereditary spherocytosis	SA	0–2	+	1+	1+	0	1–4+	2+
Thalassemia minor	AA₂	0–8	0	1+	2–3+	2–3+	1+	±

Thalassemia major	AF	10–100	0	10–35	2–4+	2–4+	3–4+	4+
Hb C–thalassemia	CA	0–2	0	3+	1+	1+	0–1+	0
Hb E–thalassemia	EF	20–40	0	10–40	2+	2+	1+	3+
Hb G–thalassemia	EG	0–2	0	1+	1+	1+	1+	0
Hb H–thalassemia	AH	0–2	0	2+	1+	2+	2+	±
Hb C trait	AC	0–2	0	1–100	0	1+	0	0
Hb C disease	CC	0–5	0	30–100	0–1+	3+	1+	2+
Hb C–elliptocytosis	AC	0–2	0	1+	1+	2+	0–1+	0
Hb D trait	AD	0–2	0	0	0	0	0	0
Hb E trait	AE	0–2	0	0	0	0	0	0
Hb E disease	EE	0–9	0	25–60	2+	0	0–1+	±
Hb G trait	AG	0–2	0	0	0	0	0	0
Hb G disease	GG	0–2	0	0	0	0	0	0
Hb I trait	AI	0–2	0	0–2	0	0	0	0

1+ to 4+ = degree present on a scale of 1–4.

WBC is increased (10,000–30,000/cu mm), with normal differential or shift to the left.

Platelet count is increased (300,000–500,000/cu mm), with abnormal forms.

Bone marrow shows hyperplasia of all elements.

Decreased ESR becomes normal after blood is aerated.

Osmotic fragility is decreased (more resistant RBCs).

Mechanical fragility of RBCs is increased.

RBC survival time is decreased.

Indirect serum bilirubin is increased ($\leqq 6$ mg/100 ml).

Urine contains increased urobilinogen but is negative for bile.

Urobilinogen in stool is increased.

Hemosiderin appears in urine sediment.

Hematuria is frequent.

Renal concentrating ability is decreased, leading to a fixed specific gravity in virtually all patients after the first few years of life.

Serum uric acid may be increased.

Serum alkaline phosphatase is increased during crisis, representing vaso-occlusive bone injury as well as liver damage.

Leukocyte alkaline phosphatase activity is decreased.

Laboratory findings due to complications

Infarction of lungs, spleen, brain, bowel, etc.

Stasis and necrosis of liver—increased bile in urine, increased direct serum bilirubin $\leqq 40$ mg/100 ml, other findings of obstructive type of jaundice. Chronic cholecystitis and cholelithiasis in one-third of adults.

Salmonella osteomyelitis (see p. 464).

Anemia and hemolytic jaundice are present throughout life after age 3–6 months; hemolysis and anemia are not increased during crises.

Hemoglobin SC disease (occurs in 1:833 American blacks)

Hemoglobin electrophoresis: Hemoglobin A is absent; hemoglobin S predominates (30–60%) with hemoglobin C present; hemoglobin F is 2–15%.

Blood smear shows tetragonal crystals within RBC in 70% of patients.

Other findings are the same as for sickle cell anemia, but there is less marked destruction of RBC's, anemia, etc., and the disease is less severe clinically. *Crises may cause a more marked fall in RBC than occurs in hemoglobin SS disease.*

Sickle cell–thalassemia disease (occurs in 1:1667 American blacks)

Hemoglobin electrophoresis: Hemoglobin S is 20–80%; hemoglobin F is 2–20%; hemoglobin A is 0–50%.

Anemia is hypochromic microcytic; target cells are prominent; serum iron is normal.

Other findings resemble those of sickle cell anemia.

Sickle cell-persistent high fetal hemoglobin (occurs in 1 : 25,000 American blacks)

Hemoglobin electrophoresis: Hemoglobin F is 20–40%; decreased hemoglobin A and A_2 and combined hemoglobin S.

Findings are intermediate between those of sickle cell anemia and of sickle cell trait.

Sickle cell-hemoglobin D disease (occurs in 1 : 20,000 American blacks)

Findings are intermediate between those of sickle cell anemia and of sickle sickle cell trait.

THALASSEMIAS

Thalassemia trait

There are decreased hemoglobin and hematocrit values, with normal or increased RBC (5–7 million/cu mm) causing slight hypochromic microcytic anemia.

RBC >5.7 million/cu mm and MCV <75 cu μ are most often due to thalassemia trait; MCH is decreased and MCHC is normal or slightly decreased.

Blood smear changes are less marked than in thalassemia major but disproportionately more marked than in anemia.

Reticulocyte count is increased (2–10%).

Cellular marrow contains stainable iron.

Serum iron is normal or increased.

Osmotic fragility is decreased.

Beta type of thalassemia minor has increased A_2 hemoglobin (3–6%) on starch or agar electrophoresis and a slight increase in hemoglobin F (2–10%); A_2 and F hemoglobins are absent in the alpha type of thalassemia.

Thalassemia major

Fetal hemoglobin is 10–90%; hemoglobin A is decreased; hemoglobin A_2 is not increased.

There is marked hypochromic microcytic regenerative hemolytic anemia.

Blood smear shows marked anisocytosis, poikilocytosis, target cells, spherocytes, and hypochromic, fragmented, and bizarre RBCs; also many nucleated RBCs—basophilic stippling, Cabot's rings, siderocytes.

Reticulocyte count is increased.

WBCs are often increased, with normal differential or marked shift to the left.

Platelets are normal.

Bone marrow is cellular and shows erythroid hyperplasia and contains stainable iron.

Serum iron and TIBC are increased.

Indirect serum bilirubin is increased (1–3 mg/100 ml).

Urine urobilinogen is increased without bile.

Stool urobilinogen is increased.

RBC survival time is decreased.

Osmotic fragility is decreased.

Mechanical fragility is increased.

Laboratory findings due to secondary hypersplenism are present.

Hemoglobin E–thalassemia

The laboratory findings resemble those in thalassemia major.

HEMOGLOBIN C DISEASE

Hemoglobin C trait (occurs in 2% of American blacks, less frequently in other Americans)

    Hemoglobin electrophoresis demonstrates the abnormal hemoglobin.

    Blood smear shows variable number of target cells.

    No other abnormalities are seen.

Hemoglobin C disease

    Hemoglobin electrophoresis demonstrates the abnormal hemoglobin.

    Mild hypochromic hemolytic anemia is present.

    Blood smear shows many target cells, variable number of microspherocytes, occasional nucleated RBCs, a few tetragonal crystals within RBCs that increase following splenectomy.

    Reticulocyte count is increased (2–10%).

    Osmotic fragility is decreased.

    Mechanical fragility is increased.

    RBC survival time is decreased.

    Hemoglobin F is slightly increased.

    Increase in serum bilirubin is minimal.

    Normoblastic hyperplasia of bone marrow is present.

HEMOGLOBIN D DISEASE

Homozygous hemoglobin D disease

    Hemoglobin electrophoresis demonstrates the abnormal hemoglobin at acid pH.

    Mild microcytic anemia.

    Target cells and spherocytes.

    Decreased RBC survival time.

Heterozygous hemoglobin D trait

    Hemoglobin electrophoresis demonstrates the abnormal hemoglobin at acid pH.

    There are no other laboratory findings.

Sickle cell–hemoglobin D disease

    Hemoglobin electrophoresis demonstrates the abnormal hemoglobin at acid pH.

    Findings are intermediate between those of sickle cell anemia and sickle cell trait.

HEMOGLOBIN E DISEASE

Homozygous hemoglobin E disease

    Mild hypochromic hemolytic anemia

    Target cells (25–60%)

    Decreased osmotic fragility

    Hemoglobin F sometimes slightly increased

Heterozygous hemoglobin E trait

    There are no laboratory findings.

Hemoglobin E–thalassemia

    The laboratory findings resemble those in thalassemia major.

METHEMOGLOBINEMIA

Due To

Drugs and chemicals, especially aniline derivatives (e.g.,

acetanilid, phenacetin, certain sulfonamides, various clothing dyes)

Abnormal hemoglobin M (several different Ms)

Inherited enzyme deficiency (e.g., methemoglobin reductase)

Laboratory Findings

Freshly drawn blood is chocolate-brown; does not become red after exposure to air.

Starch block electrophoresis identifies the hemoglobin M.

Spectroscopic absorption analysis. Band at 630 mμ disappears on addition of 5% KCN.

RBC is slightly increased; no other hematologic abnormalities are found; there is no jaundice.

Patient is cyanotic clinically but in apparent good health.

SULFHEMOGLOBINEMIA

Due To

Drugs, especially phenacetin (including Bromo-Seltzer) and acetanilid

Laboratory Findings

Spectroscopic absorption analysis. Band at 618 mμ does not disappear on addition of 5% KCN.

Laboratory findings due to associated bromide intoxication. Bromide intoxication and sulfhemoglobinemia may be due to excessive intake of Bromo-Seltzer.

HEREDITARY ELLIPTOCYTOSIS (OVALOCYTOSIS)

Blood smear shows 25–90% of RBCs are oval.

No other hematologic abnormalities are seen in most patients; about 12% of patients show a chronic congenital hemolytic anemia with decreased RBC survival time, moderate anemia, increased serum bilirubin, and increased reticulocyte count, increased osmotic fragility, and autohemolysis.

Hemoglobin electrophoresis is normal.

Osmotic fragility and autohemolysis are normal in patients without hemolytic anemia.

Mechanical fragility is increased.

HEREDITARY SPHEROCYTOSIS

Defective RBC membrane is abnormally permeable to sodium, causing water inflow and rupture.

Anemia (hemolytic type) is moderate (RBC = 3–4 million/cu mm), microcytic (MCV = 70–80 cu μ) and hyperchromic (MCHC = 36–40 gm/100 ml).

Anisocytosis is marked; poikilocytosis is slight.

Spherocytes are present.

Osmotic fragility is increased; when normal in some patients, the incubated fragility test shows increased hemolysis

Autohemolysis (sterile defibrinated blood incubated for 48 hours) is increased (10–20% compared to normal of <4% of cells).

Abnormal osmotic fragility and autohemolysis are reduced by 10% glucose.

Mechanical fragility is increased.

Reticulocytes are increased.

WBC and platelet counts are usually normal; they may be increased during hemolysis.

Bone marrow shows marked erythroid hyperplasia; moderate hemosiderin is present.

Indirect serum bilirubin is increased.

Stool urobilinogen is usually increased.

Haptoglobins are decreased or absent.

Coombs' test is negative.

RBCs show Howell-Jolly bodies, Pappenheimer bodies. Heinz

Laboratory findings due to gallstones.

Diagnosis should be questioned if splenectomy does not cause a complete response.

HEREDITARY NONSPHEROCYTIC HEMOLYTIC ANEMIAS

This is a heterogeneous group. Some are due to deficiency of G-6-PD; others to unknown cause or to other rare congenital enzyme defects (e.g., glutathione).

Anemia is of the hemolytic type; may be severe; may begin in newborn; may be precipitated by certain drugs.

RBCs show Howell-Jolly bodies, Pappenheimer bodies, Heinz bodies, basophilic stippling; there may be slight macrocytosis.

Increase in reticulocyte count is marked, even with mild anemia.

Bone marrow shows marked erythroid hyperplasia; normal hemosiderin is present.

WBC, platelet count, hemoglobin electrophoresis, osmotic fragility, and mechanical fragility are normal.

Autohemolysis is present in some cases but not in others; reduction by glucose is less than in normal blood.

GLUCOSE-6-PHOSPHATE DEHYDROGENASE (G-6-PD) IN RBCS

Decreased In

American black males (13%)

American black females (3%) (20%) are carriers)

Some other ethnic groups (e.g., Greeks, Sardinians, Sephardic Jews)

May be associated with at least 4 clinical syndromes
> Some drug-induced acute hemolytic anemias (e.g., primaquine, sulfonamides, antipyretics)
> Favism
> Nonimmunologic hemolytic disease of the newborn
> Some cases of congenital nonspherocytic hemolytic anemia

Other Findings

Higher frequency of coronary heart disease and of cholelithiasis

Higher risk in presence of some other diseases (e.g., diabetes mellitus, viral hepatitis, pneumonia)

Increased In

Pernicious anemia to 3 times normal level; remains elevated for several months, even after administration of vitamin B_{12}

ITP (Werlhof's disease); becomes normal soon after splenectomy

Also reported in hepatic coma, hyperthyroidism, myocardial infarction (first week after), other megaloblastic anemias, and chronic blood loss

ERYTHROCYTE PYRUVATE KINASE DEFICIENCY

Congenital inherited nonspherocytic hemolytic anemia showing
  Icterus
  Anemia that varies from mild to profound
  Reticulocytosis
  Macrocytosis
  Few or no spherocytes
  Occasional "tailed poikilocytes"
  Varying abnormalities of incubated RBC osmotic fragility
  Deficiency of erythrocyte pyruvate kinase

Acquired type may be due to
  Drug ingestion
  Metabolic diseases of liver

PAROXYSMAL NOCTURNAL HEMOGLOBINURIA (MARCHIAFAVA-MICHELI SYNDROME)

Hemoglobinemia is present; increases during sleep.

Hemoglobinuria is evident on arising.

Serum haptoglobin is absent during an episode.

Chronic hemolytic anemia is well developed.

Urine contains hemoglobin, hemosiderin (in WBCs and epithelial cells of sediment), and increased urobilinogen.

Osmotic fragility is normal.

Serum iron may be decreased.

WBC is usually decreased.

Leukocyte alkaline phosphatase activity is decreased.

Platelet count is usually decreased but shows thrombotic rather than hemorrhagic complications.

Autohemolysis is increased.

RBC fragility is increased in acid medium (Ham test) and in hydrogen peroxide; amount of change is related to clinical severity.

RBC acetylcholinesterase activity is decreased.

PAROXYSMAL COLD HEMOGLOBINURIA

Sudden hemoglobinuria follows exposure to cold environment.

Findings are of acute hemolytic anemia.

Cold autohemolysin is present in blood.

Positive direct Coombs' test is present only during the attack.

There may be a biologic false positive test for syphilis, or the attack may be due to congenital syphilis.

ACQUIRED HEMOLYTIC ANEMIA

Laboratory findings due to increased destruction of RBCs

RBC survival time differentiates intrinsic RBC defect from factor outside RBC.

Blood smear often shows marked spherocytosis. Anisocytosis, poikilocytosis, and polychromasia are seen.

Slight abnormality of osmotic fragility is shown.

There is increased indirect serum bilirubin (less than 6 mg/100 ml because of compensatory excretory capacity of liver).

Urine urobilinogen is increased (may vary with liver function; may be obscured by antibiotic therapy altering intestinal flora). Bile is absent from urine.

Stool urobilinogen is increased.

Hemoglobinemia and hemoglobinuria are present when hemolysis is very rapid.

Haptoglobins are decreased or absent in chronic hemolytic diseases (removed following combination with free hemoglobin in serum).

WBC is usually elevated.

Laboratory findings due to compensatory increased production of RBCs

There is a degree of anemia. MCV reflects immaturity of circulating RBCs. Polychromatophilia is present.

Reticulocyte count is increased.

Erythroid hyperplasia of bone marrow is evident.

Laboratory findings due to mechanism of RBC destruction

Coombs' tests are positive.

Warm antibodies are found.

Cold agglutinins are found.

There is a biologic false positive test for syphilis.

Laboratory findings due to underlying conditions

Malignant lymphoma

Collagen diseases (e.g., disseminated lupus erythematosus)

Disseminated intravascular coagulation (see p. 337)

Idiopathic pulmonary hemosiderosis (see p. 188)

Infections, especially viral pneumonia

Drug-induced hemolytic anemia associated with a positive Coombs' test

Other

LABORATORY FINDINGS DUE TO INTRAVASCULAR HEMOLYSIS

Plasma hemoglobin increases transiently with return to normal in 8 hours. Determinations lack accuracy and precision.

Plasma haptoglobin level decreases in 6–10 hours and lasts for 2–3 days after lysis of 20–30 ml blood. Determination is relatively reliable and very sensitive.

Urine hemosiderin occurs 3–5 days after hemolysis with positive Prussian blue staining of renal tubular epithelial cells. It may be difficult to detect a single episode. Urine hemosiderin is commonly found in paroxysmal nocturnal hemoglobinuria.

Hemoglobinuria occurs 1–2 hours after severe hemolysis and lasts ≤ 24 hours. It is a transient finding and is relatively insensitive. False positive is due to myoglobinuria or to lysis of RBCs in urine.

Schumm's test for methemalbuminemia becomes positive 1–6 hours after hemolysis of 100 ml blood and lasts 1–3 days. Methemalbuminemia also occurs in hemorrhagic pancreatitis.

Serum bilirubin increase depends on liver function and amount of hemolysis. With normal liver function, it is increased 1 mg/100 ml in 1–6 hours to maximum in 3–12 hours following hemolysis of 100 ml blood.

Fecal urobilinogen may be increased but not useful because of wide normal range and variability.

Urine urobilinogen is similarly insensitive and unreliable as an index of hemolysis.

Extravascular hemolysis may cause increases in serum bilirubin and urine and fecal urobilinogen and a decrease in serum haptoglobin.

HEMOLYTIC DISEASE OF THE NEWBORN (ERYTHROBLASTOSIS FETALIS)
(due to destruction of fetal RBCs by maternal antibodies caused by isoimmunization of pregnant mother)

Serum indirect bilirubin shows rapid rise to high levels. May rise 0.3–1.0 mg/hour to level of 30 mg/100 ml in untreated infants to maximum in 3–5 days unless they die. Increased urine and fecal urobilinogen parallels serum levels.

Direct Coombs' test is strongly positive on cord blood RBC when due to Rh, Kell, Kidd, Duffy antibodies but is usually negative or weakly positive when due to anti-A antibodies. It becomes negative within a few days of effective exchange transfusion, but may remain positive for weeks in untreated infants. Indirect Coombs' test on cord blood may be positive because of "free" immune antibody.

At birth there is little or no anemia. In severe cases anemia may develop rapidly (RBC may decrease by 1 million/cu mm/day) to maximum by third or fourth day.

MCHC is normal; MCV and MCH are increased.

Nucleated RBCs in peripheral blood are markedly increased (10,000–100,000/cu mm) during first 2 days (normal = 200–2000/cu mm) and are usually very large. They tend to decrease and may be absent by third or fourth day. Normoblastosis is mild or absent when due to other antigens than Rh_o.

Peripheral smear shows marked polychromatophilia, macrocytic RBCs, increased reticulocyte count. In ABO incompatibility, spherocytosis may be marked, with associated increased osmotic fragility; *spherocytosis is slight or absent in Rh incompatibility*.

Hemoglobin F is decreased, and adult hemoglobin is increased.

WBC is increased (usually 15,000–30,000/cu mm).

Platelet count is usually normal; may be decreased in severe cases but returns to normal after 1 week. With decreased platelets, one may find increased bleeding time, poor clot retraction, and purpura. Prothrombin and fibrinogen deficiencies may occur.

Disease terminates in 3–6 weeks with elimination of maternal antibodies from infant's serum.

Late anemia occurs during second to fourth week of life in 5% of those receiving exchange transfusion. Reticulocyte count is low, and marrow may not show erythroid hyperplasia.

Exchange Transfusion

Use mother's serum for crossmatch.

Use Rh-negative donor unless mother and baby are both Rh-positive.

Use indirect Coombs' test for crossmatch.

Indications for Exchange Transfusion

Serum bilirubin in normal newborn is 1–3 mg/100 ml on first day.

May peak $\leqq$ 6 mg/100 ml of third to fifth day (mild jaundice may be evident)

Declines to normal 1.5 mg/100 ml over 2-week period.

In smaller, more premature infants, "physiologic" jaundice tends to last longer (see p. 228).

Peak $\leqq$ 10–12 mg/100 ml on fifth to seventh day.

Decline to normal may take 4–5 weeks.

Clinical jaundice before the third day is more marked than usual; after sixth day it is pathologic.

Hyperbilirubinemia is most likely to produce CNS damage (kernicterus) in infants that are

Most premature

Lightest weight

Afflicted with dehydration, hypoglycemia, acidosis, hypoxia, hypoalbuminemia, sepsis

Kernicterus is caused only by unconjugated (not conjugated) hyperbilirubinemia.

Exchange transfusion is indicated if

Birth weight is	*and serum bilirubin in first 48 hours is*	*or thereafter is*
(grams)	*(mg/100 ml)*	*(mg/100 ml)*
<1000	10	12
1000–1499	12	14
1500–2000	14	16
2001–2500	16	18
>2500	18	20

Transfuse at one step earlier in presence of

Serum protein <5 gm/100 ml

Metabolic acidosis (pH <7.25)

Respiratory distress (with O_2 <50 mm Hg)

Certain clinical findings (e.g., hypothermia, CNS or other clinical deterioration)

Other criteria for exchange transfusion are suddenness and rate of bilirubin increase and when it occurs; e.g., an increase of 3 mg/100 ml in 12 hours, especially after bilirubin has already leveled off, must be followed with frequent serial determinations, especially if it occurs on first or on seventh day rather than on third day. Beware of rate of bilirubin increase >1 mg/100 ml during first day. In ABO hemolytic disease, rate of bilirubin increase is not as great as in Rh disease; if danger level for exchange transfusion is not reached by third day, it is unlikely that it will be reached.

Criteria	*Continue to Follow Patient*	*Consider Exchange*	*Perform Exchange*
Rh antibody titer in mother	<1:64	>1:64	
Cord hemoglobin	>14 gm/100 ml	12–14 gm/100 ml	<12 gm/100 ml
Cord bilirubin	>4 mg/100 ml	4–5 mg/100 ml	>5 mg/100 ml
Capillary blood hemoglobin	>12 gm/100 ml	<12 gm/100 ml	<12 gm/100 ml and decreasing in first 24 hours
Serum bilirubin	<18 mg/100 ml	18–20 mg/100 ml	20 mg/100 ml in first 24 hours; after 48 hours 22 mg/100 ml on two tests 6–8 hours apart

In sick premature infants, 15 mg/100 ml is upper limit to indicate exchange transfusion.

Phototherapy of Coombs' positive infants decreases exchange transfusions (from 25 to 10% of these infants); follow effect of therapy with serum bilirubin every 4–8 hours. Phototherapy is usually not begun until serum bilirubin is 10 mg/100 ml. Skin color is disguised by phototherapy, so serum bilirubin determination is even more important. Beware of untreated anemia in these infants.

ABO ERYTHROBLASTOSIS
Mother is Group O with Group A_1 or B infant; rarely is mother Group A_2 with Group A_1 or B infant.
Infant's serum shows positive indirect Coombs' test with adult RBCs of same group.
Infant's RBCs show a negative direct Coombs' test (by standard methods).
Both Coombs' reactions have disappeared after the fourth day.
Marked microspherocytosis is present.
Osmotic fragility is increased.
Anti-A or anti-B titer in mother's serum is not useful since there is no correlation between the occurrence of hemolytic disease and the presence or height of the titer. If mother's serum does not hemolyze RBCs of same type as infant's, the diagnosis should be questioned.
Rapidly developing anemia is rare; serial bilirubin determinations

are indicators for exchange transfusion to prevent a level of 20 mg/100 ml.

For exchange transfusion, use Group O, Rh-type specific blood or Group O, Rh-negative blood.

Infants born subsequently to same parents do not have more serious disease, and they may have less serious disease.

Indications for Amniocentesis

Prior immunized pregnancy with maternal antibody titer >1:8 in albumin

History of hemolytic disease of newborn

Repeat amniocentesis every 2–3 weeks to measure presence and increase in bilirubin pigments; rise in these pigments according to age of fetus correlates with severity of disease and is indication for intrauterine transfusion, repeat examination, or immediate delivery (see p. 33).

Severe jaundice during first day of life indicates hemolytic disease, most probably Rh or ABO hemolytic disease. If Coombs' test is negative, the following must be ruled out

  Hereditary spherocytosis (blood smear is not helpful since hemolytic disease of the newborn also shows spherocytes)

  Elliptocytosis (blood smear shows elliptocytes, is diagnostic)

Only erythroblastosis causes a positive Coombs' test in the newborn.

If jaundice appears later, other causes of hemolytic disease to be ruled out are

  Glucose-6-phosphate deficiency and, less frequently, pyruvate kinase deficiency

  Slowly developing hemolytic disease

  Sepsis

If jaundice persists or peaks late, rule out

  Hemolytic disease   Hepatitis

  Sepsis   Biliary obstruction

Rare causes of later-appearing jaundice (second to third week) are

  Pyloric stenosis

  Galactosemia

See also pp. 224–229, Crigler-Najjar syndrome, Gilbert's disease, etc.

CRITERIA FOR SELECTION OF PATIENTS FOR IMMUNOSUPPRESSION OF Rh SENSITIZATION

Mother must be Rh_O (D) negative and D^u negative.

Mother's serum must have no Rh antibodies.

Baby must be Rh_O (D) positive.

Baby must have negative direct Coombs' test (cord blood).

Crossmatch of mother's RBC and Rh_O Gam (1:1000) must be compatible.

ANEMIA DUE TO ACUTE BLOOD LOSS

RBC, hemoglobin, and hematocrit level are not reliable initially because of compensatory vasoconstriction and hemodilution. They decrease for several days after hemorrhage ceases. RBC returns to normal in 4–6 weeks. Hemoglobin returns to normal in 6–8 weeks.

Anemia is normocytic. (*If hypochromic or microcytic, rule out iron deficiency due to prior hemorrhages.*)

Reticulocyte count is increased after 1–2 days, reaches peak in 4–7 days ($\leq 15\%$). Persistent increase suggests continuing hemorrhage.

Increased WBC (usually $\leq 20,000$/cu mm) reaches peak in 2–5 hours, becomes normal in 3–4 days. Persistent increase suggests continuing hemorrhage, bleeding into a body cavity, or infection. Differential count shows shift to the left.

Platelets are increased (≤ 1 million/cu mm) within a few hours; coagulation time is decreased.

BUN is increased if hemorrhage into lumen of GI tract occurs.

Serum indirect bilirubin is increased if hemorrhage into a body cavity or cystic structure occurs.

Laboratory findings due to causative disease (e.g., peptic ulcer, esophageal varices, leukemia) are noted.

ANEMIAS IN PARASITIC INFESTATIONS
Anemia due to blood loss, malnutrition, specific organ damage
Malaria
    Hemolytic anemia
Diphyllobothrium latum (fish tapeworm)
    Macrocytic anemia
Hookworm
    Hypochromic microcytic anemia due to chronic blood loss
Schistosoma mansoni
    Hypochromic microcytic anemia due to blood loss from intestine
    Macrocytic anemia due to cirrhosis of schistosomiasis
Amebiasis
    Due to blood loss and malnutrition

"ANEMIA" IN PREGNANCY
This is a normal physiologic change due to hemodilution—total blood volume and plasma volume increase more than red cell mass.

Onset is at eighth week; full development by 16th to 22d week; rapid return to normal in puerperium.

Hemoglobin averages 11 gm/100 ml; hematocrit value averages 33.

RBC morphology is normal.

RBC indices are normal.

If hemoglobin is <10 gm/100 ml or there are hypochromic microcytic indices, rule out iron deficiency anemia, which may occur frequently during pregnancy.

See Megaloblastic Anemia of Pregnancy, p. 292.

ANEMIA IN CHILDREN

Due To
Iron deficiency
Blood loss
Hemorrhagic disease of the newborn (hypoprothrombinemia)
Hemolytic disease of the newborn (erythroblastosis fetalis)
Hemolytic anemias (*more acute in children and show more marked anemia, erythroblastosis, reticulocytosis, jaundice, leukocytosis*)
 Thalassemia
 Hemoglobinopathies
 Hereditary spherocytosis
 Other
Anemias of chronic diseases
Megaloblastic anemia of infancy
Other hematologic diseases
 Leukemias
 Histiocytoses (e.g., Gaucher's disease, Niemann-Pick disease, histiocytosis X)
 Osteopetrosis
 Gargoylism

POLYCYTHEMIA VERA
RBC is 7–12 million; may increase to >15 million/cu mm.
Hemoglobin is 18–24 gm/100 ml.
Hematocrit value is increased.
MCV, MCH, and MCHC are normal or decreased.
Blood volume and red cell mass are increased; plasma volume is variable.
ESR is decreased.
Blood viscosity is increased.
Osmotic fragility is decreased (increased resistance).
Platelet count is increased (often >1 million).
Moderate polynuclear leukocytosis is present (usually >15,000/cu mm; sometimes there is a leukemoid reaction).
Peripheral blood smear may show macrocytes, microcytes, polychromatophilic RBCs, normoblasts, large masses of platelets, neutrophilic shift to the left.
Reticulocyte count is normal unless there has been some recent hemorrhage.
Bone marrow shows general hyperplasia of all elements.
Serum uric acid may be increased.
Leukocyte alkaline phosphatase may be greatly increased.
Serum vitamin B_{12} is increased.
Oxygen saturation of arterial blood is normal.
BMR is increased.
Bleeding time and coagulation time are normal but clot retraction may be poor.
Urine may contain increased urobilinogen, and occasionally albumin is present.
Laboratory findings of associated diseases
 Gout
 Duodenal ulcer

Cirrhosis
Hypertension
Laboratory findings due to complications
Thromboses (e.g., cerebral, portal vein)
Intercurrent infection
Hemorrhage
Myelofibrosis
Chronic myelogenous leukemia (develops in 20% of patients)

SECONDARY POLYCYTHEMIA
Results from hypoxia with decreased oxygen saturation of arterial blood due to
Decreased atmospheric pressure (e.g., high altitudes)
Chronic heart disease
Congenital (e.g., pulmonary stenosis, septal defect, patent ductus arteriosus)
Acquired (e.g., chronic rheumatic mitral disease)
Arteriovenous aneurysm
Impaired pulmonary ventilation
Alveolar-capillary block (e.g., Hamman-Rich syndrome, sarcoidosis, lymphangitic cancer)
Alveolar hypoventilation (e.g., bronchial asthma, kyphoscoliosis)
Restriction of pulmonary vascular bed (e.g., primary pulmonary hypertension, mitral stenosis, chronic pulmonary emboli, emphysema)
Abnormal hemoglobin pigments (methemoglobinemia or sulfhemoglobinemia due to chemicals, such as aniline and coal tar derivatives)
Associated with tumors and miscellaneous conditions
Renal disease (hypernephroma, benign tumors, hydronephrosis, polycystic kidneys)
Pheochromocytoma
Cushing's syndrome
Hemangioblastoma of cerebellum
Uterine fibromyoma
Other

The polycythemia may be relative.

See Table 43, p. 314.

RELATIVE POLYCYTHEMIA
Relative polycythemia is not secondary to hypoxia but results from a decrease in plasma volume due to decreased fluid intake (e.g., dehydration) and/or excess loss of body fluids (e.g., burns, shock).

ACUTE LEUKEMIA
Peripheral blood
WBC is rarely > 100,000/cu mm. It may be normal and is commonly less than normal. Peripheral smear shows many cells that resemble lymphocytes; it may not be possible to differ-

Table 43. Laboratory Tests in Differential Diagnosis of Polycythemia Vera, Secondary Polycythemia, and Relative Polycythemia

Test	Polycythemia Vera	Secondary Polycythemia	Relative Polycythemia
Hematocrit	I	I	I
Blood volume	I	I	D or N
Red cell mass	I	I	D or N
Plasma volume	I or N	N or I	D or N
Platelet count	I	N	N
WBC with shift to left	I	N	N
Nucleated RBC, abnormal RBC	I	N	N
Serum uric acid	I	I	N
Serum vitamin B_{12}	I	N	N
Leukocyte alkaline phosphatase	I	N	N
Oxygen saturation of arterial blood	N	D	N
Bone marrow	Hyperplasia of all elements	Erythroid hyperplasia	N

I = increased; D = decreased; N = normal.

entiate the very young forms as lymphoblasts or myeloblasts. Peroxidase-positive granules may be found in some cells in acute myeloblastic but not in acute lymphoblastic leukemia. Prognosis is better when initial WBC is < 10,000/cu mm and worse when > 100,000/cu mm.

Anemia is almost always present at clinical onset. Usually normocytic and sometimes macrocytic, it is progressive and may become severe. Normoblasts and polychromatophilia are common.

Platelet count is usually decreased at clinical onset and becomes progressively severe. May show poor clot retraction, increased bleeding time, positive tourniquet test, etc.

Bone marrow smear

Blast cells are present even when none are found in peripheral blood. (*This finding is useful to differentiate from other causes of pancytopenia.*)

There is progressively increasing infiltration with earlier cell types (e.g., blasts, myelocytes).

The myeloid-erythroid ratio is increased.

Erythroid and megakaryocyte elements are replaced.

In acute myelogenous leukemia, serum LDH and MDH are frequently but inconstantly increased; there is normal to slight increase in SGOT, SGPT, ALD.

Laboratory findings due to complications

Meningeal leukemia occurs in 25–50% of children with acute leukemia; CSF shows pleocytosis and increased pressure and LDH (see p. 291).

Urate nephropathy (see Chronic Myelogenous Leukemia, p. 316).

Infection causes 90% of deaths. Most important pathogens are gram-negative rods (especially *Pseudomonas aeruginosa*) and fungi (especially *Candida albicans*).

Hemolytic anemia (see pp. 305–306).

Complete remission is possible with drug therapy (e.g., prednisone in acute lymphoblastic leukemia).

WBC falls (or rises) to normal in 1–2 weeks with replacement of lymphoblasts by normal polynuclear leukocytes and return of RBC and platelet counts to normal; bone marrow may become normal. Maximum improvement in 6–8 weeks.

Amethopterin toxicity causes a macrocytic type of anemia with megaloblasts in marrow compared to leukemic normocytic anemia with blast cells in marrow.

PRELEUKEMIA

(poorly defined hematologic syndrome that sometimes precedes acute nonlymphocytic leukemia; overt leukemia seen in one-third of these patients by 6 months, 50% by 12 months, and 74% by 24 months)

Anemia, leukopenia, and thrombocytopenia in various combinations are most common findings.

Leukocytosis, monocytosis, and immature granulocytes may occur.

Anisocytosis, poikilocytosis, oval macrocytes, nucleated RBCs, and normochromia are most common changes in RBC morphology.

Atypical and bizarre platelets are seen in most cases.

Bone marrow is usually hypercellular, and erythroid hyperplasia occurs in 50% of patients.

Erythroid maturation defects with bizarre (e.g., multinucleated) forms and megaloblastic features unresponsive to folic acid, vitamin B_{12}, and iron.

Megakaryocytes are often atypical or bizarre.

Variable increase in mature granulocyte precursors (usually myelocytes) and monocytosis occur frequently.

CHRONIC MYELOGENOUS LEUKEMIA

Peripheral blood

Increased WBC due to increase in myeloid series is earliest change. In earlier stages the more mature forms predominate with sequentially fewer cells of the younger forms; in the later, more advanced stages the younger cells become predominant.

Eosinophilic, basophilic leukocytes may increase. Monocytes are normal or only slightly increased.

Lymphocytes are normal in absolute number but relatively decreased.

WBC is usually 100,000–500,000/cu mm when disease is discovered.

Decreased number of granulocytes show positive alkaline phosphatase staining reaction.

Anemia is usually normocytic; absent in early stage and severe in late stage. Blood smear shows few normoblasts, slight polychromatophilia, occasional stippling. Reticulocyte count is usually <3%. Anemia is due to myelophthisis; also due to bleeding (skin and GI tract), hemolysis (autoimmune hemolytic anemia is rare), and insufficient compensatory hematopoiesis. Degree of anemia is a good index of extent of leukemic process and therefore of prognosis. Anemia improves with appropriate therapy or becomes more marked as the disease progresses.

Platelet count is normal or, commonly, increased; decreased in terminal stages with findings of thrombocytopenic purpura. Low count may increase with therapy. Bleeding manifestations are usually due to thrombocytopenia.

Bone marrow
> Hyperplasia of granulocytic elements occurs, with increase in myeloid-erythroid ratio.
> Granulocytes are more immature than in the peripheral blood.
> The number of eosinophils and basophils is increased.
> Hemosiderin deposits are increased.

Needle aspiration of spleen
> The number of immature leukocytes is increased.
> Normoblastosis is present.
> Megakaryopoiesis is increased.

Serum and urine uric acid is increased, especially with high WBC and antileukemic therapy. Urinary obstruction may develop on account of intrarenal and extrarenal uric acid crystallization.

Serum LDH is increased; rises several weeks prior to relapse and falls several weeks prior to remission.
> Increased serum LDH, MDH, SGOT, SGPT, and ALD show less elevation than in acute leukemia. SGOT, SGPT, and ALD are normal in half the patients. LDH is useful for following course of therapy.

Serum protein electrophoresis shows decreased albumin with increased alpha and gamma globulins.

BMR is increased; thyroid ^{131}I uptake normal; PBI normal.

Coombs' test is positive in one-third of patients.

Serum vitamin B_{12} level is increased (often >1000 μg/ml).

Philadelphia chromosome (small satellite of chromosome 22 is found in 85% of patients and in asymptomatic relatives.

Laboratory findings due to leukemic infiltration of organs (e.g., kidney [hematuria common; uremia rare], heart, liver)

CHRONIC LYMPHOCYTIC LEUKEMIA

Peripheral blood
> WBC is increased (usually 50,000–250,000/cu mm) with 90% lymphocytes. These are uniformly similar, producing a monotonous blood picture of small lymphocytes with minimal cytoplasm. Blast cells are uncommon.
> Anemia—see Chronic Myelogenous Leukemia, pp. 315–316.
> Autoimmune hemolytic anemia occurs in 25% of patients.
> Platelet count is less likely to increase with therapy than in myelogenous leukemia.

Bone marrow
> Infiltration with earlier cell types is progressively increased. There is replacement of erythroid, myeloid, and megakaryocyte series.

Lymph node aspirate or imprint. The number of immature leukocytes, predominantly blast cells, is increased.
Uric acid levels are not increased.
Philadelphia chromosome is not found.
Serum enzyme levels are less frequently elevated and show a lesser increase than in chronic myelogenous leukemia. Even serum LDH is frequently normal.

PLASMA CELL LEUKEMIA
WBC usually >15,000, with >50% plasma cells varying from typical plasmacytes to immature and atypical forms
Other findings (see under Multiple Myeloma, pp. 322–323).

INFECTIOUS MONONUCLEOSIS
Leukopenia and granulocytopenia are evident during first week. Later, WBC is increased (usually 10,000–20,000/cu mm) because of increased lymphocytes ($\geq 50\%$), many of which are characteristically atypical. Peak changes occur in 7–10 days; may persist for 1–2 months.
Heterophil agglutination (Paul-Bunnell test) is usually more than 1:112; this is not decreased by more than 1 tube dilution following absorption with guinea pig kidney antigen but usually completely absorbed by beef red blood cell antigen (the reverse is true in normal persons and in serum sickness). Peak titer occurs in 2–3 weeks; duration is for 4–8 weeks. The agglutination is not related to lymphocytosis or to clinical severity.
Evidence of mild hepatitis (e.g., increased serum transaminase, increased urine urobilinogen) is very frequent at some stage but may be transient. Clinical jaundice occurs in <10% of patients.
Serologic test for syphilis is transient false positive.
Occasional RBCs and albumin are seen in urine.
Hemolytic anemia and thrombocytopenia are rare.

See Cytomegalic Inclusion Disease, pp. 488–489.

ACUTE INFECTIOUS LYMPHOCYTOSIS
Markedly increased WBC ($\geq 40,000$/cu mm) is due to lymphocytosis (normal appearance, small-sized lymphocytes).
Heterophil agglutination is negative.

LEUKEMIC RETICULOENDOTHELIOSIS
This is a rare condition of splenomegaly and absence of lymphadenopathy with characteristic pathologic changes in marrow and spleen that often respond to splenectomy but not to chemotherapy.
Diagnosis is established by finding the characteristic cells in the peripheral blood or bone marrow. These cells show a characteristic histochemical reaction of tartrate-resistant acid phosphatase (isoenzyme 5) activity. This isoenzyme 5 may also be increased in the serum.
Hypersplenism causing thrombocytopenia, anemia, and leukopenia of varying degrees is present.

Increased ESR may be present.
Abnormal platelet function may be found.
Leukocyte alkaline phosphatase activity is markedly increased in
  some patients.

	Leukemic Reticuloendotheliosis	Sézary Syndrome
Involvement of		
Bone marrow	Constant	Exceptional
Skin and lymph node	Uncommon	Constant
Characteristic cell	Hairy cell	Sézary cell

SÉZARY SYNDROME

Syndrome of skin lesion due to infiltration of Sézary cells as-
  sociated with presence of these cells in peripheral blood
Increased peripheral blood lymphocyte count, >10% of which are
  atypical lymphocytes (Sézary cells)
Total WBC often increased.
ESR, hemoglobin, and platelet counts usually normal
Bone marrow, lymph nodes, and liver biopsy usually normal.

CHRONIC GRANULOMATOUS DISEASE

This is a heterogeneous, genetically determined disorder of leuko-
  cyte function that appears at an early age and results in death
  due to repeated severe bacterial infections (leukocytes ingest
  bacteria normally but kill them at a slower rate).
WBCs appear normal.
Neutrophils fail to reduce nitroblue tetrazolium dye.
Serum complement and immunoglobulin levels are normal.
Leukocytosis, anemia, increased ESR, elevated gamma globulin
  levels are noted.
Infections with organisms that usually have low virulence (e.g.,
  Escherichia coli, Enterobacteriaceae, *Salmonella, Candida al-
  bicans, Serratia marcescens*).

CHÉDIAK-HIGASHI SYNDROME

This is a rare autosomal recessive genetic disease that causes
  hypopigmentation of skin, hair, and uvea.
Neutrophils contain coarse, deeply staining large granulations in
  cytoplasm and are present less frequently in other WBCs.
Pancytopenia appears during the (accelerated) "lymphomalike"
  phase.
Laboratory findings due to frequent severe pyogenic infections and
  hemorrhage (which cause early death) are noted.

AGRANULOCYTOSIS

In acute fulminant form, WBC is decreased to ≦2000/cu mm—
  sometimes as low as 50/cu mm. Granulocytes are 0–2%.
  Granulocytes may show pyknosis or vacuolization.
In chronic or recurrent form, WBC is down to 2000/cu mm with
  less marked granulocytopenia.
There is relative lymphocytosis and sometimes monocytosis.
Bone marrow shows absence of cells in granulocytic series but
  normal erythroid and megakaryocytic series.
ESR is increased.

Hemoglobin and RBC count and morphology, platelet count, and coagulation tests are normal.

Laboratory findings due to infection are noted.

Laboratory findings due to underlying causes (see Aplastic Anemia, p. 289) are noted.

PERIODIC (CYCLIC) NEUTROPENIA

In this rare condition there is a regular periodic occurrence of neutropenia.

WBC is 2000–4000/cu mm and granulocytes are as low as 0%.

Monocytosis may occur.

Eosinophilia may occur during recovery.

Bone marrow appearance is variable.

MAY-HEGGLIN ANOMALY

This is an inherited dominant abnormality of WBCs and platelets.

Large, poorly granulated platelets are associated with anomalous area in cytoplasm of all granulocytes. Usually no other hematologic abnormalities are present.

The lesion is an asymptomatic familial one.

PELGER-HUËT ANOMALY

This is an autosomal-dominant, usually heterozygous, anomaly of WBCs.

Nuclei of granulocytes lack normal segmentation but are shaped like eyeglasses, rods, dumbbells, or peanuts. Coarse chromatin is evident in nuclei of granulocytes, lymphocytes, and monocytes. These cells are present in peripheral blood and bone marrow.

No other hematologic or clinical abnormality is present.

Occasionally cells resembling those in this anomaly are seen following administration of myelotoxic agents in acute and chronic myelogenous leukemia.

ALDER-REILLY ANOMALY

Heavy azurophilic granulation of granulocytes and some lymphocytes and monocytes associated with mucopolysaccharidoses (see p. 369) are seen.

HEREDITARY HYPERSEGMENTATION OF NEUTROPHILS (simple dominant abnormality)

Hypersegmentation of neutrophils resembles that seen in pernicious anemia but is a permanent abnormality. Most neutrophils have four or more lobes.

There is a similar condition that affects only the eosinophilic granulocytes (hereditary constitutional hypersegmentation of the eosinophil).

There is also an inherited giant multilobed abnormality of neutrophilic leukocytes.

CONGENITAL ABSENCE OF SPLEEN

Presence of Heinz bodies in 5–20% of RBCs is the most characteristic finding.

Erythroblastosis (2000–40,000/cu mm) may be present, with increased frequency of Howell-Jolly bodies and target cells.
Decreased osmotic fragility may be found.

HYPERSPLENISM

The disease is either secondary to enlarged spleen (see next section) or "primary" (with no detectable underlying disease).

There are various combinations of anemia, leukopenia, thrombocytopenia associated with bone marrow showing normal or increased cellularity of affected elements (includes primary splenic pancytopenia and primary splenic neutropenia).

Chromium[51]-tagged RBCs from normal person or from patient are rapidly destroyed after transfusion, and radioactivity accumulates in spleen.

SOME CAUSES OF SPLENOMEGALY
(see appropriate separate sections)

Congestion (Banti's disease)
    Cirrhosis of the liver
    Congestive heart failure
    Thrombosis or partial occlusion of the portal or splenic veins
Hematologic diseases
    Infectious mononucleosis
    Polycythemia vera
    Leukemias and lymphomas
    Multiple myeloma, macroglobulinemia
    Myelofibrosis with myeloid metaplasia (*teardrop RBCs are pathognomonic*)
    Hemolytic anemias (e.g., thalassemias, hereditary spherocytosis, acquired hemolytic anemia, hemolytic disease of newborn)
    Thrombocytopenic purpuras
    Pernicious anemia and related macrocytic anemias
    Primary hypersplenism (see preceding section)
Infections
    Bacterial (e.g., endocarditis, septicemia, *Salmonella;* granulomas, e.g., tuberculosis, tularemia, brucellosis)
    Viral (e.g., hepatitis)
    Rickettsial (e.g., Rocky Mountain spotted fever, typhus)
    Protozoal (e.g., malaria, kala-azar)
    Metazoal (e.g., schistosomiasis)
    Mycotic (e.g., histoplasmosis, blastomycosis, coccidioidomycosis)
Collagen diseases (e.g., SLE, polyarteritis nodosa, Felty's syndrome)
Histiocytoses
    Gaucher's disease
    Nieman-Pick disease
    Histiocytosis X (Hand-Schüller-Christian disease, Letterer-Siwe disease)
Miscellaneous (e.g., sarcoidosis, amyloidosis, gargoylism, hemochromatosis)
Tumors of spleen
    Cysts (e.g., echinococcus, neoplastic)

Primary tumors (e.g., hemangioma, lymphangioma, lymphangiosarcoma)

Needle aspiration of spleen

May be useful in diseases without other manifestations, especially tuberculosis, sarcoidosis, Hodgkin's disease, carcinoma, lipid storage diseases (Niemann-Pick and Gaucher's diseases)

Contraindicated in hemorrhagic conditions, in patients with septic or tender spleen, or in unconscious patients

Caution in presence of leukopenia or mild thrombopenia

See Spleen Scanning, pp. 157–158.

Spontaneous rupture of spleen may occur in (see appropriate separate sections)

Malaria

Chronic myelogenous leukemia

Infectious mononucleosis

Splenitis

HODGKIN'S DISEASE AND OTHER MALIGNANT LYMPHOMAS

On biopsy of lymph node, the histologic findings establish diagnosis.

Blood findings may vary from completely normal to marked abnormalities.

Moderate normocytic anemia occurs, occasionally of the hemolytic type; may become severe.

WBC is variable and may be normal, decreased, or slightly or markedly increased (25,000/cu mm). Leukopenia, marked leukocytosis, anemia are bad prognostic signs. Eosinophilia occurs in $\cong 20\%$ of patients. Relative and absolute lymphopenia may occur. *If lymphocytosis is present, look for another disease.* Neutrophilia may be found. Monocytosis may be found. These changes may all be absent or may even be present simultaneously or in various combinations. Rarely, Reed-Sternberg cells are found in marrow or peripheral blood smears.

Serum protein electrophoresis. Albumin is frequently decreased. Increased alpha$_1$ and alpha$_2$ globulins suggest disease activity. Decreased gamma globulin is less frequent in Hodgkin's disease than in lymphosarcoma. Gamma globulins may be increased, with macroglobulins present and evidence of autoimmune process (e.g., hemolytic anemia, cold agglutinins, positive LE test).

ESR and CRP are increased during active stages; may be normal during remission.

BMR is increased.

Laboratory findings due to involvement of other organ systems (e.g., liver, kidney) are noted.

Beware of complicating infections, especially disseminated tuberculosis and fungal and viral (especially herpes zoster and varicella) infections.

See ^{67}Ga scanning, p. 159.

MYCOSIS FUNGOIDES

Biopsy of lesion (usually skin) shows microscopic findings that parallel clinical findings.

Laboratory findings are generally not helpful.

Bone marrow may show increase in reticuloendothelial cells, monoblasts, lymphocytes, plasma cells.

Peripheral blood may occasionally show increased eosinophils, monocytes, and lymphocytes.

CLASSIFICATION OF PLASMA CELL DYSCRASIAS

	% Frequency
Plasma cell myeloma	
Multiple myeloma—symptomatic	65
Multiple myeloma—asymptomatic and indolent	2
Localized plasmacytoma	5
Benign idiopathic monoclonal gammopathy	20
Waldenström's macroglobulinemia	8
Heavy-chain diseases	<1
Primary amyloidosis	<1

LOCALIZED PLASMACYTOMA

Myeloma proteins are low or normal concentration in serum.

Nonmyeloma immunoglobulin concentration in serum is generally normal.

Following local radiotherapy, level of any myeloma protein is reduced and level of nonmyeloma immunoglobulins may be increased above normal.

IDIOPATHIC ("BENIGN," "ASYMPTOMATIC") MONOCLONAL GAMMOPATHY
(found in 0.5% of normal persons over age 30)

The following changes are present for a period of >5 years

Monoclonal serum protein concentration <3 gm/100 ml; IgG type in 90% of patients; normal immunoglobulins not depressed

Normal serum albumin

<5% plasma cells in bone marrow

Absence of Bence Jones protein, anemia, myeloma bone lesions

May be associated with aging, cholecystitis, neoplasms, many chronic diseases.

MULTIPLE MYELOMA

Very elevated serum total protein is due to increase in globulins (with decreased A/G ratio) in 50% to two-thirds of the patients.

Serum protein immunoelectrophoresis reveals abnormal proteins in 80% of patients.

60% of patients	IgG myeloma protein
20% of patients	IgA myeloma protein
10–20% of patients	Bence Jones protein only
1–10% of patients	No abnormal protein
<1% of patients	IgD myeloma protein*

*IgD myeloma is difficult to recognize because serum levels are relatively low; specific antiserum is required to demonstrate IgD; on electrophoresis, IgD is often included in beta globulin peak, and clinical features are the same as in other types of myeloma. *Bence Jones proteinuria is almost always present, and total protein is often normal.*

Bence Jones proteinuria occurs in 35–50% of patients. (Paper-strip tests for urine protein will miss Bence Jones protein.)

Urinary electrophoresis is positive in 50% of patients.

Electrophoresis of serum or urine or both is abnormal in almost all patients. If only serum electrophoresis is performed, kappa and some lambda light-chain myelomas will be missed.

Bone marrow aspiration usually shows 20–50% plasma cells or myeloma cells; multiple sites may be required.

Hematologic findings

 Anemia (normocytic, normochromic) in 60% of patients.

 Rouleaux formation (due to serum protein changes) occasionally causing difficulty in crossmatching blood, in 85% of patients.

 Increased ESR in 90% of patients and other abnormalities due to serum protein changes

 Usually normal WBC count and platelet count; 40–55% lymphocytosis frequently present on differential count, with variable number of immature lymphocytic and plasmacytic forms

 Cold agglutinin or cryoglobulins

Laboratory findings of repeated bacterial infections, especially those due to *Diplococcus pneumoniae, Staphylococcus aureus,* and *Escherichia coli.*

See bone diseases, calcium, and phosphorus, Table 56, p. 386.

 Serum calcium is markedly increased in 25–50% of patients.

 Serum phosphorus is usually normal.

 Serum alkaline phosphatase is normal or slightly increased. Increase may reflect amyloidosis of liver rather than bone disease.

See Kidney in Multiple Myeloma, p. 448.

 BUN is increased.

 Uric acid is increased.

 Renal function is decreased.

 Urine abnormalities appear—albumin, casts, etc.

Renal failure is usually present when there is a marked increase of Bence Jones protein in blood.

Presymptomatic phase (may last up to many years) may show only

 Unexplained persistent proteinuria

 Increased ESR

 Myeloma protein in serum or urine

 Repeated bacterial infections, especially pneumonias

 Amyloidosis (see p. 520)

High tumor mass is present when *any* of the following are present:

 Hemoglobin <8.5 gm/100 ml

 Corrected calcium >11.5 mg/100 ml

 Serum IgG peak >7 gm/100 ml or IgA peak >5 gm/100 ml

Low tumor mass is present when *all* the following are present:

 Hemoglobin >10.5 gm/100 ml

 Corrected calcium <11.5 mg/100 ml

 Serum IgG peak <5 gm/100 ml or IgA peak >3 gm/100 ml

Corrected calcium (mg/100 ml) = serum calcium (mg/100 ml) − serum albumin (gm/100 ml) + 4.0.

MACROGLOBULINEMIA

Electrophoresis of serum shows an intense sharp peak in globulin fraction, usually in the gamma zone, and takes PAS stain. The pattern is indistinguishable from that in multiple myeloma.

Acrylic gel electrophoresis shows no penetration by abnormal globulin (therefore it is a macroglobulin).

Ultracentrifugation confirms the macroglobulinemia when $> 5-10\%$ of serum components have a sedimentation constant of > 16 Svedberg units (normally such components are $<2\%$)

Total serum protein and globulin are markedly increased. Immunoelectrophoresis identifies IgM as a component of increased globulin.

ESR is very high.

Rouleaux formation is marked.

There is severe anemia, usually normochromic normocytic, occasionally hemolytic.

WBC is decreased, with relative lymphocytosis; monocytes or eosinophils may be increased.

Bone marrow sections are always hypercellular and show extensive infiltration with atypical "lymphocytes" and also plasma cells.

Lymph node biopsy shows invasion of capsule and loss of architecture as seen in lymphosarcoma in $\cong 50\%$ of patients.

Spleen and liver involvement occurs in $\cong 50\%$ of patients.

Persistent oronasal hemorrhage occurs in $\cong 75\%$ of patients.

Coagulation abnormalities. There may be decreased platelets, abnormal bleeding time, coagulation time, prothrombin time, prothrombin consumption, etc.

Macroglobulinemia may be primary Waldenström's or may be associated with neoplasms, collagen diseases, cirrhosis, chronic infections.

HEAVY-CHAIN DISEASE
(This is a lymphomalike disease with excessive production of heavy-chain proteins.)

Serum protein electrophoresis
  Marked decrease in albumin
  Gamma globulin almost absent
  Narrow band of abnormal protein in region of beta or gamma globulin that is similar in serum and urine
  Immunoelectrophoresis—marked decrease of IgG, IgA, IgM

Serum tests
  Reversed A/G ratio
  Positive cephalin flocculation test
  Increased uric acid (>8.5 mg/100 ml)
  Increased BUN (30–50 mg/100 ml)

Hematologic findings
  Anemia almost always present
  Leukopenia and thrombocytopenia common
  Eosinophilia sometimes marked; relative lymphocytosis
  Vacuolated mononuclear cells sometimes seen

Bone marrow aspiration—many atypical plasma cells and
   lymphocytes (some patients)
Urine tests
   Trace to 1+ protein
   Negative for Bence Jones protein
   Identical to abnormal serum protein on electrophoresis

WISKOTT-ALDRICH SYNDROME
This is a rare immunologic sex-linked recessive condition featuring
   eczema, repeated infections, and thrombocytopenia.

Platelet count is decreased, with bleeding tendency.
There is marked susceptibility to infections (e.g., bacteria, viruses,
   fungi, *Pneumocystis carinii*)
Serum IgM is decreased.
Serum IgA is normal or may be markedly increased.
Serum IgG is normal or increased.
Blood lymphocytes are usually decreased in number, especially
   the small lymphocytes.
Incidence of malignancy of the lymphoid system is increased.

HEREDITARY ANGIOEDEMA
CBC and ESR are usually normal when the manifestation is
   peripheral or facial angioedema, but they may be abnormal when
   the manifestation is diarrhea and abdominal pain.
Serum complement-1-esterase inhibitor is either decreased or is
   functionally inactive. (Test is performed only at reference
   laboratories.)

BISALBUMINEMIA
Two albumin bands are present on serum protein electrophoresis
   in clinically healthy homozygotes or carriers.

ALPHA₁-ANTITRYPSIN DEFICIENCY
This is a congenital inherited deficiency associated with familial
   pulmonary emphysema and liver disease. The heterozygous
   state occurs in 1:20 persons with serum levels of alpha₁-
   antitrypsin in ≅60% of normal; homozygous state occurs 1:2000
   persons with serum levels ≅ 10% of normal.

Pulmonary emphysema occurs in family of 25% of patients; occurs
   in heterozygotes and homozygotes. Secondary bronchitis and
   bronchietasis may occur.
Liver disease occurs in 10–20% of children with this deficiency.
   Clinical picture may be neonatal hepatitis, prolonged obstructive
   jaundice during infancy, juvenile cirrhosis, or abnormal liver
   functions tests (e.g., SGPT) in 50% of apparently healthy
   asymptomatic patients. Liver biopsy (in both heterozygotes and
   homozygotes) shows characteristic intracytoplasmic inclusions;
   these may be found in patients with emphysema without liver
   disease and in asymptomatic heterozygous relatives, but these

Table 44. Classification of Primary Immunologic Defects

Syndrome	Number of Circulating Lymphocytes	Number of Plasma Cells	Immunoglobulin Changes	Thymus	Lymph Node Germinal Center	Lymph Node Paracortical Zone	Other Laboratory Findings
Infantile sex-linked agammaglobulinemia (Bruton's disease)	N	O	Markedly D in all	N	O	N	X; increased frequency of malignant lymphoma
Selective inability to produce IgA	N	IgA-producing plasma cells, especially in lamina propria	IgA is O; others are usually N	N	N	N	May have malabsorption syndrome, steatorrhea, bronchitis
Transient hypogammaglobulinemia of infancy	N	D	IgG is D		O or rare		X
Non-sex-linked primary immunoglobulin deficiencies (e.g., dysgammaglobulinemias—acquired, congenital)	N	V (usually D)	Present, but type and amount are V	N	Usually O Reticulum hyperplasia	Often D	X, Z; increased frequency of malignant lymphoma and autoimmune diseases
Agammaglobulinemia with thymoma (Good's syndrome)	Progressively D, often to very low levels	D or O	Markedly D in all	Enlarged (stromal epithelial spindle-cell type)	D or O	May be D	X, Z; thymoma (see p. 290); pure red cell aplasia may occur; eosinophils O or markedly D
Wiskott-Aldrich syndrome (immune deficiency with thrombopenia and eczema)	Usually progressively D	N	Usually present, but type and amount is V (frequently IgM is D and IgA is I)	N	May be D	Progressively D in lymphocytes	X, Z; eczema and thrombocytopenia; increased frequency of malignant lymphoma

Ataxia-telangiectasia (Louis-Bar syndrome)	V (usually slightly D)	V (usually present)	Usually present, but type and amount are V (frequently IgA and IgE are D or O)	Embryonic type (no Hassall's corpuscles or cortical medullary organization)	May be D	Lymphocytes D	Progressive cerebellar ataxia; telangiectasia in tissues; ovarian dysgenesis; increased frequency of malignant lymphoma; frequent pulmonary infections when IgA is D
Primary lymphopenic immunologic deficiency (Gitlin's syndrome)	V–D	V	Always present, but type and amount are V	Hypoplastic (Hassall's corpuscles and lymphoid cells D)		Marked D in tissue lymphocytes; foci of lymphocytes may be present in spleen and lymph nodes	Z
Autosomal recessive alymphocytic agammaglobulinemia (Swiss type agammaglobulinemia; Glanzmann and Riniker's lymphocytophthisis)	Markedly D	O	Markedly D in all	Hypoplastic (Hassall's corpuscles and lymphoid cells O)		Lymphocytes O or markedly D	X, Z; increased frequency of malignant lymphoma
Autosomal recessive lymphopenia with normal immunoglobulins (Nezelof's syndrome)	D	Present	N	Hypoplastic (Hassall's corpuscles and lymphoid cells O)	May be present	Lymphocytes markedly D	Z
DiGeorge's syndrome (thymic aplasia)	v (usually N)	Present	N	Absent	Present	Rare paracortical lymphocytes present	Z; absent parathyroids (tetany of the newborn); frequent cardiovascular malformations

N = normal; O = absent; D = decreased; V = variable; X = recurrent infections with pyogenic organisms; Z = frequent virus, fungus, or *Pneumocystis* infection.

Source: Adapted from M. Seligmann, H. H. Fudenberg, and R. A. Good, A proposed classification of primary immunologic deficiencies. *Am. J. Med.* 45:818, 1968.

inclusions must be searched for and stained specifically, since the rest of the pathology in the liver is not specific.
Decreased serum alpha₁ antitrypsin

HYPOANABOLIC HYPOALBUMINEMIA
This is an inherited disorder present from birth, without kidney or liver disease. Growth and development are normal. The patient is unaffected except for periodic peripheral edema.

Serum albumin is <0.3 gm/100 ml.
Total globulins are 4.5–5.5 gm/100 ml.
Serum cholesterol is increased.
Albumin synthesis is decreased, with decreased catabolism of IV injected albumin.

CLASSIFICATION OF HEMORRHAGIC DISORDERS
Vascular abnormalities
    Congenital (e.g., hereditary hemorrhagic telangiectasia)
    Acquired (see Nonthrombocytopenic Purpura, pp. 333–334)
        Infection (e.g., bacterial endocarditis, rickettsial infection)
        Immunologic (e.g., allergic purpura, drug sensitivity)
        Metabolic (e.g., scurvy, uremia)
        Miscellaneous (e.g., neoplasms, amyloidosis)
Connective tissue abnormalities
    Congenital (e.g., Ehlers-Danlos syndrome)
    Acquired (e.g., Cushing's syndrome)
Platelet abnormalities (see sections on thrombocytopenic purpura, thrombocythemia, thrombocytopathies)
Plasma coagulation defects
    Causing defective thromboplastin formation
        Hemophilia (Factor VIII deficiency)
        PTC (Factor IX) deficiency (Christmas disease)
        PTA (Factor XI) deficiency
        von Willebrand's disease
    Causing defective rate or amount of thrombin formation
        Vitamin K deficiency (due to liver disease, prolonged bile duct obstruction, malabsorption syndrome, hemorrhagic disease of the newborn, anticoagulant therapy)
        Congenital deficiency of Factor II (prothrombin), Factor V (proaccelerin, labile factor), Factor VII (proconvertin, stable factor), Factor X (Stuart factor)
    Decreased fibrinogen due to intravascular clotting and/or fibrinolysis
        Obstetric abnormalities (e.g., amniotic fluid embolism, premature separation of placenta, retention of dead fetus)
        Congenital deficiency of Factor XIII (fibrin-stabilizing factor), congenital afibrinogenemia, hypofibrinogenemia, etc.
        Neoplasms (leukemia, carcinoma of prostate, etc.)
        Transfusion reactions
        Gram-negative septicemia, meningococcemia

(Continued on p. 333)

Table 45. Summary of Coagulation Studies in Three Main Types of Hemorrhagic Conditions[a]

Condition	Platelet Count	Capillary Fragility (Rumpel-Leede tourniquet test)	Bleeding Time	Coagulation Time	Clot Retraction	Prothrombin Time	Partial Thromboplastin Time (PTT)[b]	Prothrombin Consumption Time
Platelet								
Thrombocytopenic purpura	(D)	I	(I)	N	P	N	N	I
Thrombocytopathy, etc.	(N)	N or I	(I)	N	V	N	(N or I)	N or I
Coagulation disorders	N	N	N	I	N	N	(I)	I
"Vascular" disorders	N	N	N	N	N	N	N	N

◯ = most useful diagnostic tests; D = decreased; I = increased; N = normal; P = poor; V = variable.

[a]See Table 46, pp. 330–332, for further details of subcategories of hemorrhagic conditions.

[b]PTT is the *best* single screening test for disorders of coagulation. When it is used with platelet count, prothrombin time, and bleeding time, virtually all hemorrhagic disorders will be detected.

Table 46. Summary of Coagulation Studies in Hemorrhagic Conditions

Condition	Platelet Count	Capillary Fragility (Rumpel-Leede tourniquet test)	Bleeding Time	Coagulation Time	Clot Retraction	Prothrombin Time	Partial Thromboplastin Time (PTT)	Prothrombin Consumption Time	Thromboplastin Generation Test (TGT)
Thrombocytopenic purpura	D	+	I	N	Poor	N	N	I	I
Nonthrombocytopenic purpura	N	V	N	N	N	N	N	N	N
Glanzmann's thrombasthenia	N[a]	+ or N	N or I	N	Poor	N	N	I — Corrected by platelet substitute	I
von Willebrand's disease	N	N + in severe	I or N	V	N	N	N or I	I	V Corrected by absorbed plasma
AHG (Factor VIII) deficiency (hemophilia)	N	N	N	I N in mild	N	N	I	I	I Corrected by absorbed plasma

PTC (Factor IX) deficiency (hemophilia B; Christmas disease)	N	N	N	(I) N in mild	N	N	I	(I)	(I) Corrected by serum
Factor X (Stuart) deficiency	N	N	N	N or slightly I	I	I	I	I	I
PTA (Factor XI) deficiency	N	N	N I in severe	(I)	N	N	I	I	(I) Corrected by serum or plasma
Factor XII (Hageman) deficiency	N	N	N	(I)	N	N	I	(I)	(I)
Factor XIII deficiency	N	N	N	N	N	N	N	N	N
Fibrinogen deficiency	N	N	N I in severe	I	N	(I)	I	N	N
Hypoprothrombinaemia	N	N	N or I	I	N	(I)	I	N	N
Excess dicumarol therapy	N	N + in severe	N I in severe	I N in mild	N	(I)	I	N	N
Heparin therapy	N	N	N to I	I	N				

Table 46 (Continued)

Condition	Platelet Count	Capillary Fragility (Rumpel-Leede tourniquet test)	Bleeding Time	Coagulation Time	Clot Retraction	Prothrombin Time	Partial Thromboplastin Time (PTT)	Prothrombin Consumption Time	Thromboplastin Generation Test (TGT)
Vascular purpura (e.g., Schönlein-Henoch, hereditary hemorrhagic telangiectasia)	N	N	N	N	N	N	N	N	N
Increased anti-thromboplastin	N			I		I	N	I	May be I and not corrected by absorbed plasma or aged serum
Increased anti-thrombin	N	N	N	N May be I in severe	N	I	N	N[b]	N
Increased fibrinolysin	N	N	N or I	N or I	Lysis of clot	N	N	N[b]	N

$\bigcirc$ = most useful diagnostic tests; D = decreased; I = increased; N = normal; V = variable.

[a]Platelets appear abnormal.

[b]Not useful; may be difficult to do.

Circulating anticoagulants
Heparin therapy
Dysproteinemias, SLE, postpartum state, some cases of
hemophilia, etc.

THROMBOCYTOPENIC PURPURA

Due To
Idiopathic thrombocytopenic purpura (ITP; Werlhof's disease;
purpura hemorrhagica)
Hematologic disorders
Leukemias
Anemias (aplastic, myelophthisic, pernicious anemia, ac-
quired hemolytic)
Hypersplenism (e.g., Gaucher's disease, Felty's syndrome,
sarcoidosis, congestive splenomegaly)
Thrombotic thrombocytopenic purpura
Massive blood transfusions
May-Hegglin anomaly
Other
Infections (e.g., subacute bacterial endocarditis, septicemia,
typhus)
Other diseases (e.g., disseminated lupus erythematosus)
Marrow suppressive agents (e.g., ionizing radiation, benzol, nitro-
gen mustards and other antitumor drugs)
Drug senstivity reactions (e.g., chloramphenicol and other an-
tibacterial drugs, tranquilizers, antipyretic drugs, heavy metals)

Laboratory Findings
Decreased platelet count—no bleeding until <60,000/cu mm
Positive tourniquet test
Increased bleeding time
Poor clot retraction
Normal coagulation time
Normal partial thromboplastin time
Normal prothrombin time
Bone marrow: normal or increased number of megakaryocytes but
without marginal platelets
Blood smear—decreased number of platelets, abnormal appear-
ance of platelets (small or giant or deeply stained)
Normal WBC
Laboratory findings due to hemorrhage
Increased WBC with shift to left
Anemia proportional to hemorrhage, with compensatory in-
crease in reticulocytes, polychromatophilia, etc.

NONTHROMBOCYTOPENIC PURPURA
Abnormal platelets
Thrombocytopathies
Thrombasthenia
Thrombocythemia
Other
Abnormal serum globulins
Multiple myeloma

    Macroglobulinemia
    Cryoglobulinemia
    Hyperglobulinemia
    Other
Infections (e.g., meningococcemia, subacute bacterial endocarditis, typhoid, Rocky Mountain spotted fever)
Other diseases (e.g., amyloidosis, Cushing's syndrome, polycythemia vera, hemochromatosis, diabetes mellitus, uremia)
Drugs and chemicals (e.g., mercury, phenacetin, salicylic acid, chloral hydrate)
Allergic reaction (e.g., Schönlein-Henoch purpura, serum sickness)
Diseases of the skin (e.g., Osler-Weber-Rendu disease, Ehlers-Danlos syndrome)
von Willebrand's disease
Avitaminosis (e.g., scurvy)
Miscellaneous (e.g., mechanical, orthostatic)
Blood coagulation factors (e.g., hemophilia)

THROMBOTIC THROMBOCYTOPENIC PURPURA
Thrombocytopenic purpura (see p. 333)
Hemolytic anemia with
    Increased indirect bilirubin
    Increased reticulocytes
    Microspherocytes present
    Erythroid hyperplasia of marrow
    Negative Coombs' test
Various bizarre RBC (burr cells) in peripheral blood smear
Increased WBC and neutrophils
Urine findings due to renal miliary infarcts (see p. 445)
Biopsy of lymph node

PRIMARY HEMORRHAGIC THROMBOCYTHEMIA
Platelets >800,000/cu mm
No evidence of leukemia or polycythemia in peripheral blood or marrow
Bone marrow—hyperplasia of all elements, with predominance of megakaryocytes and platelet masses, eosinophilia, basophilia
Iron deficiency anemia due to bleeding
Thrombohemorrhagic disease (bleeding—skin, gastrointestinal tract, nose, gums)

GLANZMANN'S THROMBASTHENIA
Probably represents a heterogeneous group of conditions incompletely studied and delineated
Normal platelet count with abnormal platelet morphology (e.g., variation in platelet size, increased platelet size, abnormal clumping and spreading)
Poor clot retraction and increased bleeding time may be present.
Normal coagulation time
TGT and prothrombin consumption tests abnormal but corrected by adding platelet substitute
Capillary fragility sometimes abnormal

VASCULAR ABNORMALITIES CAUSING HEMORRHAGE
Hereditary telangiectasia (Osler-Weber-Rendu disease)
Anaphylactoid purpura (Schönlein-Henoch)
Vascular purpura (associated with uremia, diabetes mellitus, chronic infection, hypertension, postirradiation, etc.) (other conditions, including "vascular pseudohemophilia")
Pigmented purpuric eruptions (e.g., angioma serpiginosum)

ALLERGIC PURPURA
This is called Henoch's purpura when abdominal symptoms are predominant and Schönlein's purpura when joint symptoms are predominant.
Platelet count, bleeding time, coagulation time, and clot retraction are normal.
Tourniquet test may be negative or positive.
WBC and neutrophils may be increased; eosinophils may be increased.
Stool may show blood.
Urine usually contains RBCs and slight to marked protein.
Renal biopsy shows positive immunohistologic findings and typical glomerular histologic changes.

VON WILLEBRAND'S DISEASE
This is probably the same disease as pseudohemophilia, angiohemophilia, and vascular hemophilia. It is an autosomal dominant hereditary deficiency of unknown plasma substance needed for Factor VIII synthesis and capillary hemostasis.
Bleeding time is prolonged.
Factor VIII deficiency is indicated with abnormal TGT but level of Factor VIII is extremely variable.
Platelet count is normal.
Clot retraction is normal.
Coagulation time may be normal or increased, depending on level of Factor VII.
Tourniquet test may be positive.
Platelet adhesiveness to glass beads is decreased.
Characteristic triad of prolonged bleeding time, Factor VIII deficiency, and decreased platelet adhesiveness may be present in any combination; presence or absence of these abnormalities correlates poorly with history of bleeding.

HEMOPHILIA (FACTOR VIII DEFICIENCY; AHG DEFICIENCY)
Classic hemophilia (assay of Factor VIII <2%) shows increased bleeding time, coagulation time, prothrombin consumption time, and partial thromboplastin time.
Moderate hemophilia (assay of Factor VIII <3%) shows normal coagulation time and normal prothrombin consumption time but increased partial thromboplastin time.
In mild hemophilia (assay of Factor VIII <16%) and "sub-hemophilia" (assay of Factor VIII 20–30%), these laboratory tests may be normal.
Abnormal TGT is corrected by absorbed plasma.
Laboratory findings due to hemorrhage and anemia are noted.

PTC (FACTOR IX) DEFICIENCY (CHRISTMAS DISEASE; HEMOPHILIA B)
In mild deficiency, only the TGT may be abnormal.

In more severe cases, increased coagulation time, bleeding time, prothrombin consumption time, and partial thromboplastin time are found.

Defect is corrected by frozen plasma just as well as by bank blood.

FACTOR X (STUART-PROWER) DEFICIENCY
This infrequent autosomal recessive defect resembles Factor VII deficiency; heterozygotes show mild or no clinical manifestations.

Increased prothrombin time (not corrected by use of viper venom as thromboplastin) is not corrected by administration of vitamin K. Heterozygotes may have only slight increase in prothrombin time.

Acquired form may be associated with amyloidosis.

PTA (FACTOR XI) DEFICIENCY
In mild form, coagulation may be normal, prothrombin consumption time is slightly increased, and TGT is abnormal.

In severe cases, increased coagulation time, increased prothrombin consumption time, and abnormal TGT are found.

Postoperative bleeding may not begin until several days after surgery.

FACTOR XII (HAGEMAN FACTOR) DEFICIENCY
Coagulation time and prothrombin consumption time are increased; TGT is abnormal.

No hemorrhagic symptoms occur.

CONGENITAL DEFICIENCY OF FACTOR XIII (FIBRIN-STABILIZING FACTOR)
This is an unusual disease with severe coagulation defect.

All standard clotting tests appear normal.

Patient's fibrin clot is soluble in 5M urea.

Whole blood clot is qualitatively friable.

Acquired type may occur in
    Acute myelogenous leukemia
    Liver disease
    Association with hypofibrinogenemia in obstetrical complications

FIBRINOGEN DEFICIENCY
Congenital
    Afibrinogenemia, hypofibrinogenemia, dysfibrinogenemia
Acquired (see Disseminated Intravascular Coagulation, pp. 337–338)
    Obstetric (amniotic fluid embolism, meconium embolism, abruptio placentae, septic abortion, missed abortion with prolonged retention, eclampsia)
    Surgical procedures (e.g., prostate, T and A, open heart, lung)

Neoplasms (e.g., carcinoma of prostate, carcinoma of lung)
Hematologic conditions (e.g., leukemia, lymphomas, multiple myeloma, acquired hemolytic anemias, hemolytic transfusion reaction, thrombotic thrombocytopenic purpura)
Other (e.g., cirrhosis, fat embolism, shock, burns, septicemia, drugs, snake bite)
Often associated with depletion of other coagulation factors (e.g., Factors V and VIII, platelets) and presence of circulating anticoagulants
Severe bleeding with failure of blood to clot, abnormal prothrombin time and thrombin time, lysis of clot, decreased platelets, etc.
Fibrinolysis (lysis of sterile whole blood clot in 24 hours)
    Acute hemorrhage
    Severe burns
    Postoperative, obstetric states
    Drug poisoning (e.g., phenobarbital)
    Cirrhosis of liver
    Shock
Inhibition of fibrin formation
    Dysproteinemia and paraproteinemia (e.g., multiple myeloma, macroglobulinemia, cryoglobulinemia)

CONGENITAL AFIBRINOGENEMIA
This is a rare inherited autosomal recessive congenital condition.
Plasma fibrinogen is absent.
Bleeding time is often increased (one-third of patients).
Prothrombin and thrombin times are abnormal.
Platelet-to-glass adhesiveness is abnormal unless fibrinogen is added.

CONGENITAL (CONSTITUTIONAL) HYPOFIBRINOGENEMIA
Plasma fibrinogen is decreased.
Bleeding and coagulation times are normal.
Blood clots are soft and small.

CONGENITAL DYSFIBRINOGENEMIA
A rare congenital familial condition; it may have no bleeding diathesis.
Blood clot formation is abnormally slow.

DISSEMINATED INTRAVASCULAR COAGULATION (DIC)
See Table 47, p. 339.

Not only is the clinical picture very variable, but the laboratory findings in a particular patient differ from the textbook composite, depending on the underlying disease, duration (acute or chronic), and compensatory or overreactive coagulation mechanisms.
Many of the laboratory abnormalities may be present in patients with predisposing conditions (e.g., carcinoma of prostate, inop-

erable lung carcinoma) in whom DIC is latent; these abnormalities may predict development of DIC precipitated by surgery.

In addition to the findings listed in Table 47 (p. 339), the following abnormalities often occur

Schistocytes may be seen in the peripheral blood smear; other evidence of intravascular hemolysis may be present (e.g., increased serum LDH, decreased serum haptoglobin).

Ethanol gelation and protamine gelation tests (that reflect fibrinogen degradation products but are less specific) may be positive and may be useful for screening purposes.

Cryofibrinogen may be present.

Observation of the blood clot may show the clot that forms to be small, friable, and wispy because of the hypofibrinogenemia.

Plasma Factors V, VIII, and XIII are usually significantly decreased but are not used for primary diagnosis because of time and technical complexity.

Survival time of radioiodine-labeled fibrinogen and rate of incorporation of ^{14}C-labeled glycine ethyl ester into soluble "circulating fibrin" are sensitive indicators of DIC.

Clotting time determinations are used to monitor heparin therapy.

Underlying conditions:

Tissue injury—pregnancy and obstetric complications (e.g., abruptio placentae, intrauterine fetal death, amniotic fluid embolism), extensive surgery, neoplasms (especially prostate), leukemias, chemotherapy of neoplasia, large traumatic injuries and burns

Endothelial injury—infections, prolonged hypotension

Injury of platelets or RBCs—immunologic hemolytic anemias

Reticuloendothelial system injury—liver disease (cirrhosis, hepatitis), postsplenectomy

Vascular malformations—giant hemangiomas, aortic aneurysm

Suspect clinically in patients with underlying conditions who show bleeding (frequently acute and dramatic), purpura or petechiae, acrocyanosis, arterial or venous thrombosis.

HEMORRHAGIC DISEASE OF THE NEWBORN
(due to lack of vitamin K)

Prothrombin time is markedly increased.

Bleeding time and coagulation time are normal; may be slightly increased.

Capillary fragility, clotting time, prothrombin consumption, and platelet count are normal.

Laboratory findings due to blood loss are noted.

CONGENITAL HYPOPROTHROMBINEMIA

This is a very rare condition possibly representing autosomal recessive defect.

Increased prothrombin time (prothrombin level $\cong 10\%$ of normal) is not corrected by administration of vitamin K.

Clotting time may be normal or increased.

Table 47. Disseminated Intravascular Coagulation (DIC; Consumption Coagulopathy)

Determination	% of Cases Abnormal	Abnormal Level for DIC	Mean Values for DIC	Response to Heparin Therapy	Tests
Decreased platelet count (per cu mm)	93	<150,000	52,000	None or may take weeks	Platelet count, prothrombin time, fibrinogen level are performed first as screening tests; if all three are positive, diagnosis is considered established. If only two of these are positive, diagnosis should be confirmed by at least one of the tests for fibrinolysis.
Increased prothrombin time (seconds)	90	>15	18.0	Becomes normal or falls >5 sec in few hours to 1 day	
Decreased fibrinogen level (mg/100 ml)	71	<160	137	Rises significantly (>40 mg) in 1–3 days	
Latex test for fibrinogen degradation products (titer)	92	>1:16	1:52	Begins to fall in 1 day; if very high, may take >1 week to become normal	Tests for fibrinolysis
Prolonged thrombin time (seconds)	59	>25	27		
Euglobulin clot lysis time (minutes)	42	<120	27	Returns to normal	

[a]Platelet count is not a satisfactory indicator of response to heparin therapy.

Source: Adapted from R. W. Colman, S. J. Robboy, and J. D. Minna, Disseminated intravascular coagulation (DIC): An approach. *Am. J. Med.* 52:679, 1972.

CONGENITAL FACTOR V DEFICIENCY (PARAHEMOPHILIA)
This is an infrequent autosomal recessive defect in which bleeding occurs only in the homozygote.
Variable increase in prothrombin time, prothrombin consumption, and coagulation time is not corrected by administration of vitamin K.

CONGENITAL FACTOR VII DEFICIENCY
With this infrequent autosomal trait bleeding occurs when the gene is homozygous; heterozygotes have little or no manifestations.
Increased prothrombin time (*normal when viper venom is used as thromboplastin; this does not correct prothrombin time in Factor X deficiency*) is not corrected by administration of vitamin K.
Bleeding time, coagulation time, clot retraction, prothrombin consumption, and TGT are normal.

CIRCULATING ANTICOAGULANTS
Various types of anticoagulants may interfere with coagulation at different stages, especially Factor VIII, heparinlike activity, antithromboplastins.

See Classification of Hemorrhagic Disorders, pp. 328, 333, and Table 46, pp. 330–332.

CRYOFIBRINOGENEMIA
Plasma precipitates when oxalated blood is refrigerated at 4 °C overnight.
May cause erroneous WBC count when performed on electronic cell counter.
May be associated with increased alpha$_1$ antitrypsin, haptoglobin, alpha$_2$ macroglobulin (by immunodiffusion technique), and with increased plasma fibrinogen. Not associated with cryoglobulins.
Has been reported in association with many conditions, especially
    Neoplasms
    Thromboembolic conditions

CRYOGLOBULINEMIA
May be associated with
    Immunoproliferative diseases (e.g., multiple myeloma, Waldenström's macroglobulinemia, chronic lymphatic leukemia or lymphoma)
    Collagen disease (e.g., systemic lupus erythemastosus, polyarteritis nodosa, rheumatoid arthritis)
    Autoimmune diseases (e.g., hemolytic anemia)
    Idiopathic
Cryoprecipitate may be seen in serum.
May cause erroneous WBC count when performed on electronic cell counter.
Rouleaux formation may occur.
ESR may be increased at 37 °C but is normal at room temperature.
Laboratory findings of renal disease may occur.
Laboratory findings of associated conditions.

DANGERS OF BLOOD TRANSFUSIONS

Transfusion reaction due to mismatch of donor and recipient bloods

Hyperkalemia (due to breakdown of stored RBCs); rise in serum potassium to 15–20 mEq/L 10–14 days after blood is drawn from donor

Citrate toxicity due to anticoagulant—from rapid transfusion or liver disease; sometimes decreased serum ionized calcium or acidosis followed by metabolic alkalosis

Bleeding due to decreased platelets and alteration of other coagulation factors

Infections (e.g., serum hepatitis, syphilis, malaria, brucellosis)

Gram-negative toxemia due to administration of contaminated blood

Hemosiderosis due to excessive number of blood transfusions

Other (e.g., allergic, circulatory)

METABOLIC AND HEREDITARY DISEASES

In analysing acid-base disorders, several precautions should be kept in mind

Determination of pH and blood gases should be performed on *arterial* blood.

Determination of electrolytes, pH, and blood gases ideally should be performed on blood specimens obtained *simultaneously*, since the acid-base situation is very labile.

Repeated determinations may often be indicated because of the development of complications, the effect of therapy, and other factors.

Acid-base disorders are often mixed rather than in the pure form usually described in textbooks. These mixed disorders may represent simultaneously occurring diseases, complications superimposed on the primary condition, or the effect of treatment. The clinician is referred elsewhere for more detailed information about the use of "confidence bands" to distinguish pure and mixed disorders.

Changes in chronic forms may be notably different from those in the acute forms.

METABOLIC ACIDOSIS

Due To

Increased formation of acids

Ketosis (e.g., diabetes mellitus, starvation, hyperthyroidism, high-fat and low-carbohydrate diet, after trauma)

Cellular hypoxia, including lactic acidosis (e.g., due to pulmonary disease in which respiratory acidosis often obscures the metabolic acidosis, decreased cardiac output, cardiopulmonary bypass, shock)

Decreased excretion of H^+

Renal failure (e.g., prerenal, renal, postrenal)

Renal tubular acidosis, Fanconi syndrome

Acquired (drugs, hypercalcemia)

Inherited (cystinosis, Wilson's disease)

Addison's disease

Increased acid intake (e.g., ion exchange resins, salicylates, ammonium chloride, ACD in stored blood)

Increased loss of alkaline body fluids

Intestine (e.g., diarrhea, fistulas, aspiration of contents)

Biliary (biliary and pancreatic fluids)

Renal (carbonic anhydrase inhibitors)

Secondary to other metabolic disorders (excess potassium, alkalosis)

Laboratory Findings

Serum pH is decreased ($<7.3–7.4$)

Total plasma CO_2 content is decreased; less than 15 mEq/L almost certainly rules out respiratory alkalosis.

In evaluating acid-base disorders, calculate the anion gap, which is the concentration of sodium minus (bicarbonate + chloride) (normal = < 12 mEq/L). The metabolic acidosis with a normal anionic gap is hyperchloremic and may be due to loss of alkaline body fluids, renal tubular acidosis, or the effect of certain drugs that are potassium-sparing diuretics (e.g., spironolactone) or carbonic anhydrase–inhibiting diuretics (e.g., acetazolamide). When the anion gap is > 12–14 mEq/L, diabetic ketoacidosis is the most common cause, uremic acidosis is the second most common cause, and drug ingestion (e.g., salicylates, methyl alcohol, ethylene glycol, ethyl alcohol) is the third most common cause; lactic acidosis (see below) should always be considered when these three causes are ruled out. (*Abnormal proteins, as in myeloma, are positively charged and lower the anionic gap.*)

Serum potassium is frequently increased; it is decreased in renal tubular acidosis, diarrhea, or carbonic anhydrase inhibition.

Azotemia suggests metabolic acidosis due to renal failure.

There is decreased pCO_2 when acidosis becomes well established.

Urine is strongly acid (pH = 4.5–5.2) if renal function is normal.

LACTIC ACIDOSIS

Condition of increased blood lactic acid, with evidence of acidosis and abnormal lactate-pyruvate ratio (normal ratio is 10:1) (normal = 1.0 mEq/L and 0.1 mEq/L, respectively)

Type I (increased blood lactic acid but without significant acidosis and with a normal lactate-pyruvate ratio)

Muscular exercise
Hyperventilation
Glucagon
Glycogen storage disease
Anemia, severe
Pyruvate infusion
HCO_3 infusion
Glucose and insulin infusion

Type II-A (conditions associated with hypoxia and known to cause lactic acidosis)

Acute hemorrhage
Circulatory collapse
Cyanotic heart disease
Severe acute congestive heart failure
Acute anoxemia
Extracorporeal circulation
Epinephrine

Type II-B (idiopathic)

Mild uremia
Infections, especially pyelonephritis
Septicemia
Cirrhosis
Acute pancreatitis (?)
Pregnancy (third trimester)

Severe vascular disease
Leukemia
Anemia
Chronic alcoholism
Subacute bacterial endocarditis
Poliomyelitis
Diabetes ⎫
Phenformin ⎭ cause in 50% of patients

Type II-B (usually has a typical clinical picture [e.g., acute onset following nausea and vomiting, altered state of consciousness, hyperventilation], high mortality, and the following laboratory findings)
Decreased serum bicarbonate
Low serum pH, usually 6.98–7.25
Increased serum potassium, often 6–7 mEq/L
Serum chloride, normal or low with increased anion gap
Increased blood lactate with a lactate-pyruvate ratio >10:1
Increased WBC
Increased SGOT, LDH, and phosphorus in serum

METABOLIC ALKALOSIS

Due To
Loss of acid
     Vomiting, gastric suction, gastrocolic fistula
     Diarrhea in mucoviscidosis (rarely)
     Aciduria secondary to potassium depletion
Excess of base due to administration of
     Absorbable antacids (e.g., sodium bicarbonate)
     Salts of weak acids (e.g., sodium lactate, sodium or potassium citrate)
Some vegetable diets
Potassium depletion (causing sodium and H^+ to enter the cells)
     Gastrointestinal loss (e.g., chronic diarrhea)
     Lack of potassium intake (e.g., anorexia nervosa, IV fluids without potassium supplements for treatment of vomiting or postoperatively)
     Diuresis (e.g., mercurials, thiazides, osmotic diuresis)
     Adrenal steroids (e.g., primary aldosteronism, Cushing's disease, administration of steroids, large amounts of licorice)
     Glycogen deposition
     Chronic alkalosis
     Potassium-losing nephropathy

Laboratory Findings
Serum pH is increased.
Total plasma CO_2 is increased (bicarbonate >30 mEq/L).
pCO_2 is normal or slightly increased.
Serum potassium is usually decreased, which condition is the chief danger in metabolic alkalosis.
Serum chloride is relatively lower than sodium.
BUN may be increased.

Table 48. Illustrative Serum Electrolyte Values in Various Conditions

Electrolyte	Normal	Metabolic Acidosis							Metabolic Alkalosis			Respiratory Acidosis	Respiratory Alkalosis
		Diabetic Acidosis	Fasting	Severe Diarrhea	Hyperchloremic Acidosis	Addison's Disease	Nephritis	Nephrosis	Vomiting	Pyloric Obstruction	Duodenal Obstruction		
pH	7.35–7.45	7.2	7.2	7.2	7.2	7.2	7.2	7.2	7.6	7.6	7.6	7.1	7.6
Bicarbonate	24–26	10	16	12	12	22	8	20	38	58	42	30	14
Potassium	3.5–5.0	5.6	5.2	3.2	5.2	6.5	4	5.5	3.2	3.2	3.2	5.5	5.5
Sodium	136–145	122	142	128	142	111	129	138	150	132	138	142	136
Chloride	100–106	80	100	96	116	72	90	113	94	42	49	80	112

Table 49. Laboratory Findings in Some Syndromes Associated with Persistent Hypokalemia[a]

	Serum Sodium	Serum Renin	Serum Aldosterone	Hypertension Present
Primary hyperaldosteronism	N or I	D	I	+
Secondary hyperaldosteronism	N or I	I	I	+
Pseudoaldosteronism	N	D	N or D	+
Bartter's syndrome	N or D	I	I	N
Cushing's syndrome	N or D	D	N	+
17-Hydroxylase deficiency	N	D	D	+
Periodic paralysis	N	N		N
Fanconi's syndrome	D		N	N
Renal tubular acidosis	N	I	N	N
Salt-losing nephritis	D		I	+
Renal tumor	N	N	N	N
Renin-secreting tumor	N	I		+
Familial hypokalemia with renal interstitial fibrosis	N or D	I	N	N

N = normal; I = increased; D = decreased; + = hypertension.

[a] See elsewhere in text for other findings in these conditions.

Source: Adapted from W. Z. Potter et al., *Am. J. Med.* 57:971, 1974.

Urine pH is >7.0 (≦7.9) if potassium depletion is not severe and concomitant sodium deficiency (e.g., vomiting) is not present.

When the urine chloride is low (<10–20 mEq/L) and the patient responds to NaCl treatment, the cause is more likely loss of gastric juice, diuretic therapy, or relief of chronic hypercapnia.

When the urine chloride is high (>10–20 mEq/L) and the patient does not respond to NaCl treatment, the cause is more likely hyperadrenalism or severe potassium deficiency.

RESPIRATORY ACIDOSIS
Laboratory findings differ in acute and chronic condition.

Acute
Due to decreased alveolar ventilation (e.g., pulmonary edema, bronchoconstriction, plugs). Acidosis is severe (pH of 7.05–7.10), but bicarbonate concentration is only 29–30 mEq/L.

Severe mixed acidosis is common in cardiac arrest when respiratory and circulatory failure causes marked respiratory acidosis and severe lactic acidosis.

Chronic
Due to chronic obstructive or restrictive pulmonary disease.

Acidosis is not usually severe.

Beware of commonly occurring mixed acid-base disturbances (e.g., chronic respiratory acidosis with superimposed acute hypercapnia resulting from acute infection, such as bronchitis or pneumonia).

Superimposed metabolic alkalosis (e.g., due to diuretics or vomiting) may exacerbate the hypercapnia.

RESPIRATORY ALKALOSIS

Due To
Pulmonary emboli
Asthma
Central nervous system disorders
Salicylate intoxication
Liver disease
Bacteremia

Laboratory Findings
Acute hypocapnia—usually only a modest decrease in plasma bicarbonate concentrations and marked alkalosis

Chronic hypocapnia—usually only a slightly alkaline pH

KWASHIORKOR
(most severe form of protein-calorie malnutrition that includes marasmus and nutritional dwarfism)

Serum albumin is decreased (usually 1.5–2.5 gm/100 ml but may be <1.0 gm/100 ml). Correlates with the degree of fatty liver and of edema; becomes normal after 3 weeks of normal diet; is standard test for diagnosis of kwashiorkor and to monitor response to treatment. Serum total protein shows corresponding low level.

No significant proteinuria is present.

Plasma nonessential amino acids are increased, especially glycine, alanine, serine.

Plasma essential amino acids are markedly decreased, especially tyrosine, tryptophan, and branched-chain amino acids.

BUN is decreased.

Serum cholesterol, triglycerides, amylase, lipase, alkaline phosphatase are decreased.

Beta globulins, transferrin, ceruloplasmin, copper, iron, and folic acid are decreased; serum vitamin B_{12} is usually increased.

Serum immunoglobulins are usually increased but may be normal.

Anemia is moderate and normochromic, with macrocytosis.

Laboratory changes due to complications (e.g., decreased prothrombin time and increased serum bilirubin due to liver involvement, decreased platelet count due to severe infection, rickets, infections with measles or gram-negative bacilli) are present.

Biopsy of liver reveals increased fat and glycogen and later cirrhotic changes.

MARASMUS

Serum albumin is normal or slightly decreased; globulin is normal or slightly increased.

Plasma amino acids show normal pattern or resemble that in kwashiorkor.

BUN is decreased unless dehydration is present.

Anemia is moderate.

Serum immunoglobulins are usually normal.

Laboratory changes due to associated conditions (e.g., malabsorption, chronic infections) are present.

NUTRITIONAL DWARFISM

Serum proteins, amino acids, and BUN are usually normal.

Anemia is not prominent.

Laboratory changes due to underlying conditions (e.g., intestinal malabsorption, chronic vomiting, congenital heart disease, chronic infections, chronic renal insufficiency) are present.

SCURVY (VITAMIN C DEFICIENCY)

Plasma level of ascorbic acid is decreased—usually 0 in frank scurvy. Normal is 0.5–1.5 mg/100 ml but lower level does not prove diagnosis.

Ascorbic acid in buffy coat is decreased—usually absent in clinical scurvy. Normal is 30 mg/100 ml.

Tyrosyl compounds are present in urine (detected by Millon's reagent) in patients with scurvy but are absent in normal persons after protein meal or administration of tyrosine.

Serum alkaline phosphatase is decreased; serum calcium and phosphorus are normal.

Rumpel-Leede test is positive.

Microscopic hematuria is present in one-third of patients.

Stool may be positive for occult blood.

Laboratory findings due to associated deficiencies (e.g., anemia due to folic acid deficiency) are present.

BERIBERI (THIAMINE DEFICIENCY)

Increased blood pyruvic acid level.

Decreased thiamine level in blood and urine. Becomes normal within 24 hours after therapy begins (thus baseline levels should be established first).

Laboratory findings due to complications (e.g., heart failure).

Laboratory findings due to underlying conditions (e.g., chronic diarrhea, inadequate intake).

VITAMIN A DEFICIENCY

Decreased plasma level of vitamin A. <25 IU/ml is significantly low. *Elevated carotenoids may cause false low values for vitamin A.*

RIBOFLAVIN DEFICIENCY

Decreased riboflavin level in plasma, RBCs, WBCs

PELLAGRA (NIACIN DEFICIENCY)

Decreased excretion of niacin metabolites (nicotinamide) in 6- or 24-hour urine sample

Plasma tryptophan level markedly decreased

PYRIDOXINE (VITAMIN B$_6$) DEFICIENCY

Decreased pyridoxic acid in urine

Decreased serum levels of vitamin B$_6$

FOLIC ACID DEFICIENCY

See pp. 292, 293.

CLASSIFICATION OF SOME INHERITED METABOLIC CONDITIONS

Disorders of carbohydrate metabolism
    Diabetes mellitus
    Pentosuria
    Fructosuria
    Familial lactose intolerance
    Galactosemia
    Glycogen storage diseases
    Mucopolysaccharidoses
    Other
Disorders of amino acid metabolism
    Phenylketonuria
    Tyrosinosis
    Maple syrup urine disease
    Alkaptonuria
    Other
Disorders of purine and pyrimidine metabolism
    Gout
    Orotic aciduria
    Beta-aminoisobutyric aciduria
    Other
Disorders of lipid metabolism
    Essential familial hypercholesterolemia
    Inherited deficiency of lipoprotein lipase

Disorders of porphyrin metabolism
Disorders of metabolism involving metals
    Wilson's disease
    Hemochromatosis
    Periodic paralysis
    Adynamia episodica hereditaria
    Other
Disorders of renal tubular function
    Fanconi syndrome of cystinosis
    Vitamin D–resistant rickets of primary hypophosphatemia
    Cystinuria
    Renal glycosuria
    Other
Disorders of serum enzymes
    Hypophosphatasia
    Other
Disorders of plasma proteins
    Analbuminemia
    Agammaglobulinemia
    Atransferrinemia
    Other
Disorders of blood
    Coagulation diseases (e.g., hemophilias)
    RBC G-6-PD deficiency
    Hemoglobinopathies and thalassemias
    Hereditary spherocytosis
    Hereditary nonspherocytic hemolytic anemia
    Other

DETECTING HETEROZYGOUS CARRIERS OF SOME DISORDERS*

Disorder	*Abnormality*
Duchenne type of muscular dystrophy	Increased serum CPK
Gout	Increased serum uric acid
Wilson's disease	Abnormality detected by [48]Cu studies
G-6-PD deficiency	Decreased G-6-PD in RBCs
Orotic aciduria	Decreased orotidylic decarboxylase in RBCs
Hemoglobinopathies (e.g., thalassemia)	Abnormality detected by hemoglobin electrophoresis
Tay-Sachs disease	Decreased serum fructose 1-phosphate aldolase
Glycogen storage disease (Type III)	Decreased amylo-1, 6-glucosidase in leukocytes
Glycogen storage disease (von Gierke's, Type I)	Decreased glucose-6-phosphate in intestinal mucosa

*D.Y.Y.Hsia, The diagnosis of carriers of disease-producing genes. *Ann. N.Y. Acad. Sci.* 134:946, 1966.

Phenylketonuria	Prolonged increase in serum phenylalanine after phenylalanine load
Argininosuccinic aciduria	Decreased argininosuccinase in RBCs and increased argininosuccinic acid in urine
Cystathioninuria	Increased cystathionine in urine
Cystinuria	Increased cystine and lysine in urine
Homocystinuria	Decreased cystathionine synthetase in liver
Histidinemia	Decreased histidase in skin
Hyperoxaluria	Abnormality detected by special radioisotope study
Galactosemia	Decreased galactose-1-p-uridyl transferase in RBCs

DETECTING INBORN ERRORS OF METABOLISM BY AMNIOTIC FLUID CELLS*

Amino acid metabolism
    Argininosuccinicaciduria
    Citrullinemia
    Cystinosis
    Homocystinuria
    Hyperammonemia, Type 2
    Maple syrup urine disease
    Methylmalonic acidemia
    Methylmalonic aciduria
    Ornithine alpha-ketoacid transaminase deficiency
    Propionic acidemia
Carbohydrate metabolism
    Galactosemia
    Glycogen storage disease, Type II (Pompe's disease)
Lipid metabolism
    Fabry's disease
    Gaucher's disease
    G_{M_1} gangliosidosis, Type 1
    G_{M_1} gangliosidosis, Type 2
    G_{M_2} gangliosidosis, Type 1 (Tay-Sachs disease)
    G_{M_2} gangliosidosis, Type 2 (Sandhoff's disease)
    G_{M_2} gangliosidosis, Type 3
    Krabbe's disease
    Metachromatic leukodystrophy
    Niemann-Pick disease
Miscellaneous
    I-cell disease
    Lesch-Nyhan syndrome
    Lysosomal acid phosphatase deficiency
Mucopolysaccharide metabolism
    Mucopolysaccharidoses

*A. B. Gerbie and J. L. Simpson, Antenatal detection of genetic disorders. *Postgrad. Med.* 59(6):131, 1976.

Table 50. Comparison of Types of Hyperlipoproteinemia

Point of Comparison	Type I (rarest)	Type IIa (relatively common)	Type IIb (relatively common)
Origin	Exogenous hyperlipidemia		Overindulgence hyperlipidemia
Definition	Familial fat-induced hyperglycidemia	Hyper-beta-lipoproteinemia (hypercholesterolemia)	Combined hyperlipidemia (mixed hyperlipidemia)
Age	Usually under age 10		
Gross appearance of plasma	On standing: supernatant creamy, infranatant clear	Clear (no cream layer on top)	No cream layer on top; clear to turbid infranatant
Serum cholesterol	Normal or slightly increased	Markedly increased (300–600 mg/100 ml)	Markedly increased (300–600 mg/100 ml)
Serum triglycerides	Markedly increased (usually > 2000 mg/100 ml)	Normal	Increased ≤ 400 mg/100 ml
Appearance of lipoprotein components visualized by electrophoresis			
Chylomicron[a]	Marked I	0	0
Beta-lipoprotein[b]	N or D	I	I
Pre-beta lipoprotein[c]	N or D	N	I
Alpha-lipoprotein[d]			
Other laboratory abnormalities	Glucose tolerance usually normal		
Triglyceride-cholesterol ratio	8	1	Variable

Type III (relatively uncommon)	Type IV (most common)	Type V (uncommon)
	Endogenous hyperlipidemia	Mixed endogenous and exogenous hyperlipidemia
Carbohydrate-induced hyperglyceridemia with hypercholesterolemia	Carbohydrate-induced hyperglyceridemia without hypercholesterolemia	Combined fat and carbohydrate-induced hyperglyceridemia
Not known under age 25	Only occasionally seen in children	
Clear, cloudy, or milky	Slightly turbid to cloudy Unchanged on standing	Markedly turbid On standing: supernatant creamy, infranatant milky
Markedly increased (300–1000 mg/100 ml)	Normal or slightly increased	Increased (250–500 mg/100 ml)
Markedly increased (200–1000 mg/100 ml)	Markedly increased (200–2000 mg/100 ml)	Markedly increased (500–3000 mg/100 ml)
0	0	1
I Floating beta	N or I	N or I
I	I	I
Hyperglycemia; glucose tolerance often abnormal; serum uric acid often increased	Glucose tolerance often abnormal; serum uric acid often increased	Glucose tolerance usually abnormal; serum uric acid usually increased
<2	1–5	>5

Table 50 (Continued)

Point of Comparison	Type I (rarest)	Type IIa (relatively common)	Type IIb (relatively common)
Lipid changes resembling primary hyperlipidemias			
Diet		Very high cholesterol diet	Same as Type IIa
Drugs		Triglyceride-lowering drugs in Types III and IV	Same as Type IIa
Primary disease		Myxedema Nephrosis Obstructive liver disease Stress Porphyria Anorexia nervosa Idiopathic hypercalcemia	Same as Type IIa

0 = absent; N = normal; I = increased; D = decreased.

[a]Chylomicrons represent exogenous triglyceride concentration.

[b]Beta-lipoproteins (low-density lipoproteins, or LDL) represent major portions of cholesterol concentration.

[c]Pre-beta lipoproteins (very-low-density lipoproteins, or VLDL) represent endogenous triglyceride concentration.

[d]Alpha-lipoproteins (high-density lipoproteins, or HDL) are not known to have pathologic significance in hyperlipoproteinemia.

Obtain blood only after at least 12–14 hours' fasting and when patient has been on usual diet for at least 2 weeks.

Rule out diabetes and pancreatitis in all groups.

Type III (relatively uncommon)	Type IV (most common)	Type V (uncommon)
	Caffeine or alcohol before testing	
Triglyceride-lowering drugs in Type IV	Cholesterol-lowering drugs Chlorthiazide Birth control pills or estrogens	
Myxedema Dysgammaglobulinemia Liver disease	Nephrotic syndrome Hypothyroidism Pregnancy Glycogen storage dis- ease	Myeloma Macroglobulinemia Nephrosis

Increased susceptibility to coronary artery disease occurs in Types II, III, IV. Accelerated peripheral vascular disease in Type III.

Xanthomas appear in Types I, II, III.

Abdominal pain occurs in Types I, V.

If dietary or drug treatment has begun, it may not be possible to classify the lipoproteinemia or the classification may be erroneous.

Type IIb is overindulgence hyperlipemia; shows increased cholesterol and triglycerides, with increased beta and pre-beta; can only be distinguished from Type III by detecting abnormal beta-migrating lipoprotein in serum fraction with density >1.006.

Table 51. Summary of Primary Overflow Aminoacidurias (increased blood concentration with overflow into urine)

Disease	Increased Blood Amino Acids	Urine Abnormalities[a]	Other Laboratory Findings
Phenylketonuria	Phenylalanine	o-hydroxyphenylacetic acid; phenylpyruvic, acetic, and lactic acids	Blood tyrosine does not rise after phenylalanine load
Maple syrup urine disease Severe infantile form	Valine, leucine, isoleucine, alloisoleucine	Branched chain keto acids in great excess; urine has odor of maple syrup	
Intermittent form	Same	Ketoaciduria and urine odor present only during attacks	
Hypervalinemia	Valine		
Homocystinuria	Methionine; homocystine slightly increased	Homocystine in great excess in urine	Blood cystine low; vascular accidents, Marfan-like syndrome, osteoporosis
Tryptophanemia	Tryptophan	Decreased excretion of kynurenin after tryptophan load	
Hyperlysinemia	Lysine	Ornithine, gamma-aminobutyric acid, and ethanolamine in excess	
Congenital lysine intolerance	Lysine, arginine		Ammonia intoxication
Tyrosinosis	Tyrosine; methionine may be markedly increased	p-hydroxyphenylpyruvic, acetic, and lactic acids; methionine may be prominent	Generalized aminoaciduria, renal glycosuria, renal rickets, cirrhosis; Fanconi syndrome

Disorder	Plasma	Urine	Comments
Cystathioninuria	Cystathionine slightly increased	Cystathionine (may be > 1 gm/day)	Congenital acidosis, thrombocytopenia, pituitary gland abnormalities
Hyperglycinemia Severe infantile	Glycine (other amino acids may be elevated)	Acetone	May have ammonia intoxication, ketosis, neutropenia, and osteoporosis
With hypo-oxaluria	Glycine	Decreased oxalate excretion	
Argininosuccinic aciduria	Argininosuccinic acid ($\cong$4 mg/100 ml)	Argininosuccinic acid (2.5–9.0 gm/day)	Ammonia intoxication
Citrullinemia	Citrulline		Liver disease, ammonia intoxication; may have low BUN
Ornithinemia	Ornithine	Ornithine may be normal	Ammonia intoxication
Histidinemia	Histidine (alanine may also be increased)	Alanine may be increased; imidazolepyruvic, acetic, and lactic acids	Urocanic acid absent in sweat and urine after oral histidine load
Carnosinuria		Carnosine (20–100 mg/day)	
Hyper-beta-alaninemia	Beta-alanine, gamma-aminobutyric acid (GABA)	Beta-aminoisobutyric acid, GABA, and taurine in excess	Beta-alanine and GABA increased in CSF
Hyperprolinemia Type I	Proline	Hydroxyproline, glycine elevated	May have hereditary nephritis
Type II	Proline	Δ^1-pyrroline-5-carboxylate, hydroxyproline, glycine elevated	No nephritis

(Continued)

Table 51 (Continued)

Disease	Increased Blood Amino Acids	Urine Abnormalities[a]	Other Laboratory Findings
Hydroxyprolinemia	Hydroxyproline	No excretion of Δ^1-pyrroline-3-hydroxy-5-carboxylate or gamma-hydroxyglutamic acid after hydroxyproline load	
Hypophosphatasia	Phosphoethanolamine slightly elevated ($\cong 0.4$ mg/100 ml)	Phosphoethanolamine ($\geqq 150$ mg/day)	Bone disease

[a]In addition to overflow aminoaciduria:

Mental retardation is often present in these patients.

For proper interpretation of aminoaciduria: Avoid all drugs and medications for 3–4 days (unless immediate diagnosis is required) since they may cause renal tubular damage with aminoaciduria or may produce confusing spots on chromatograms. Use fresh urine specimens without urinary tract infection or else amino acid pattern may be abnormal. Since aminoaciduria may occur with various acute illnesses, repeat amino acid chromatogram after recovery from acute illness to avoid misdiagnosis.

Some aminoacidurias may not be clinically significant (e.g., newborn aminoaciduria, glycinuria, beta-aminoisobutyric aciduria).

Source: M. D. Efron and M. G. Ampola, The aminoacidurias. *Pediatr. Clin. North Am.* 14:881, 1967.

INCIDENCE OF METABOLIC DISORDERS DETECTED BY URINE SCREENING IN NEWBORNS

Disorder	*Incidence*
Phenylketonuria	1 : 15,000
Iminoglycinuria	1 : 10,000
Cystinuria	1 : 15,000
Histidinemia	1 : 18,000
Hartnup disease	1 : 18,000
Argininosuccinic acidemia	1 : 100,000
Cystathioninemia	1 : 100,000
Hyperglycinemia (nonketotic)	1 : 150,000
Fanconi syndrome (renal)	1 : 150,000
Propionic acidemia	< 1:300,000
Hyperlysinemia	< 1:300,000
Hyperornithinemia	< 1:300,000
Hyperprolinemia	< 1:300,000

PHENYLKETONURIA

Inherited absence of phenylalanine hydroxylase activity in liver causes increased blood and urine phenylalanine along with metabolites; associated with mental retardation.

For screening of newborns, urine amounts of phenylpyruvic acid may be insufficient for detection by colorimetric methods when blood level is <15 mg/100 ml. May not appear in urine until 2–3 weeks of age.

Preliminary blood-screening tests (inhibition assay, fluorometry, paper chromatography) detect levels >4 mg/100 ml.

To confirm diagnosis of phenylketonuria, administer 100 mg of ascorbic acid and collect blood and urine 24 hours later.

Phenylketonuria
   Serum phenylalanine is >15 mg/100 ml.
   Serum tyrosine is <5 mg/100 ml (*is never increased in phenylketonuria*).
   Urine phenylalanine is >100 μg/ml.
   Orthohydroxyphenylacetic acid is present in urine.
   Phenylpyruvic acid in urine is significant (gives positive ferric chloride test) but may not be present in some patients.

Abnormalities of tyrosine metabolism (e.g., incomplete development of tyrosine oxidizing system, especially in premature or low-birth-weight infants)
   Serum phenylalanine is >4 mg/100 ml (5–20 mg/100 ml).
   Serum tyrosine is between 10 and 75 mg/100 ml.
   Tyrosine metabolites in urine are ≦1 mg/ml (parahydroxyphenyl-lactic and parahydroxyphenylacetic acids can be distinguished from orthohydroxyphenylacetic acid by paper chromatography).
   Orthohydroxyphenylacetic acid is absent from urine.

Without administration of ascorbic acid, 25% of premature infants may have increased serum phenylalanine and tyrosine for several weeks (but reversed in 24 hours after ascorbic acid administration) and increased urine tyrosine and tyrosine derivatives.

Table 52. Summary of Renal Transport Aminoacidurias (blood amino acids normal or low)

Disease	Amino Acids Increased in Urine
Oasthouse urine disease (methionine malabsorption syndrome)	Methionine (may not be much increased on normal diet but is on high-methionine diet); smaller amounts of valine, leucine, isoleucine, tyrosine, and phenylalanine
Hartnup disease	Neutral (monoamine, monocarboxylic) amino acids; basic amino acids, methionine, proline, hydroxyproline, and glycine normal or only slightly increased
Glycinuria (may be harmless; may be heterozygolous, for benign prolinuria; may be associated with many conditions)	Glycine
Severe prolinuria (Joseph's syndrome)	Proline, hydroxyproline, and glycine in great excess ($\leqq 3$ gm/day proline)
Benign prolinuria	Proline, hydroxyproline, and glycine ($\leqq 600$ mg/day proline)
Cystine-lysinuria Type I (renal calculi) Type II Type III	Cystine and dibasic amino acids
Isolated cystinuria (familial hypoparathyroidism—incidental?)	Cystine

Source: M. D. Efron and M. G. Ampola, The aminoacidurias. *Pediatr. Clin. North Am.* 14:881, 1967.

Similar blood and urine findings not reversed by administration of ascorbic acid may occur in untreated galactosemia, tyrosinemia, congenital cirrhosis, and giant-cell hepatitis; jaundice occurs frequently.

Serum serotonin (5-hydroxytryptophan) is decreased.

Urine 5-HIAA excretion is decreased.

MAPLE SYRUP URINE DISEASE (KETOACIDURIA)
(metabolic block in degradation of ketoacids of branched chain amino acids)

Urine has maple syrup odor.

Chromatography of urine shows greatly increased urinary excretion of ketoacids of leucine, isoleucine, and valine.

The disease may be severe or intermittent.

HOMOCYSTINURIA

This is an inborn error of methionine metabolism with deficient cystathionine synthetase in liver and brain with inability to change homocystine to cystathionine.

Urine excretion of homocystine is increased (positive nitroprusside screening test).

Level of homocystine and methionine is increased in serum and also increased in CSF.

Laboratory findings due to associated clinical conditions (e.g., mental retardation, Marfan's syndrome, osteoporosis, thromboembolic accidents, mild variable hepatocellular dysfunction) are noted.

TYROSINOSIS

There is increased urinary excretion of p-hydroxyphenylpyruvic acid (due to deficiency of p-hydroxyphenylpyruvic oxidase) (chromatography of urine). *Also increased in myasthenia gravis, liver disease, ascorbic acid deficiency, malignancies.*

Acetic and lactic acids and methionine may be increased in urine.

Increased blood tyrosine; methionine may be markedly increased.

Laboratory findings due to Fanconi syndrome and hepatic cirrhosis are noted.

CYSTATHIONINURIA
(rare disorder of intermediate metabolism of methionine)
Increased cystathionine in urine

HYPERGLYCINEMIA

Long-chain ketosis (without hypoglycemia) and ketonuria accentuated by leucine ingestion

Neutropenia

Thrombocytopenia

Hypogammaglobulinemia

Increased glycine in blood and urine

Osteoporosis

ARGININOSUCCINIC ACIDURIA

Argininosuccinic acid is increased in urine; may also be increased in blood and CSF.

Serum alkaline phosphatase may be increased.

Fasting blood ammonia is normal but may be markedly increased after eating.

Heterozygous carriers show increased argininosuccinic acid in urine and decreased argininosuccinase in RBCs.

CITRULLINEMIA
(rare condition of metabolic block in citrulline utilization and associated mental retardation)
Increased citrulline in blood and also CSF and urine
Laboratory findings due to liver disease

HISTIDINEMIA
(rare inherited disorder)
Blood histidine is increased.
Histidine, imidazole acetic, imidazole lactic, and imidazole pyruvic acids are increased in urine; alanine may be increased.

Urine may show positive Phenistix test because of imidazole pyruvic acid.
With oral histidine load, no FIGLU appears in urine.

HYPERPROLINEMIA
Increased proline in blood
Increased glycine and hydroxyproline in urine

HYDROXYPROLINEMIA
Increased hydroxyproline in blood

OASTHOUSE URINE DISEASE
(distinctive odor of urine)
Increase of various amino acids in blood and also in urine (e.g., phenylalanine, tyrosine, methionine, valine, leucine, isoleucine)

HARTNUP DISEASE
(hereditary abnormality of tryptophan metabolism)
Urine chromatography shows greatly increased amounts of indolacetic acid, alpha-N (indole-3-acetyl) glutamine, and tryptophan.

JOSEPH'S SYNDROME (SEVERE PROLINURIA)
Urine shows marked increase in proline, hydroxyproline, and glycine.
Heterozygotes may show mild prolinuria.

BENIGN PROLINURIA
Increased proline, hydroxyproline, and glycine appear in urine.
Heterozygotes may show glycinuria but not prolinuria.
Prolinuria may occur in association with various diseases; may be harmless.

CYSTINURIA
(failure of renal tubular reabsorption and of intestinal uptake of cystine and of dibasic amino acids)
Increased cystine in urine (20–30 times normal)
Increased urinary arginine, lysine, and ornithine
Cystine renal stones

BETA-AMINOISOBUTYRIC ACIDURIA
(familial recessive disorder of thymine metabolism)
Increased beta-aminoisobutyric acid in urine (50–200 mg/24 hours)

May also occur in leukemia due to increased breakdown of nucleic acids.

FAMILIAL IMINOGLYCINURIA
(inherited autosomal defect of renal transport; may be associated with mental retardation)
Increased urine glycine
Increased urine imino acids (proline, hydroxyproline)

METHYLMALONIC ACIDURIA
(very rare inborn error of metabolism with neonatal metabolic acidosis and mental and somatic retardation)
Metabolic acidosis
Increased methylmalonic acid in urine and blood
Long-chain ketonuria
Intermittent hyperglycinemia
All findings accentuated by high-protein diet or supplemental ingestion of valine or isoleucine
Neutropenia
Possibly, thrombocytopenia
Methylmalonic aciduria also occurs in vitamin B_{12} deficiency.

"ODOR-OF-SWEATY-FEET" SYNDROME
(rare inborn error of short-chain fatty acid metabolism; begins soon after birth with death at about age 1 month)
Laboratory findings due to dehydration, acidosis, gram-negative sepsis
Pancytopenia

FAMILIAL LECITHIN–CHOLESTEROL ACYLTRANSFERASE DEFICIENCY
(rare genetic disorder of adults)
Anemia with large RBCs that are frequently target cells
Proteinuria
Serum cholesterol level normal but cholesterol esters virtually absent

PRIMARY OXALOSIS
(rare familial disease)
Increased serum and urinary oxalic acid
Increased urinary glycolic and glyoxylic acid
Calcium oxalate renal calculi and nephrocalcinosis with extrarenal deposition of calcium oxalate
Uremia causes death.
Manifestations of hyperoxaluria are the same but extrarenal calcium oxalate deposits are absent.*

L-GLYCERIC ACIDURIA
(genetic variant of primary hyperoxaluria; autosomal trait that causes disease only when homozygous)
Renal calculi composed of calcium oxalate
Increased urinary oxalic acid (3–5 times normal)
L-Glyceric acid in urine (not found in normal urine)

CYSTINOSIS
Children
  Renal Fanconi syndrome
    Phosphaturia

*L. Boquist, B. Lindqvist, Y. Ostberg, and L. Steen, Primary oxalosis. *Am. J. Med.* 54:673, 1973.

Decreased serum phosphorus

Decreased serum calcium (usually normal)

Decreased serum potassium due to high urine potassium

Hyperchloremic acidosis (*Renal calcinosis develops in renal tubular acidosis but not in cystinosis.*)

Generalized aminoaciduria (similar to that seen in lead and other heavy-metal poisoning, Wilson's disease, and vitamin D deficiency)

Glycosuria with normal blood sugar; frequently ketonemia and ketonuria

Vitamin D–resistant rickets (*In vitamin D–resistant rickets of primary hypophosphatemia, there is no aminoaciduria; severe rickets develops before azotemia appears.*)

(*Renal hypophosphatemia, aminoaciduria, and glycosuria begin at age 6 months.*)

Polyuria with low specific gravity; proteinuria sometimes present

Progressive loss of glomerular function with increasing azotemia and death from uremia, usually before age 10

Cystine crystals in bone marrow and in tissues (especially reticuloendothelial system)

Serum uric acid sometimes decreased

Adults (benign disease)

Urinary tract calculi

Cystinuria (cystine crystals in urine; >200 mg of cystine in 24-hour urine)

SECONDARY AMINOACIDURIA

Severe liver disease

Renal tubular damage due to

Lysol

Heavy metals

Maleic acid

Burns

Galactosemia

Wilson's disease

Scurvy

Rickets

Fanconi syndrome (e.g., outdated tetracycline, multiple myeloma, inherited)

Neoplasm

Cystathionine excretion in neuroblastoma of adrenal gland; ethanolamine excretion in primary hepatoma

GALACTOSEMIA

(inherited defect of galactose-1-phosphate uridyl transferase in liver and in RBCs that converts galactose to glucose; therefore accumulation of galactose-1-phosphate)

Jaundice (onset at age 4–10 days)

Liver biopsy—dilated canaliculus filled with bile pigment with surrounding rosette of liver cells

Galactosuria—detected by nonspecific reducing tests; identified by chromatography

General ammoaciduria—identified by chromatography

Proteinuria

Galactosemia (equal to total reducing sugar minus glucose-oxidase sugar)

Serum glucose—*apparently* elevated in fasting state but falls as galactose increases; development of hypoglycemia possible

Galactose tolerance test—positive but is unnecessary for diagnosis and may be hazardous because of induced hypoglycemia and hypokalemia

Lack of RBC galactose-1-phosphate uridyl transferase

CONGENITAL FRUCTOSE INTOLERANCE

This is a severe familial genetic disease of infancy due to defect involving fructose-1-phosphoaldolase and fructose-1, 6-diphosphoaldolase; it resembles galactosemia.

Fructose in urine of 100–300 mg/100 ml gives a positive test for reducing substances (Benedict's reagent, Clinitest) but not with glucose-oxidase methods (Clinistix, Tes-Tape). Identify fructose by paper chromatography.

Aminoaciduria and proteinuria may be present.

Fructose tolerance test shows prolonged elevation of blood fructose and marked decrease in serum glucose. Serum phosphorus shows rapid prolonged decrease.

Hypoglycemia with convulsions and coma follows ingestion of fructose.

Increased serum bilirubin and cirrhosis may occur.

BENIGN FRUCTOSURIA

This is a benign asymptomatic disorder due to fructokinase deficiency.

Large amount of fructose in urine gives a positive test for reducing substances (Benedict's reagent, Clinitest) but not with glucoseoxidase methods (Clinistix, Tes-Tape).

Identify fructose by paper chromatography.

Fructose tolerance test shows that blood fructose increases to 4 times more than in normal persons, blood glucose increases only slightly, and serum phosphorus does not change.

ALKAPTONURIA

Recessive inherited absence of liver homogentisic acid oxidase causes excretion of homogentisic acid in urine.

Urine becomes brown-black on standing and reduces Benedict's solution and Fehling's solution but glucose-oxidase methods are negative.

Ferric chloride test is positive.

An oral dose of homogentisic acid is largely recovered in the urine of affected patients but not in normal persons.

SUCROSURIA

Urine specific gravity is very high ($\leqq 1.070$).

Urine tests for reducing substances are negative.
Sucrosuria may follow IV administration of sucrose or the purposeful addition of cane sugar to urine.

PENTOSURIA

Pentosuria is due to a block in oxidation of glucuronic acid; the patient can metabolize only the sixth carbon, excreting the 5-carbon fraction as pentose.

Urinary excretion of L-xylulose is increased (1–4 gm/day), and the increase is accentuated by administration of glucuronic acid and glucuronogenic drugs (e.g., aminopyrine, antipyrine, menthol).

Differential Diagnosis

Alimentary pentosuria—arabinose or xylose excreted after ingestion of large amount of certain fruits (e.g., plums, cherries, grapes)

Healthy normal persons—small amounts of D-ribose in urine.

Healthy normal persons—trace amounts of ribulose in urine

Muscular dystrophy—small amounts of D-ribose in urine (some patients)

MANNOHEPTULOSURIA

Mannoheptulose in urine after the eating of avocados occurs in some persons; not clinically important.

LACTOSURIA

This is a transient disorder of infancy with chronic diarrhea and failure to thrive due to interference with or inhibition of or late development of intestinal lactase.

Lactose in urine produces positive test for reducing sugars (Benedict's reagent, Clinitest) but negative test with glucose-oxidase methods (Tes-Tape, Clinistix).

In the oral lactose tolerance test, serum glucose curves are nearly normal.

Stools are acid.

PHYSIOLOGIC LACTOSURIA

Occurs near the end of pregnancy and during lactation.

INTESTINAL DEFICIENCY OF SUGAR-SPLITTING ENZYMES (MILK ALLERGY; MILK INTOLERANCE; CONGENITAL FAMILIAL LACTOSE INTOLERANCE; LACTASE DEFICIENCY; DISACCHARIDASE DEFICIENCY)

Familial disease which often begins in infancy with diarrhea, vomiting, failure to thrive, malabsorption, etc.; patient becomes asymptomatic when lactose is removed from diet.

Oral lactose tolerance test shows a rise in blood sugar of <20 mg/100 ml (dose of 100 gm of lactose).

A dose of 50 gm each of glucose and galactose produces a rise in blood sugar of >25 mg/100 ml.

In diabetics, lactose ingestion may cause a greater increase in blood sugar.

After ingestion of milk or 50–100 gm of lactose, stools have a pH of 4.5–6.0 (normal pH is >7.0) and are sour and frothy.

Lactose in urine amounts to 100–2000 mg/100 ml. It produces a positive test for reducing sugars (Benedict's reagent, Clinitest) but a negative test with glucose-oxidase methods (Tes-Tape, Clinistix).

CLASSIFICATION OF PORPHYRIAS

I. Congenital erythropoietic porphyria (due to excess production of free uroporphyrin I by marrow RBCs; very rare; autosomal recessive; onset usually before age 2; extreme photosensitivity)

Urine is burgundy red and fluoresces; composed chiefly of uroporphyrin I.

Stool contains large amounts of coproporphyrin I.

Excretion of porphobilinogen and delta-aminolevulinic acid is normal.

Hypersplenism is present.

There is severe normochromic normocytic anicteric hemolytic anemia, which is improved by splenectomy.

Teeth fluoresce.

Skin shows abundant melanin in deeper epidermis.

II. Hepatic porphyria

A. Acute intermittent type is the most frequent and most severe form in the United States. The disease is mendelian dominant, has its onset in adults, and is characterized by abdominal pain and nervous system manifestations; no photosensitivity. Symptoms are due to demyelinization of nervous system. Variation is from latent to very severe.

Urine

Marked increase in porphobilinogen is seen (also usually increased in latent form).

Usually there is an increase in delta-aminolevulinic acid (also increased in latent form).

Coproporphyrin and uroporphyrin may be increased.

May be normal color when fresh and become brown, red, or black on standing.

Proteinuria may accompany the abdominal pain.

Fecal protoporphyrin and coproporphyrin are usually normal.

Slight leukocytosis may be present.

BSP retention is abnormal.

Serum magnesium level may be decreased during acute attack.

Serum sodium and chloride may be decreased during acute attack.

Syndrome of inappropriate secretion of antidiuretic hormone may occur.

Other laboratory abnormalities that occur frequently are increased serum cholesterol, hyper-beta-lipoproteinemia (Type IIa), increased serum iron, increased serum PBI and T-4 without hyperthyroidism, increased TBG, abnormal glucose tolerance.

Level of uroporphyrinogen I synthetase in RBCs is 50% of mean value in normal persons.

Laboratory findings and symptoms may be precipitated by drugs (especially barbiturates, alcohol, sulfonamides), certain steroids, starvation, and infections.

B.   Hereditary mixed types may be cutaneous with few or no acute manifestations, acute intermittent without cutaneous symptoms, various combinations, or latent. Cutaneous manifestations are due to excess production of porphyrins in liver. On postmorten examination, tissues show pink fluorescence under ultraviolet light.

Laboratory findings in porphyria variegata

Urine delta-aminolevulinic acid, porphobilinogen, uroporphyinuria, and coproporphyrin are usually increased during attacks and normal during remission.

Characteristically stool shows increased uroporphyrin, coproporphyrin and protoporphyrin, even during asymptomatic period.

C.   Acquired

Due to hepatoma, cirrhosis, chemicals (an epidemic in Turkey was caused by contamination of wheat by hexachlorobenzene and mercury).

Urine contains predominantly increased uroporphyrin and coproporphyrins; protoporphyrinogen is normal; delta-aminolevulinic acid may occasionally be increased.

Fecal porphyrins are usually normal.

Abnormal liver function tests

Fluorescence of liver tissue under ultraviolet light, hepatic siderosis, and histologic evidence of liver disease are very common.

III.   Erythropoietic protoporphyria (infrequent autosomal dominant condition with photosensitivity)

RBC protoporphyrin and coproporphyrin are increased.

Fecal protoporphyrin and coproporphyrin are increased.

Plasma protoporphyrin is increased.

Urine uroporphyrin and coproporphyrin are not increased.

Usually no significant anemia is seen and serum iron and TIBC are normal.

No fluorescence of teeth is found.

Increased frequency of associated gallstones

RBC, but not plasma, protoporphyrins are also increased in iron deficiency anemia and lead intoxication. Screening tests using fluorescence microscopy of RBCs or Wood's lamp viewing of treated whole blood may also be positive in iron deficiency anemia, lead intoxication, and other dyserthyropoietic states.

GENETIC MUCOPOLYSACCHARIDOSES

Mucopolysaccharide Type	*Mucopolysaccharide Excreted in Urine*
I (Hurler's syndrome)	Chondroitin sulfate B and heparitan sulfate
II (Hunter's syndrome)	Chondroitin sulfate B and heparitin sulfate
III (Sanfilippo's syndrome)	Heparitin sulfate
IV (Morquio-Ulrich syndrome)	Keratosulfate
V (Schei's syndrome)	Chondroitin sulfate B
VI (Maroteaux-Lamy syndrome)	Chondroitin sulfate B
VII (I-cell disease)	—
VIII (Lipomucopolysaccharidoses)	—

All mucopolysaccharide diseases show metachromatically staining inclusions of mucopolysaccharides in circulating polynuclear leukocytes (Reilly granulations) or lymphocytes, cells of inflammatory exudate, and bone marrow cells (most consistently in clasmatocytes). Mucopolysaccharide is also deposited in various parenchymal cells.

GENETIC DISEASES OF MUCOPOLYSACCHARIDE METABOLISM

Morquio-Ulrich syndrome
> Excess excretion of keratosulfate in urine associated with aortic valvular disease, osteochondrodystrophy, and cloudy cornea

Schei's syndrome
> Excess excretion of chondroitin sulfate B in urine associated with aortic valve disease (usually regurgitation) and cloudy cornea

Hurler's syndrome (gargoylism)
> Excess excretion of chondroitin sulfate B and mucopolysaccharide in urine Alder-Reilly anomaly—azurophil granules in cytoplasm of myeloid cells (occasionally lymphocytes and monocytes)
> Fibrosis of heart valves with functional changes

CLASSIFICATION OF GLYCOGENOSES (GLYCOGEN STORAGE DISEASES—GSD)

Frequency of Types (GSD%)	*Type*	*Clinical Name*	*Enzyme Defect*
20	I	Classic von Gierke's disease	Deficiency of liver glucose-6-phosphatase
20	II	Pompe's disease	Defect in lysosomal alpha-1, 4-glucosidase
30	III	Forbes' disease (debrancher deficiency, limit dextrinosis)	Deficiency of amylo-1, 6-glucosidase (debranching enzyme)
<1	IV	Andersen's disease (brancher deficiency, amylopectinosis)	Absence of amylo-$(1,4 \rightarrow 1,6)$-transglucosidase (branching enzyme)
5	V	McArdle's disease of muscle	Absence of muscle phosphorylase
25	VI		Deficiency of liver phosphorylase
	VII		Deficiency of muscle phosphofructokinase

VON GIERKE'S DISEASE (TYPE I GLYCOGEN STORAGE DISEASE; GLUCOSE-6-PHOSPHATASE DEFICIENCY)

Blood glucose is markedly decreased.

Blood triglycerides, cholesterol, and serum free fatty acids are markedly increased.

Mild anemia is present.

There is increased serum uric acid (due to depressed renal tubular function by increased blood lactic acid) causing clinical gout.

Serum phosphorus and alkaline phosphatase are decreased.

Urine glucose is increased.

Urinary nonspecific amino acids are increased, without increase in blood amino acids.

Other renal function tests are relatively normal.

Liver function tests (other than related to carbohydrate metabolism) are relatively normal.

Glucose tolerance may be normal or diabetic type; diabetic type is more frequent in older children and adults.

Functional tests

Administer 1 mg of glucagon intravenously after 8-hour fast. A 50–60% increase in blood glucose appears in 10–20 minutes in the normal person. No increase occurs in infants or young children with von Gierke's disease; delayed response may occur in older children and adults.

Administer the galactose or fructose intravenously. No rise in blood glucose occurs in von Gierke's disease but normal rise occurs in limit dextrinosis (Type III GSD).

Biopsy of liver

Histology is not diagnostic; shows vacuolization of hepatic cells and abundant glycogen granules. Confirm with Best's stain.

Biochemical studies

Glycogen content >4% by weight.

Glucose-6-phosphatase is absent or markedly decreased.

Glycogen is biochemically normal.

Other enzymes (other GSD) are present in normal amounts.

Biopsy of jejunum

Intestinal glucose-6-phosphatase is decreased or absent.

Biopsy of muscle shows no abnormality of enzyme activity or glycogen content.

Type IB

Shows all the changes of von Gierke's disease except that liver biopsy does not show deficiency of glucose-6-phosphatase.

POMPE'S DISEASE (TYPE II GLYCOGEN STORAGE DISEASE; GENERALIZED GLYCOGENOSIS; ALPHA-GLUCOSIDASE DEFICIENCY GLYCOGENOSIS)

Features of the disease are imbecility, varying neurologic defects, muscle hypotonia, cardiac enlargement, and frequent liver enlargement.

Fasting blood sugar, GTT, glucagon responses, and rises in blood glucose after fructose infusion are normal. No acetonuria is present.

General hematologic findings are normal.

Staining of circulating leukocytes for glycogen shows massive deposition.

Confirm diagnosis by muscle biopsy, specific enzymatic assays, glycogen structure analysis (these are special studies).

TYPE III GLYCOGEN DEPOSITION DISEASE (FORBES' DISEASE; DEBRANCHER DEFICIENCY; LIMIT DEXTRINOSIS)

This is a familial disease with enlarged liver, retarded growth, chemical changes, and benign course.

Serum cholesterol is increased.

Acetone appears in urine.

Fasting hypoglycemia occurs.

There is a diabetic type of glucose tolerance curve with associated glucosuria.

Infusions of galactose and fructose cause a normal hyperglycemic response.

Fasting blood sugar does not show expected rise after administration of subcutaneous glucagon or epinephrine but does increase 2 hours after high-carbohydrate meal.

Confirm diagnosis by biochemical findings of increased liver glycogen, abnormal glycogen structure, absence of detectable amylol, 6-glucosidase activity with normal phosphorylase and glucose-6-phosphatase. RBC glycogen is often increased.

Serum uric acid is normal or slightly increased.

TYPE IV GLYCOGEN DEPOSITION DISEASE (ANDERSEN'S DISEASE; BRANCHER DEFICIENCY; AMYLOPECTINOSIS)

This extremely rare fatal condition is due to absence of amylo-(1,4 → 1.6)-transglucosidase.

Liver function tests may be altered (e.g., slight increase in bilirubin, reversed A/G ratio, increased SGOT, decreased serum cholesterol).

There may be a flat blood glucose response to epinephrine and glucagon.

There may be increased WBC and decreased hemoglobin.

Biopsy of liver may show a cirrhotic reaction to the presence of polysaccharide of abnormal structure, which stains with Best's carmine and periodic acid-Schiff stain but has a very low glycogen content.

TYPE V GLYCOGEN DEPOSITION DISEASE (MCARDLE'S SYNDROME; MCARDLE-SCHMID-PEARSON DISEASE; MYOPHOSPHORYLASE DEFICIENCY)

This is a familial autosomal recessive disease showing very limited ischemic muscle exercise tolerance in the presence of normal appearance of muscle.

Epinephrine or glucagon causes a normal hyperglycemic response.

Biopsy of muscle is microscopically normal in youth; vacuolation and necrosis are seen in later years. Increased glycogen is present. Absence of phosphorylase is demonstrated by various techniques.

Following exercise that quickly causes muscle cramping and

weakness, the regional blood lactate and pyruvate does not increase (in a normal person it increases 2–5 times). Similar abnormal response occurs in Type III involving muscle and in
Types VII, VIII, X.
Myoglobulinuria may occur after strenuous exercise.

TYPE VI GLYCOGEN STORAGE DISEASE (HEPATIC PHOSPHORYLASE DEFICIENCY)

Enlarged liver present from birth is associated with hypoglycemia.
Hypoglycemia is mild to moderate.
Serum cholesterol and lactic acid are mildly increased.
Serum uric acid is moderately increased.
Liver function tests are normal, except for mobilization of glyco-
gen.
Fructose tolerance is normal.
Response to glucagon and epinephrine is variable but tends to be
poor.
Leukocyte phosphorylase activity is decreased, but muscle phos-
phorylase is normal. Liver phosphorylase is decreased.

TYPE VII GLYCOGEN STORAGE DISEASE (MUSCLE PHOSPHOFRUCTOKINASE DEFICIENCY)

Fasting hypoglycemia is marked.
Other members of family may have reduced tolerance to glucose.
RBCs show 50% decrease in phosphofructokinase activity.
Biopsy of muscle shows marked decrease (1–3% of normal) in
phosphofructokinase activity.

TYPE O GLYCOGEN STORAGE DISEASE

This is a very rare condition.
Blood glucose is markedly decreased, causing hypoglycemic seizures and mental retardation.
Glucagon administration causes no increase in blood glucose (see
von Gierke's disease, p. 370) but ingestion of food causes a
rise in 2–3 hours.
Biopsy of liver shows marked decrease in glycogen synthetase.

FAMILIAL PAROXYSMAL PERITONITIS (FAMILIAL MEDITERRANEAN FEVER; "PERIODIC DISEASE")

WBC is increased (10,000–20,000/cu mm), and there may be in-
creased eosinophils during an attack but a return to normal be-
tween attacks.
ESR is increased during an attack but normal between attacks.
Mild normocytic normochromic anemia is occasionally seen.
Serum glycoprotein is increased in patients and their relatives.
Increased alpha$_2$ globulin and fibrinogen are common.
Amyloidosis develops in 10–40% of patients; it is not related to
frequency or severity of clinical attacks.
Etiocholanolone is increased in urine and blood during attacks in a
few patients.

LESCH-NYHAN SYNDROME

The syndrome appears in children, with choreoathetosis, mental
retardation, tendency to self-mutilating biting and scratching.

Serum uric acid levels are very high (because of complete absence of hypoxanthine-guanine phosphoribosyltransferase).

FAMILIAL DYSAUTONOMIA (RILEY-DAY SYNDROME)

This condition is due to an autosomal recessive trait occurring in Ashkenazi Jews, who show difficulty in swallowing, corneal ulcerations, insensitivity to pain, motor incoordination, excessive sweating, diminished gag reflex, lack of tongue papillae, progressive kyphoscoliosis, pulmonary infections, etc.

Urine vanillylmandelic acid (VMA) (3-methoxy-4-hydroxymandelic acid) may be low and homovanillic acid (HVA) increased.

In asymptomatic carriers, urine VMA may be lower than in healthy adults.

BATTEN'S DISEASE (BATTEN-SPIELMEYER-VOGT DISEASE) (autosomal recessive type of juvenile amaurotic idiocy)

Azurophilic hypergranulation of leukocytes occurs in patients and in heterozygous and homozygous members of their families. In Giemsa- and Wright-stained smears, it resembles toxic granulation but differs by the absence of supravital staining in Batten's disease and by normal leukocyte alkaline phosphatase activity (markedly increased in toxic granulation). This granulation occurs in $\geqq 15\%$ of neutrophils.

TAY-SACHS DISEASE (GM$_2$ GANGLIOSIDOSIS)

This condition is due to an autosomal recessive trait found predominantly (but not exclusively) in Ashkenazi Jews and is characterized by the appearance during infancy of psychomotor deterioration, blindness, "cherry-red spot" in the macula, and an exaggerated extension response to sound.

Accumulation of GM$_2$ is due to deficiency or absence of hexosaminidase A (in a variant of Tay-Sachs disease called Sandhoff's disease, both hexosaminidase A and B are defective).

There is early marked increase of serum LDH and SGOT and decrease of serum fructose 1-phosphate aldolase. (Serum fructose 1-phosphate aldolase is also decreased *in heterozygotes*.) Serum LDH and SGOT return to normal if patient survives 3–4 years.

CSF GOT parallels serum GOT.

Occasional vacuolated lymphocytes are seen.

Serum aldolase is normal during first few months, then increases (reflecting muscle atrophy); peaks (2 times the normal value) at age 12–24 months; becomes normal in next 3–12 months.

CSF aldolase rises early and then declines slowly as disease progresses; does not parallel serum level since it originates from a different source.

Liver function tests are normal.

Serum acid phosphatase is normal.

LANDING'S DISEASE (GM$_1$ GANGLIOSIDOSIS; SYSTEMIC LATE INFANTILE LIPIDOSIS)

This is a rare familial disorder due to an autosomal recessive gene with no racial predilection, characterized by psychomotor dete-

Table 53. Classification of Gangliosidoses

Clinical Name	Enzyme Defect	Major Lipid Accumulation	Signs and Symptoms
Gaucher's disease	Beta-glucosidase	Glucocerebroside	Spleen and liver enlargement Erosion of long bones and pelvis Mental retardation only in infantile form
Niemann-Pick disease	Sphingomyelinase	Sphingomyelin	Liver and spleen enlargement Mental retardation About 30% with red spot in retina
Krabbe's disease (globoid leukodystrophy)	Beta-galactosidase	Galactocerebroside	Mental retardation Almost total absence of myelin Globoid bodies in white matter of brain Increased CSF protein (150–300 mg/100 ml)
Metachromatic leukodystrophy	Sulfatidase	Sulfatide	Mental retardation Psychological disturbances in adult form Nerves stain yellow-brown with cresyl violet dye CSF normal or increased CSF protein ($\leqq$200 mg/100 ml) (see p. 254)
Ceramide lactoside lipidosis	Beta-galactosidase	Ceramide lactoside	Slowly progressing brain damage Liver and spleen enlargement

Fabry's disease	Alpha-galactosidase	Ceramide trihexoside	Reddish-purple skin rash Kidney failure Pain in lower extremities
Tay-Sachs disease	Hexosaminidase A	Ganglioside GM_2	Mental retardation Red spot in retina Blindness Muscular weakness
Tay-Sachs variant (Sandhoff's disease)	Hexosaminidase A and B	Globoside (and ganglioside GM_2)	Same as Tay-Sachs disease but progresses more rapidly
Generalized gangliosidosis	Beta-galactosidase	Ganglioside GM_1	Mental retardation Liver enlargement Skeletal deformities About 50% with red spot in retina
Fucosidosis	Alpha-fucosidase	H-isoantigen	Cerebral degeneration Muscle spasticity Thick skin

rioration, enlargement of liver and/or spleen, and roentgenographic findings resembling those in Hunter and Hurler syndromes.

Vacuolated lymphocytes may be found.

Abnormal leukocytic granulations (Alder-Reilly bodies) may be present.

Serum LDH, SGOT, and fructose-1-phosphate aldolase are normal.

Foam cell histiocytes (resembling Niemann-Pick cells) may be seen in biopsy from bone marrow, liver, or rectum.

GAUCHER'S DISEASE

Gaucher's cells appear in bone marrow aspiration, needle biopsy, or aspiration of spleen, liver, or lymph nodes.

Serum acid phosphatase is increased (if substrate for test is different from that for prostatic acid phosphatase; i.e., use phenyl phosphate or p-nitrophenylphosphate instead of glycerophosphate). It may return to normal following splenectomy.

Serum cholesterol and total fats are normal.

Laboratory findings due to involvement of specific organs

Spleen. Hypersplenism occurs with anemia (normocytic normochromic), leukopenia (with relative lymphocytosis; monocytes may be increased), and/or thrombocytopenia.

Bone. Serum alkaline phosphatase may be increased.

Liver. Serum SGOT may be increased.

Spinal fluid. GOT may be increased.

NIEMANN-PICK DISEASE

Foamy histiocytes may be found in bone marrow aspiration and may appear in peripheral blood terminally.

Peripheral blood lymphocytes and monocytes may be vacuolated (2–20% of cells). WBC is variable.

Rectal biopsy may show changes in ganglion cells of myenteric plexus.

Laboratory findings due to involvement of specific organs

Anemia is due to hypersplenism or microcytic anemia associated with anisocytosis, poikilocytosis, and elliptocytosis.

SGOT may be increased in serum and spinal fluid.

Enzyme changes in CSF are same as in Tay-Sachs disease, except that LDH is normal (see next section).

Acid phosphatase is increased (same as in Gaucher's disease—see preceding section).

Serum aldolase is increased.

LDH is normal in serum and CSF

HISTIOCYTOSIS X

Letterer-Siwe disease

Bone marrow aspiration or biopsy of lymph node may show characteristic histiocytes and histologic changes.

Progressive normocytic normochromic anemia is present.

Hemorrhagic manifestations (thrombocytopenia) occur.

Hand-Schüller-Christian disease
    Diabetes insipidus may occur.
    Histologic examination of skin, bone, etc., is diagnostic.
    Anemia, leukopenia, thrombocytopenia may or may not be present.

Eosinophilic granuloma
    Biopsy of bone is diagnostic.
    Blood is normal; eosinophilia is unusual.

Development of leukopenia and thrombocytopenia suggests poorest prognosis.

DOWN'S SYNDROME (TRISOMY 21; MONGOLISM)
Karyotyping shows 47 chromosomes with trisomy 21 in most patients (see p. 161).
Increased leukocyte alkaline phosphatase staining reaction.
Leukocytes show decreased incidence of drumsticks (see p. 160) and mean lobe counts.
Serum acid phosphatase may be decreased.
Incidence of leukemia is increased.

D₁ TRISOMY (TRISOMY 13)

D_1 TRISOMY (TRISOMY 13)
In peripheral blood smears, most of the neutrophilic leukocytes show an increased number of anomalous nuclear projections compared to those of normal persons. The nuclear lobulation may appear abnormal (nucleus may look twisted without clear separation of individual lobes, coarse lumpy chromatin, etc.).
Fetal hemoglobin may persist longer than normal (i.e., be increased).

32

ENDOCRINE DISEASES

HYPERTHYROIDISM

Serum T-3 concentration (radioimmunoassay) and uptake (resin) are increased.

Serum T-4 (total thyroxine) is increased.

Serum free thyroxine is increased.

Serum PBI is increased.

Serum BEI is increased.

Serum PB^{131}I and conversion ratio are increased.

Thyroid uptake of ^{131}I is increased. It is relatively more affected at 1, 2, or 6 hours than at 24 hours. It may be normal in presence of recent iodine ingestion.

Salivary excretion of ^{131}I is increased.

Urinary excretion of ^{131}I is increased.

Iodine tolerance test shows increased utilization of iodine.

BMR is increased.

Serum thyroxine-binding globulin (TBG) is normal.

Serum cholesterol is decreased.

Serum total lipids are usually decreased.

Hyperglycemia is present.

Glycosuria is present.

Glucose tolerance is decreased, with early high peak and early fall.

Creatine excretion in urine and creatine tolerance are increased (normal serum creatine almost excludes hyperthyroidism).

There is increased urinary and fecal excretion of calcium with normal serum phosphorus.

Serum total and ionized calcium is increased in >10% of patients. Parathormone level is not increased.

Thyroid suppression test. Triiodothyronine administration decreases ^{131}I uptake in normal persons but not in hyperthyroid persons.

Serum TSH (radioimmunoassay) is decreased in most patients. Administration of TRH does not cause a significant rise in serum TSH as it does in normal persons; a normal rise virtually excludes hyperthyroidism (see p. 77).

There is associated impairment of liver function (e.g., impaired excretion of BSP).

Triiodothyronine (T-3) toxicosis

> Should be suspected particularly in patients with clinical thyrotoxicosis (with increased BMR) in whom usual laboratory tests are normal.
>
> Serum T-4 is normal.
>
> TBG and TBPA (thyroxine-binding albumin) are normal.
>
> ^{131}I uptake is autonomous (not suppressed by T-3 administration).
>
> Serum T-3 (measured by radioimmunoassay) is increased.

Increased serum T-3 is associated with increased T-4 in
> Graves' disease
> Toxic adenoma

Toxic multinodular goiter

Factitious hyperthyroidism (self-induced hyperthyroidism by thyroxine administration)

All thyroid function tests indicate hyperthyroidism in the presence of a low radioactive iodine uptake (RAIU).

Increased serum T-3 is associated with normal or low T-4 in
T-3 hyperthyroidism
TBG deficiency with hyperthyroidism
Ingestion of T-3 alone or combined with T-4
Premonitory clinical hyperthyroidism

Decreased serum T-3 is associated with decreased T-4 in
Hypothyroidism, primary or secondary

Decreased serum T-3 is associated with normal T-4 in
Newborn (first week of life)
Fetus at term

HYPOTHYROIDISM

Serum T-4 (total thyroxine) concentration is decreased.

Serum free thyroxine concentration is decreased.

Serum T-3 concentration (radioimmunoassay) is decreased (may be normal in $\cong 20\%$ of hypothyroid patients).

Serum T-3/T-4 ratio is increased.

Serum T-3 uptake is decreased. (May be normal in $\leqq 50\%$ of hypothyroid patients.)

Serum PBI is decreased.

Serum BEI is decreased.

Serum PB^{131}I and conversion ratio are decreased.

Thyroid uptake of ^{131}I is decreased.

Serum alkaline phosphatase is increased (originates from bone).

Serum calcium is sometimes increased.

Salivary excretion of ^{131}I is decreased.

Urinary excretion of ^{131}I is decreased.

Iodine tolerance test shows decreased utilization of iodine.

BMR is decreased.

Serum thyroxine-binding globulin (TBG) is normal.

Serum cholesterol is increased (chiefly useful to follow effect of therapy, especially in children).

Fasting blood sugar is decreased.

Glucose tolerance is increased (oral GTT is flat; IV GTT is normal).

Serum TSH (radioimmunoassay) is increased in proportion to degree of hypofunction. A single determination is usually sufficient to establish the diagnosis. Administration of TRH causes a greater increase in serum TSH in primary hypothyroidism than in pituitary hypothyroidism (see p. 77 and Table 55, p. 383).

TSH stimulation (20 units/day for 3 days) increases ^{131}I uptake to $\cong$ normal (20%) in secondary (pituitary) hypothyroidism but not in primary hypothyroidism.

Normocytic normochromic anemia is found.

Serum carotene is increased.

Laboratory findings indicative of pernicious anemia and primary adrenocortical insufficiency occur with increased frequency in primary hypothyroidism.

Table 54. Thyroid Function Tests in Various Conditions

Disease	RAIU (radioactive iodine uptake)	Free Thyroxine ("normalized")	T-4 (total serum thyroxine)	Serum PBI	Serum TSH	Serum T-3 Concentration	Serum T-3 Uptake	Serum TBG (thyroxine-binding globulin)	Serum Cholesterol	BMR
Hypothyroidism[a]	D	D	D	D	I	D	D	N or I	I	D
Hyperthyroidism[b]	I	I	I	I	D	I	N	D	I	I
T-3 thyrotoxicosis	N or I	N	N	N	D	I	N or slightly I	N	D	I
Administration of Thyroxine (factitious hyperthyroidism)[c]	D	I	I	I	D	V	I	N	D	I
Inorganic iodine[d]	D	N	N	I	N	N	N	N	N	N
Radiopaque contrast media[e]	D	N	N	I	N	N	N	N	N	N
Estrogen and anti-ovulatory drugs	I	N	I	I	N	I	D	I	V	V
Testosterone	D	N	D	D	N	D	I	D	V	V

380

ACTH and corticosteroids	D	N	D	D	N or D	I	N or D	D	V	V
Dilantin or large doses of salicylates	N	N	D	D	D	I	D	D	D	V
Pregnancy	—f	N	I	I	I	D	I	I	V	V
With hyperthyroidism	—f	I	I	I	N	N	I	I	V	
With hypothyroidism	—f	D	D–N	D–N	D	D	I	I		
Hereditary increase of TBG in euthyroid state	I	N	I	I	N	D	I	I	V	V
Hereditary decrease of TBG in euthyroid state	D	N	D	D	D	I	D	D	V	V
Granulomatous thyroiditisg	D	V–I	V–I	V–I	V–D	V–I	V	V	V	V
Adenomatous thyroid goiter	N	N	N	N	N	N	N	N	N	N
Thyroid neoplasm (nonfunctional)	N	N	N	N	N	N	N	N	N	N
Nephrosish	May be I	N	D	D	N	I	D	I	I	I

(Continued)

Table 54 (Continued)

N = normal; D = decreased; I = increased; V = variable.

[a] Increased serum TSH is diagnostic of primary hypothyroidism. TRH stimulation test differentiates primary and secondary hypothyroidism. Normal T-3 does not rule out hypothyroidism, since in many hypothyroid patients it falls in the normal range.

[b] Graves' disease—long-acting thyroid stimulator (LATS) may be present. Antithyroid antibody titer may be high. Toxic nodular goiter—LATS is not found. Antithyroid antibody titer is normal. Radioactive iodine scan shows a "hot" nodule with decreased uptake in rest of thyroid. Administration of T-3 does not suppress iodine uptake by nodule. Administration of TSH increases iodine uptake in rest of thyroid.

[c] RAIU is decreased when all other thyroid function tests indicate hyperactivity.

[d] Very high PBI associated with a very low RAIU probably means ingestion of iodine.

[e] Invalidates PBI and RAIU results.

[f] Contraindicated.

[g] Increased ESR. Antithyroid antibodies are present briefly. Moderately high PBI and low RAIU suggest thyroiditis. PBI is highest when the thyroiditis is maximal. As thyroiditis progresses, patient may be transiently hypothyroid; this condition may be followed by increased serum TSH and RAIU for a period. All tests usually become normal ultimately.

[h] Thyroid function tests are altered due to loss of TBG in urine.

Source: Data in above table footnotes from K. L. Becker, Endocrine and Metabolic Disorders. In J. A. Halsted (Ed.), *The Laboratory in Clinical Medicine*. Philadelphia: Saunders, 1976.

Table 55. Laboratory Tests in Differential Diagnosis of Primary and Secondary Hypothyroidism

Test	Panhypopituitarism	Primary Myxedema
Serum TSH	Decreased	Increased
Serum TSH response to TRH administration	Absent	Normal or exaggerated
Response to administration of thyrotropic hormone	Responds with increase in ^{131}I uptake, BMR, etc.	No response
Urine 17-ketosteroids	Absent	Low
Response to insulin	Prompt decrease in sugar; fails to return to normal	Usually delayed fall in blood sugar and sometimes delayed return to normal
BMR	More marked decrease (e.g., minus 40–50)	Less marked decrease

When hypothyroid patient becomes euthyroid after treatment
   PBI is low (usually 2 μg/100 ml) when treated with tri-
      iodothyronine (Cytomel).
   PBI is often high normal or slightly increased when treated
      with thyroxine (Synthyroid).
   PBI is normal when treated with desiccated thyroid (thyroid
      U.S.P.).
   PBI may be below normal when treated with thyroglobulin
      (Proloid).
Thyroid hormone treatment of hypothyroidism is best monitored
   by determining the dosage that suppresses the serum TSH below
   the normal value; but this suppression does not indicate over-
   treatment.

THYROID FUNCTION DURING PREGNANCY
During pregnancy BMR normally increases 10–25% above nonpregnant level and serum cholesterol also increases; these are
   therefore not useful in differential diagnosis. Radioactive iodine
   uptake is contraindicated.
PBI reaches upper limit of normal 3–6 weeks after conception; if
   PBI does not rise early in pregnancy, abortion is probable. PBI
   may reach 10–12 μg/100 ml. *Beware of falsely increased PBI due
   to prior administration of x-ray contrast media (even many years
   before) and of drugs.*
In hyperthyroidism, both serum T-3 uptake and T-4 are increased,
   but in the pregnant euthyroid patient or euthyroid patient taking
   birth control pills or estrogens, the T-4 is increased and the T-3
   uptake is decreased. Hyperthyroidism may be indicated by the
   failure of the T-3 uptake to decrease during pregnancy.
T-3 uptake gradually decreases (as early as 3–6 weeks after conception) until the end of the first trimester and then remains
   relatively constant. It returns to normal 12–13 weeks postpartum. Failure to decrease by the eighth to tenth week of preg-

nancy may indicate threatened abortion (one should know the patient's normal nonpregnant level).

THYROID FUNCTION DURING NEONATAL PERIOD

Neonatal Hyperthyroidism
Laboratory findings due to present or past maternal hyperthyroidism are noted.

> If there was hyperthyroidism in the past, all laboratory tests may be normal except that administration of thyroid fails to produce the normal expected depression of thyroid function.

Laboratory findings due to increased susceptibility to infection are noted.
Laboratory findings of hyperthyroidism are noted (see pp. 378–379).

Neonatal Hypothyroidism (frequency is $\cong 1 : 8500$ newborns)
Increased serum TSH is the most useful test; can be used on cord or infant's blood.
Serum T-3 and T-4 (radioimmunoassay) may be decreased.
Serum alkaline phosphatase and PBI are decreased.
Serum cholesterol may be increased.
Occasionally RAIU may be indicated (little or no uptake shown) because of the need for early diagnosis to avoid permanent brain damage.
Laboratory findings of maternal hypothyroidism are often present.

Whenever there is suspicion of hypothyroidism (e.g., prolonged icterus neonatorum, anemia, a birth weight of >9 lbs [$\cong 4$ kg], various clinical findings), tests should always be done to establish the diagnosis as promptly as possible.

ACUTE STREPTOCOCCAL THYROIDITIS
WBC and polynuclear leukocytes are increased.
ESR is increased.
The 24-hour uptake of ^{131}I is usually decreased but sometimes is normal.
Serum PBI is usually normal but may be increased or decreased.
BEI is lower than PBI because with thyroid necrosis iodine-containing proteins enter the blood; these are included in the PBI determination but not in the BEI because they are not soluble in butanol.

HASHIMOTO'S THYROIDITIS (STRUMA LYMPHOMATOSA)
Thyroid function may be normal; 15–20% of patients develop hypothyroidism; occasionally a patient passes through a hyperthyroid stage.
Serum antithyroglobulin antibodies (tanned RBCs) are positive at a titer of 1 : 25,000, but lower titers may be significant. 50% of patients may have a significant titer.
PBI may be decreased, normal, or increased and may vary over a period of time (because of thyroid destruction and regeneration). *Suspect Hashimoto's thyroiditis when PBI is increased or nor-*

mal but BEI and T-4 are decreased (gland is making iodoprotein but decreased amounts of thyroxine). [131]I may be higher than expected in hypothyroidism.

Radioiodine scan may show involvement of only a single lobe (more common in younger patients).

Response to TSH distinguishes primary and secondary hypothyroidism. If thyroid uptake for each lobe is measured separately after TSH, a difference between the lobes may demonstrate lobar thyroiditis when total uptake is apparently normal.

Laboratory findings of hypothyroidism, when present (see pp. 379, 383), are noted.

Biopsy of thyroid may be performed.

Serum TSH is increased in one-third of persons who are clinically euthyroid and in those with clinical hypothyroidism, many of whom have normal T-4, T-3, and T-7.

DE QUERVAIN'S THYROIDITIS (SUBACUTE THYROIDITIS) (probably of viral origin)

[131]I uptake is decreased; may be zero in early stages. It is not increased by TSH administration during active phase. It may be >50% for several weeks after recovery.

PBI is normal to increased; BEI may be <80% of PBI.

ESR is increased.

WBC is normal or decreased.

Biopsy of thyroid confirms diagnosis.

Antithyroglobulin antibodies (tanned RBCs) may be present for up to several months at levels of about 1 : 320), but the titer is never as high as in Hashimoto's thyroiditis. The level falls with recovery.

RIEDEL'S CHRONIC THYROIDITIS

Biopsy of thyroid confirms diagnosis.

Some patients may have laboratory findings of hypothyroidism.

SIMPLE NONTOXIC DIFFUSE GOITER

No specific laboratory findings

SINGLE OR MULTIPLE NODULAR GOITERS

Isotope scanning of thyroid may show decreased ("cold") or increased ("hot") uptake.

Functioning solitary adenoma may produce hyperthyroidism.

CARCINOMA OF THYROID

Serum hormone levels are almost always normal in untreated patients. Rarely, evidence of hyperthyroidism may be found with large masses of follicular carcinoma.

Increased baseline serum calcitonin levels or increased level after calcium infusion is a sensitive indicator of medullary carcinoma of the thyroid. May be found even in absence of palpable mass in the thyroid.

Laboratory findings due to associated lesions (pheochromocytoma, parathyroid tumors) and to production of additional sub-

Table 56. Laboratory Findings in Various Diseases of Calcium and Phosphorus Metabolism[a]

Disease	Serum Calcium[b] (>11 mg/100 ml in 90%)	Serum Phosphorus (<3 mg/100 ml in 90%)	Serum Alkaline Phosphatase	Urine Calcium[c]	Urine Phosphorus
Hyperparathyroidism[d]	I	D	I (N if no bone disease)	I	I
Hypoparathyroidism	D	I	N	D	D[e]
Pseudohypoparathyroidism	D	I	N; occ. D	D	D[e]
Pseudopseudohypoparathyroidism	N	N	N	N	N
Secondary hyperparathyroidism (renal rickets)	V	I	I or N	D or I	D
Vitamin D excess	I	I or D	N or I	I	I
Rickets and osteomalacia	D or N	D or N	I	D	D
Osteoporosis	N	N	N	N or I	N
Polyostotic fibrous dysplasia	N	N	N or I	N	N
Paget's disease	N	N or I	I	N or I	I
Metastatic neoplasm to bone	N or I	V	N or I	V	I

Multiple myeloma	N or I	V	N or I	N or I	N or I
Sarcoidosis	N or I	N or I	N or I	I	N
Fanconi syndrome or renal loss of fixed base	D or N	D	N or I	I	I
Histiocytosis X (Letterer-Siwe, Hand-Schüller-Christian, eosinophilic granuloma)	N	N	N or I	N or I	N
Hypercalcemia and excess intake of alkali (Burnett's syndrome)	I	I or N	N	N	N
Solitary bone cyst	N	N	N	N	N

N = normal; D = decreased; I = increased; V = variable; occ. = occasionally.

[a] See Serum Parathyroid Hormone (p. 82).
[b] Serum calcium. Repeated determinations may be required to demonstrate abnormalties. Serum total protein level should always be known. See also response to corticoids on p. 92.
[c] Urine calcium. Patient should be on a low-calcium diet (e.g., Bauer-Aub).
[d] See Table 57, p. 390.
[e] See Ellsworth-Howard test on p. 92.

stances (e.g., ACTH, serotonin, histaminase) by medullary carcinoma.
RAIU is almost always normal.
Radioactive scan of thyroid (see p. 153)
Needle biopsy of thyroid nodule

PRIMARY HYPERPARATHYROIDISM

Serum calcium is increased (may be as high as 20 mg/100 ml). Repeated terminations may be required to demonstrate increased serum calcium levels. Rapid decrease after excision of adenoma may cause tetany during next few weeks, especially when serum alkaline phosphatase is increased.

Serum total protein must always be measured simultaneously as marked decrease may cause a decrease in calcium.
Normal calcium level may occur with coexistence of conditions that decrease serum calcium level (e.g., high phosphate intake, malabsorption, acute pancreatitis, nephrosis, infarction of parathyroid adenoma); also beware of laboratory error as a cause of "normal" serum calcium.
High phosphate intake can abolish increased serum and urine calcium and decreased serum phosphorus; low-phosphate diet unmasks these changes.

Serum phosphorus is decreased (less than 3 mg/100 ml). It may be normal in the presence of high phosphorus intake or renal damage with secondary phosphate retention. It may be normal in one-half of patients, even without uremia.
Serum alkaline phosphatase is normal or may be markedly increased in the presence of bone disease. There is a slow decrease to normal after excision of adenoma.
Urine calcium is increased (>400 mg on a normal diet; 180 mg on a low-calcium diet). Urine calcium increase is found in only 70% of patients with hyperparathyroidism.
Urine phosphorus is increased unless there is renal insufficiency or phosphate depletion (especially due to commonly used antacids containing aluminum). Phosphate loading unmasks the increased urine phosphorus of hyperparathyroidism.
Polyuria is present, with low specific gravity.
Cortisone administration (150 mg/day for 10 days)
    Usually does not affect the increased serum calcium of parathyroid adenoma.
    Within 2 weeks lowers the increased serum calcium of multiple myeloma, metastatic carcinoma, vitamin D intoxication, infantile hypercalcemia, sarcoidosis.
Serum chloride is increased (>102 mEq/L; <99 mEq/L in other types of hypercalcemia).
Serum alpha$_2$ and beta$_1$ globulins are slightly increased but return to normal after parathyroidectomy. *Serum protein electrophoresis should always be performed in hyperparathyroidism to rule out multiple myeloma and sarcoidosis.*
Uric acid is increased in $>15\%$ of patients. Uric acid level is not

affected by cure of hyperparathyroidism, but a postoperative gout attack may occur.

Increased hydroxyproline in serum and urine may occur with bone disease but is not as useful as serum alkaline phosphatase for detection of bone disease.

Frequently anemia, decreased WBC, and sometimes decreased platelets due to bone marrow depression are found.

Serum parathyroid hormone level (measured by radioimmunoassay) is elevated (see p. 82). Intravenous infusion of calcium sufficient to induce hypercalcemia suppresses the level of serum parathyroid hormone in primary hyperplasia of the parathyroids and in secondary hyperparathyroidism due to renal insufficiency but does not suppress the serum parathyroid hormone level due to parathyroid adenoma.

Serum parathyroid hormone level rises above baseline level after neck massage only on the side of the adenoma, thereby aiding preoperative localization of the adenoma.

Hyperparathyroidism must always be ruled out in the presence of
Renal colic and stones or calcification (2–3% have hyperparathyroidism). (See Table 70, page 442.)

Peptic ulcer (occurs in 15% of patients with hyperparathyroidism)

Calcific keratitis

Bone changes *(present in 20% of patients with hyperparathyroidism)*

Jaw tumors

Clinical syndrome of hypercalcemia (nocturia, hyposthenuria, polyuria, abdominal pain, adynamic ileus, constipation, nausea, vomiting) *(present in 20% of patients with hyperparathyroidism; only clue to diagnosis in 10% of patients with hyperparathyroidism)*

Multiple endocrine adenomatosis (e.g., islet cell tumor of pancreas, pituitary tumor, pheochromocytoma)

Relatives of patients with hyperparathyroidism or "asymptomatic" hypercalcemia

Mental aberrations

"Asymptomatic" hyperparathyroidism (tested by routine serum calcium screening) is found in 0.09% of patient population.

See sections on decreased tubular reabsorption of phosphate, increased phosphate clearance, negative calcium tolerance test, serum calcium and phosphorus changes induced by phosphate deprivation—all on pp. 92–93.

SECONDARY HYPERPARATHYROIDISM

This is a diffuse hyperplasia of parathyroid glands usually secondary to chronic advanced renal disease.

Laboratory findings due to underlying causative disease are noted.

Laboratory findings like those in primary hyperparathyroidism are noted, but

Serum calcium is usually not increased in osteomalacia, rickets, renal rickets, steatorrhea.

Table 57. Comparison of Types of Excess Parathormone Production

Laboratory tests	Ectopic Parathyroid Hormone Production	Primary Hyperparathyroidism
Cause	Epidermoid or large cell carcinoma of bronchus, hypernephroma of kidney, cancer of ovary, colon	Primary hyperplasia, adenoma, carcinoma of parathyroids
Serum calcium	Very high: >14 mg/100 ml in 75% of patients. Suppressed by cortisone in 25–50% of patients	Moderately high: >14 mg/100 ml in 25% of patients. Rarely suppressed by cortisone
Serum chloride	Low: <99 mEq/L	High: >102 mEq/L
Serum bicarbonate	Often increased	Normal or low
Serum alkaline phosphatase	Increased in 50% of patients, even when bone x-rays are negative	Seldom increased unless bone disease is present
Serum phosphorus	Normal or low	Normal or low
Urine calcium	Often >400 mg/24 hours	Usually <400 mg/24 hours
Serum parathormone	Increased but less than in primary hyperparathyroidism for the calcium level	Increased
Nephrolithiasis and x-ray changes in bone	Absent	Common
Anemia and other findings due to malignancy	Present	Absent

Serum calcium may be slightly increased in pituitary basophilism, multiple myeloma, metastatic carcinoma of bone, osteogenesis imperfecta, etc.

HYPOPARATHYROIDISM
Serum calcium is decreased (as low as 5 mg/100 ml). *More than one-third of these patients may present as "epileptics."* Hypoparathyroidism should be ruled out in presence of mental and emotional changes, cataracts, faulty dentition in children, associated changes in skin and nails (e.g., moniliasis is frequent).
Serum phosphorus is increased (usually 5–6 mg/100 ml; as high as 12 mg/100 ml).
Serum alkaline phosphatase is normal or slightly decreased.
Urine calcium is decreased (Sulkowitch's test is negative).
Urine phosphorus is decreased. Phosphate clearance is decreased (see p. 93).
Serum parathyroid hormone level is decreased (see p. 82).

Injection of potent parathyroid extract (200 units IV) causes urine phosphorus to increase $\geqq$ 10 times within 3–5 hours. In a normal person the increase in urine phosphorus is 5–6 times. In pseudohypoparathyroidism, the urine phosphorus is not increased >2 times (see Ellsworth-Howard test, p. 92).

Alkalosis is present.

Congenital form may be associated with thymic aplasia (DiGeorge's syndrome) (see p. 327).

Serum uric acid is increased.

There is a flat oral GTT (due to poor absorption).

CSF is normal, even with mental or emotional symptoms or with calcification of basal ganglia.

PSEUDOHYPOPARATHYROIDISM

Serum calcium, phosphorus, and alkaline phosphatase are the same as in hypoparathyroidism but cannot be corrected by (or they respond poorly to) administration of parathyroid hormone (see reference to Ellsworth-Howard test in the preceding section).

Serum parathyroid hormone level is normal or slightly elevated.

PSEUDOPSEUDOHYPOPARATHYROIDISM

Serum and urine calcium, phosphorus, and alkaline phosphatase are normal.

Response to parathyroid hormone is normal.

Clinical anomalies are the same as in pseudohypoparathyroidism.

PRIMARY HYPOPHOSPHATEMIA

This is a familial but occasionally sporadic condition of intrinsic renal tubular defect in phosphate resorption.

Serum phosphorus is always decreased in the untreated patient.

Serum calcium is usually normal.

Serum alkaline phosphatase is often increased.

Bone biopsy shows a characteristic pattern of demineralization around osteocyte lacunae.

HYPOPHOSPHATASIA

This rare genetic disease of bone mineralization with x-ray changes and clinical syndromes is found in infants and children, and adults.

Serum alkaline phosphatase is decreased to $\cong$ 25% of normal (may vary from $0 \leqq 40\%$ of normal); is not correlated with severity of disease.

Serum and urine levels of phosphoethanolamine are increased (may be normal in asymptomatic heterozygotes).

Serum calcium is increased in severe cases.

Serum phosphorus is normal.

Treatment with corticosteroids usually causes an increase in serum alkaline phosphatase (but it never attains normal level) with a marked fall in serum calcium; phosphoethanolamine excretion in urine continues high.

PSEUDOHYPOPHOSPHATASIA
(clinical syndrome resembling hypophosphatasia)

Serum alkaline phosphatase is normal.

IDIOPATHIC HYPERPHOSPHATASIA OF INFANCY (FAMILIAL OSTEOECTASIA)

This condition is characterized by excessive osteoblastic activity but almost no formation of normal cortical bone.
Serum alkaline phosphatase is increased.

IDIOPATHIC HYPERCALCEMIA OF INFANCY WITH FAILURE TO THRIVE

Characteristics are mental retardation, elfin face, and chemical changes.
Serum calcium is increased to $\geqq 12$ mg/100 ml.
Serum phosphorus is normal.
Serum cholesterol is increased occasionally.
Renal calcinosis may cause proteinuria, microscopic hematuria, azotemia, and hyperchloremic acidosis.

NEONATAL HYPOCALCEMIA
(age 1–4 weeks; serum calcium <8 mg/100 ml)

Age 1–2 days—associated with
  Prematurity and low birth weight (occurs in $\leqq 50\%$ of infants)
  Maternal diabetes (occurs in $\leqq 25\%$ of infants)
Age 5–10 days—associated with
  Feeding of cow's milk (increased serum phosphorus and decreased serum calcium)
Rarely associated with
  Maternal hypercalcemia or hyperparathyroidism
  Congenital absence of parathyroid glands
  Hypoproteinemia (e.g., nephrosis, liver disease)
  Maternal osteomalacia
  Renal disease (primary renal tubular defect; decreased glomerular filtration rate causing phosphate retention)
  Iatrogenic disorders (e.g., citrate administration during exchange transfusion)

When tetany syndrome is associated with a normal serum calcium or not relieved by administration of calcium, rule out decreased serum magnesium.
Serum phosphorus is >8 mg/100 ml when neonatal hypocalcemia is due to high phosphate feeding. BUN is increased when neonatal hypocalcemia is due to severe renal disease.

SYNDROME OF FAMILIAL HYPOCALCEMIA, LATENT TETANY, AND CALCIFICATION OF BASAL GANGLIA

This rare clinical syndrome has features resembling those of pseudohypoparathyroidism, pseudopseudohypoparathyroidism, and basal cell nevus syndrome.
Hypocalcemia is not responsive to parathormone administration.
Parathormone administration produces a phosphate diuresis.

DECREASED TISSUE CALCIUM WITH TETANY

The tetany, associated with normal serum calcium, magnesium, potassium, and Co_2, responds to vitamin D therapy.

Special radioactive calcium studies show decreased tissue calcium pool that returns toward normal with therapy.

VITAMIN D INTOXICATION
Serum calcium may be increased.
Serum phosphorus is usually also increased but sometimes is decreased, with increased urinary phosphorus.
Serum alkaline phosphatase is decreased.

MAGNESIUM DEFICIENCY TETANY SYNDROME
Serum magnesium is decreased (usually < 1 mEq/L).
Serum calcium is normal (slightly decreased in some patients)
Blood pH is normal.
Tetany responds to administration of magnesium but not of calcium.

DIABETES MELLITUS
When glycosuria is present, diabetes mellitus must always be ruled out.
Elevated fasting blood sugar (FBS) may be normal in mild diabetes; therefore it is not adequate for case finding.
Elevated 2-hour postprandial blood sugar alone is superior to FBS alone for routine screening for diabetes.
Glucose tolerance test (GTT) is most useful for detecting latent or incipient diabetes. If GTT is normal but diabetes mellitus is clinically suspected, test should be repeated. Cortisone GTT increases the sensitivity of the test.

With fasting hyperglycemia, prolonged increase of blood sugar follows glucose ingestion.

With normal FBS, a 1-hour blood sugar > 170 mg/100 ml and 2-hour blood sugar > 150 mg/100 ml indicates diabetes mellitus.

More severe diabetes produces a more abnormal curve.

Some cases of mild diabetes show hypoglycemia at 4–5 hours.

When only one of the blood sugar levels at 1-, 2-, or 3-hour intervals is abnormal, 50% of the patients become diabetic.

A diabetic type of GTT curve may result if the patient has had inadequate caloric and carbohydrate diet; therefore, during the preceding 3 days, he should have a carbohydrate intake of 300 gm/day.

When plasma insulin levels are measured at the same time as glucose in the GTT, several patterns of insulin response are seen.

Diabetes with full insulin response—elevated insulin curve associated with a mild diabetic curve (see Fig. 2, p. 87); occurs mainly in adult obesity, pregnancy, cirrhosis, and acromegaly.

Diabetes with partial insulin response—abnormally elevated glucose curve, with an insulin rise that is not proportionately increased and that may show a delayed peak. This curve is seen in most cases of adult-onset diabetes. Insulin response varies from almost normal to almost absent and slowly deteriorates as the disease evolves.

Diabetes without insulin response—very high glucose curve, with little change in insulin levels (which are normal in baseline state). Occurs in juvenile diabetes or severe adult-onset diabetes.

Serum sodium is inversely related to increased blood sugar (e.g., glucose of 180 mg/100 ml is associated with a decrease of serum sodium of 5 mEq/L).

Lipemia causes false decrease in all serum electrolytes.

Hypoglycemic episodes may occur in the prediabetic state. 50% of patients with hypoglycemic episodes have a positive family history of diabetes.

Primary diabetes mellitus
Inherited metabolic defect with impaired production, release, or effectiveness of insulin
Secondary diabetes
Pancreas
Chronic pancreatitis, hemochromatosis, carcinoma of pancreas, postpancreatectomy
Endocrine
Hyperthyroidism, hyperadrenalism (Cushing's syndrome, primary aldosteronism, pheochromocytoma), acromegaly

See sections on diabetic nephrosclerosis, papillary necrosis, infection of genitourinary tract, lipoproteins, etc.

PREDIABETES
Blood glucose and insulin levels are normal with fasting and during oral GTT and intravenous tolbutamide tests.

During intravenous GTT, glucose tolerance is normal but serum insulin levels are subnormal, especially in the early phase of the insulin response.

Rule out prediabetic state in patients who
Develop glycosuria during treatment with thiazide or birth control pills.
Have significant family history of diabetes mellitus
Have given birth to infants with birth weight > 10 pounds
Show premature development of arteriosclerosis

Prediabetics should be observed for the development of overt diabetes in the presence of obesity, infections, pregnancy, pancreatitis, thyrotoxicosis, Cushing's syndrome, acromegaly.

DIABETIC KETOACIDOSIS
Blood glucose is increased (usually >300 mg/100 ml).

Plasma acetone is present.

There is hemoconcentration due to dehydration and electrolyte changes.

Azotemia is present.

Blood pH is decreased.

WBC is increased (often >20,000/cu mm without infection).

Urine contains increased sugar, ketones, protein, and casts.

See Metabolic Acidosis, pp. 342–343; Lactic Acidosis, pp. 343–344; Hyperosmolar State, p. 50.

Look for precipitating factors, especially infection.

SOME HETEROGENEOUS GENETIC DISEASES ASSOCIATED WITH HYPERGLYCEMIA
Alström's syndrome
Ataxia-telangiectasia
Diabetes mellitus
Friedreich's ataxia
Hemochromatosis
Herrmann's syndrome
Hyperlipoproteinemias (three different types)
Isolated growth hormone deficiency
Laurence-Moon-Biedl-Bardet syndrome
Lipoatrophic diabetes
Myotonic dystrophy
Optic atrophy
Prader-Willi syndrome
Refsum's syndrome
Schmidt's syndrome
Werner's syndrome

PRADER-WILLI SYNDROME
This condition is characterized by mental retardation, muscular hypotonia, obesity, short stature, and hypogonadism associated with diabetes mellitus.

Diabetes mellitus frequently develops in childhood and adolescence but is insulin-resistant, responds to oral hypoglycemic drugs, and is not accompanied by adidosis.

ISLET CELL TUMORS OF PANCREAS—CLASSIFICATION
Insulin-secreting beta cell tumor (may be benign or malignant, primary or metastatic) produces hyperinsulinism with hypoglycemia (see next section for laboratory findings and differential diagnosis).

Non-insulin-secreting non-beta cell tumor (benign or malignant, primary or metastatic) may produce several types of syndromes.

Zollinger-Ellison syndrome (see next page)
Profuse diarrhea with hypokalemia and dehydration
Profuse diarrhea with hypokalemia (and sometimes periodic paralysis) may occur as a separate syndrome without peptic ulceration. (*Some of the patients have histamine-fast achlorhydria.*) Diabetic glucose tolerance curves may occur in some patients because of chronic potassium depletion. May be associated with multiple endocrine adenomas.

Nonspecific diarrhea
Steatorrhea (due to inactivation of pancreatic enzymes by acid pH)

HYPERINSULINISM
(due to hyperfunctioning islet cell tumor of pancreas or islet cell hyperplasia)

Blood glucose is $<$ 40 mg/100 ml at time of symptoms. Symptoms are relieved by administration of glucose. Frequent blood glucose determinations may be required. It may be necessary to provoke symptoms by fast for 72 hours and determining glucose levels whenever symptoms develop. *(This procedure may have to be repeated since some tumors secrete insulin intermittently.)*

Elevated fasting serum insulin level is highly suggestive but is normal in 30% of patients. May require administration of tolbutamide glucagon, or leucine to stimulate an excessive insulin response to establish the diagnosis. Only a positive response is useful; negative test results are not of diagnostic value.

Note that 24% of patients with islet cell tumor have a family history of diabetes; 25% of patients with diabetes have a family history of diabetes; and 3–6% of nondiabetics have a family history of diabetes.

Dumping syndrome shows normal blood glucose level.

See sections on advanced liver disease, hypopituitarism, hypoadrenalism, glycogen-storage disease, alcoholism, hypoglycemia associated with neoplasms, etc.

See Tolbutamide Tolerance Test, p. 89.

ZOLLINGER-ELLISON SYNDROME (GASTRINOMA)

Serum gastrin is markedly increased.

There is a large volume of highly acid gastric juice in the absence of pyloric obstruction; it is refractory to vagotomy and subtotal gastrectomy* (see Serum Gastrin, pp. 84–85; Gastric Analysis, pp. 143–144).

Hypokalemia is frequently associated with chronic severe diarrhea that may be a clue to this diagnosis.

Steatorrhea occurs rarely.

Laboratory findings due to peptic ulcer of stomach, duodenum, or proximal jejunum (e.g., performation, fluid loss, hemorrhage) are noted. *25% of these patients have ulcers in unusual locations or have multiple ulcerations. A tendency toward rapid or severe recurrence of ulcer after adequate therapy is a clue to Zollinger-Ellison syndrome.*

Gastrinomas are non-beta cell tumors arising in pancreas.

Tumors are multiple in 28% of all patients.

Adenomas are multiple in 29% of patients and may be ectopic (e.g., in duodenal wall).

Tumors are malignant in 62% of patients; 44% of patients have metastases.

Diffuse hyperplasia occurs in 10% of patients.

*12-hour nocturnal secretion shows acid of $>$100 mEq/L and volume of $>$ 1500 ml baseline secretion is $>$ 60% of the secretion caused by histamine or betazole stimulation.

This syndrome is associated with hyperparathyroidism in 20% of patients and frequently with adenomas of other endocrine glands, adrenal and pituitary (e.g., insulinoma) (see Multiple Endocrine Adenoma, p. 425).

REACTIVE (FUNCTIONAL) HYPOGLYCEMIA

Table 58. Differentiation of Hypoglycemic Symptoms

Criteria for Diagnosis	Anxiety State	Reactive Hypoglycemia[a]
5-Hour GTT	Blood glucose level not usually <50 mg/100 ml	Blood glucose level falls to <40 mg/100 ml
Symptoms	Not related to blood glucose level	Coincide with low blood glucose level
Response of plasma cortisol level to low blood glucose level	No plasma cortisol response	Plasma cortisol level doubles within 90 minutes after hypoglycemic symptoms or low blood glucose level occurs

[a]Reactive hypoglycemia refers to low blood glucose level during 5-hour GTT (not during fasting) and may be due to alimentary conditions (e.g., peptic ulcer) or diabetes mellitus, or it may be idiopathic. Fasting hypoglycemia almost always indicates organic disease.

Diagnosis of reactive hypoglycemia should not be made only on the basis of the blood glucose level. After a 100-gm glucose load in healthy asymptomatic young men, postprandial glucose levels of <60 mg/100 ml are found in 20–25% of subjects and <40 mg/100 ml in 2–3% of subjects.

Serum insulin levels rarely reach the high insulin levels seen in insulinoma patients, even after stimulation with tolbutamide.

ADRENAL FUNCTION TESTS*

Daily infusion of 50 units of ACTH for 5 days, with before and after measurement of 24-hour urines for 17-ketosteroids (KS), 17-hydroxyketosteroids (OHKS) *(Protect possible Addison's disease patient with 1 mg of dexamethasone.)*

    Complete primary adrenal insufficiency (Addison's disease)—no increase in urine steroids or increase of <2 mg/day

    Incomplete primary adrenal insufficiency—less than normal increases on all 5 days or slight increase on first 3 days that may be followed by decrease on days 4 and 5

    Secondary adrenal insufficiency due to pituitary hypofunction—"staircase" response of progressively higher values each day

    Secondary adrenal insufficiency due to chronic steroid therapy—may require prolonged ACTH testing to elicit the "staircase" response; may produce increments only in 17-OHKS but not in 17-KS

*See footnote, p. 398.

Normal = 3–5 times increase on first day and further increase next day

Do not do metyrapone test until this test proves that adrenals are sensitive to ACTH.

Measurement of circulating eosinophil count before and after ACTH stimulation (see p. 397)
    Normal
        Decrease of 80% if previous baseline was >100 cells/cu mm and no parasitic eosinophilia
    Adrenal insufficiency
        Decrease of <25%

LABORATORY TESTS FOR EVALUATION OF ADRENAL-PITUITARY FUNCTION IN PATIENTS WITH HYPERAD-RENALISM*

Adrenal-Cortical Reserve (stimulation of adrenal cortex by administration of ACTH)

Functioning adrenal cortex is indicated by increased blood and urine 17-OHKS above patient's previous baseline level.
    Normal adrenal-cortical reserve. An increase of 3–5 times is shown the first day and a further increase the next day.
    Adrenal cortical hyperplasia. Test is often not helpful in diagnosis of Cushing's syndrome.
    Hypopituitarism. A slight increase is shown the first day and a greater increase the next day.
Nonfunctioning adrenal cortex is indicated by no increase of blood and urine 17-OHKS.
    Adenoma of adrenal cortex. Lack of response almost always means autonomous tumor.
    Carcinoma of adrenal cortex. Lack of response almost always means autonomous tumor; there is an associated characteristic marked increase over baseline of urinary neutral 17-KS.
    Addison's disease.

Pituitary-Adrenal Suppression (suppression of pituitary ACTH secretion by administration of dexamethasone)

Functioning pituitary-adrenal system is indicated by decrease in blood and urine 17-OHKS.
    Normal pituitary-adrenal system. Urinary level falls to <50% of baseline level following lower or higher dose of dexamethasone. Plasma cortisol decreases ($<5\mu g$/100 ml) after both lower and higher dose schedules of dexamethasone.
    Adrenal hyperplasia. Urinary level falls to <50% only after higher but not after lower dose of dexamethasone. Plasma cortisol decreases ($<5\mu g$/100 ml) only after higher dose of

*Measurement of plasma cortisol and ACTH by radioimmunoassay has become more readily available and is more sensitive and specific and convenient then urinary 17-OHKS 24-hour urine measurements which is gradually being replaced.

dexamethasone; remains >10 μg/100 ml after low dose of dexamethasone in Cushing's syndrome.

Failure of pituitary control of adrenal-cortical secretion is indicated by *no* decrease in blood and urine 17-OHKS.

Adenoma or carcinoma of adrenal cortex. Lack of response to high and low doses of dexamethasone confirms diagnosis of Cushing's syndrome and differentiates autonomous tumor from adrenal hyperplasia due to pituitary dysfunction.

Adrenal hyperfunction due to extra-adrenal tumor (e.g., cancer of bronchus). There is a lack of response to high or low doses of dexamethasone.

Pituitary Reserve (adrenal suppression of pituitary secretion of ACTH inhibited by administration of metyrapone)

Functioning adrenal-pituitary system is indicated by increased urine 17-OHKS to twice the previous baseline level with

Normal adrenal glands

Adrenal-cortical hyperplasia

Nonfunctioning adrenal-pituitary system. (Long-standing production of excessive cortisol by adrenal tumor decreases pituitary reserve and responsiveness. Therefore ACTH is not secreted and there is no increase in urinary 17-OHKS and 17-KS.)

Adenoma or carcinoma of adrenal cortex

Adrenal hyperfunction due to extra-adrenal tumor (e.g., cancer of bronchus)

Also: Addison's disease, hypopituitarism

CUSHING'S SYNDROME*

Glucose tolerance is diminished.

GTT is frequently diabetic in type.

Glycosuria appears in 50% of patients.

Fasting blood glucose may be elevated.

Insulin tolerance is increased.

Occasional polydipsia and polyuria are seen.

Usually moderate increase in serum sodium and decrease in serum potassium are found.

Hypokalemic alkalosis occurs in ≅ 10% of patients.

Hypokalemic alkalosis may indicate extra-adrenal neoplasia such as a bronchogenic carcinoma causing increased production of ACTH with increased secretion of mineralocorticoids and glucocorticoids; occurs in 30–50% of such patients.

Urine potassium is increased; sodium is decreased.

Salivary sodium-potassium ratio is decreased.

Hematologic changes are as follows.

WBC is normal or increased.

Relative lymphopenia is frequent (differential is usually <15% of cells).

Eosinopenia is frequent (usually <100/cu mm).

*T. Nichols, C. A. Nugent, and F. H. Tyler, Steroid laboratory tests in the diagnosis of Cushing's syndrome. *Am. J. Med.* 45:116, 1968.

Hematocrit is usually normal; if increased, it indicates an androgenic component.

Osteoporosis causes changes.

Serum and urine calcium may be increased.

BUN may be increased.

Urine creatine is increased.

Serum gamma globulins may be decreased and alpha$_2$ globulin may be moderately increased.

Urinary 17-KS levels are usually increased (> 25 mg/24 hours).

Urinary 17-OHKS levels are increased (>10 mg/24 hours).

The night collection sample is equal to or greater than the day sample (opposite pattern in normal person).

ACTH stimulation produces the lowest urinary 17-OHKS in Cushing's syndrome due to adrenal carcinoma and the highest urinary 17-OHKS due to adrenal adenoma.

Plasma cortisol is increased and remains high late in day (in normal person, plasma cortisol falls by >50% late in day).

Dexamethasone suppression of adrenal cortex. In normal person given small doses of dexamethasone, the urinary 17-OHKS falls to <2.5 mg/24 hours (often <2 mg/24 hours) and the plasma cortisol level to <5 μg/100 ml. Cushing's syndrome due to adenoma or carcinoma shows little or no fall in urinary 17-OHKS; with adrenal hyperplasia large doses of dexamethasone suppress urinary 17-OHKS to <50% of baseline, but there is less or no suppression with small doses of dexamethasone. (*See below. There are cases in both categories that do not follow these general rules.*) No suppression is seen in Cushing's syndrome due to nonendocrine neoplasm even when large doses of dexamethasone are given.

Serum ACTH is high when Cushing's syndrome is of pituitary or hypothalamic origin and markedly decreased when it is due to adrenal tumor or hyperplasia. Serum ACTH level is very high and shows no diurnal variation in ectopic ACTH syndrome (e.g., carcinoma of lung).

Metyrapone test (see Table 59, pp. 402–403)

Various steroid tests are abnormal in 55–100% of patients with Cushing's syndrome and 36% of patients without Cushing's syndrome. They are >40% above normal in 28–96% of patients with Cushing's syndrome and ≦5% of patients without Cushing's syndrome.

Therefore the clinician should remember that in Cushing's syndrome, as in all other complex clinical problems, the diagnosis should not be established or ruled out on the basis of only 1 or 2 laboratory tests.

Best steroid tests for identifying patients with Cushing's syndrome are the failure of suppression of urinary 17-OHKS by low dose of dexamethasone and the suppression of plasma cortisol by a single dose of dexamethasone.

No single test can establish the cause of Cushing's syndrome with certainty.

Suppression of urinary 17-OHKS by high dose of dexamethasone is positive in 80% of patients with adrenal hyperplasia due to excessive pituitary secretion of ACTH without tumor; a positive result is very uncommon in adrenal tumors.

Increased urinary 17-OHKS by metyrapone administration is positive in
100% of adrenal hyperplasias without tumor
50% of adrenal adenomas
25% of adrenal carcinomas
Increased urinary 17-KS is >4 times normal in
50% of adrenal carcinomas
15% of extrapituitary tumors that secrete ACTH
3% of adrenal hyperplasias without tumors
Urinary 17-KS is normal or low in
70% of adrenal adenomas
50% of adrenal hyperplasias
10% of adrenal carcinomas
Increased urinary 17-OHKS is >4 times normal in
63% of patients with Cushing's syndrome
3% of patients without Cushing's syndrome
65% of Cushing's syndrome due to extrapituitary tumors that secrete ACTH
3% of Cushing's syndrome due to adrenal hyperplasia without tumor
Plasma renin activity is increased; suppressed activity suggests ectopic ACTH syndrome or adrenal adenoma or carcinoma (causing increased secretion of DOC or aldosterone).

CONGENITAL ADRENAL HYPERPLASIA (ADRENOGENITAL SYNDROMES)

Pregnanetriol is almost always elevated in all cases of adrenogenital syndrome; it is the most specific diagnostic procedure for adrenogenital syndrome.

Urinary 17-ketogenic steroids (17-KGS) are elevated in all types (17-OHKS included).

ACTH stimulation causes marked increase in 17-KGS, 17-KS, and pregnanetriol; little or no change in Porter-Silber (P-S) chromagens.

Metyrapone test causes increase in 17-KGS but subnormal increase in P-S chromagens.

See Table 60, p. 404.

COMPARISON OF ADRENOGENITAL SYNDROMES DUE TO 17-ALPHA-HYDROXYLATION AND 11-BETA-HYDROXYLATION DEFICIENCIES

	17-Alpha-Hydroxylation Deficiency	*11-Beta-Hydroxylation Deficiency*
Plasma ACTH	Increased	Increased
Plasma cortisol	Decreased	Normal
Hypokalemia	More	Less
Decreased aldosterone in plasma and urine	More marked	Less marked
Decreased plasma renin activity	More marked	Less marked
Increased plasma deoxycorticosterone	More marked	Less marked

Table 59. Laboratory Tests in Differential Diagnosis of Cushing's Syndrome of Different Etiologies

Condition	Component	Baseline	After ACTH Stimulation	Dexamethasone Suppression		Metyrapone Test
				2 mg/day	8 mg/day	
Normal	17-OHKS in urine	N	I	D	D	Markedly I
	Plasma cortisol[a]	N	I	D	D	
Adrenal hyperplasia due to Pituitary dysfunction	17-OHKS in urine	I	I	Not D	D	Markedly I
	Plasma cortisol	N or I	I	Not D	D	
Extra-adrenal tumor (e.g., cancer of bronchus)	17-OHKS in urine	I	Usually NC (may be I)	Not D	Not D	Markedly I
	Plasma cortisol	I	Usually NC (may be I)	Not D	Not D	
Adrenal adenoma	17-OHKS in urine	I	—[b]	Not D	Not D	Not I
	Plasma cortisol	I	—[b]	Not D	Not D	

Adrenal carcinoma	17-OHKS in urine	I	Not I	Not D	Not D	Not I
	Plasma cortisol	I	Not I	Not D	Not D	Not D
Steroid therapy	17-OHKS in urine	D	NC or I	Not D	Not D	Not I
	Plasma cortisol	I	NC	Not D	Not D	

I = increased; D = decreased; N = normal; NC = no change.

[a]Plasma cortisol is higher in morning than afternoon in normal person; no diurnal variation in Cushing's syndrome.

[b]NC with autonomous tumor; I with incompletely autonomous tumor.

Table 60. Comparison of Six Forms of Congenital Adrenal Hyperplasia

Form	Enzyme Deficiency	Frequency	Cortisol	Aldosterone	Adrenal Androgens[a]
Simple virilizing	Partial 21-hydroxylase	≅60%	≅N	≅ twice N	I
Salt-losing	More complete 21-hydroxylase	≅40%	D	D	I
Hypertensive	11-hydroxylase	<5%	D[b]	D[c]	I
17-OHKS deficiency	17-hydroxylase	rare	D	D[c]	D
Lethal (complete)[d]	3-β-hydroxysteroid dehydrogenase	rare	0	0	I[e]
Lethal	Prior to pregnenolone in synthesis of adrenal steroids	rare	0	0	0

N = normal; I = increased; D = decreased; 0 = absent.

[a]Especially important is androstenedione, 10% of which is transformed into testosterone.

[b]Increase of cortisol precursor (11-deoxycortisol).

[c]Increase of aldosterone precursor (deoxycorticosterone).

[d]May sometimes be partial.

[e]Increase of dehydroisoandrosterone only.

404

ADRENAL FEMINIZATION

This condition occurs in adult males with adrenal tumor (usually unilateral carcinoma, occasionally adenoma) that secretes estrogens.

Urinary estrogens are markedly increased.

17-KS are normal or moderately increased and cannot be suppressed by low doses of dexamethasone when due to adrenal tumor.

17-OHKS are normal.

Biopsy of testicle shows atrophy of tubules.

ALDOSTERONISM (PRIMARY)

Excessive mineralocorticoid hormone secretion by adrenal cortex causes renal tubules to retain sodium and excrete potassium. The classic biochemical abnormalities are urinary aldosterone, plasma renin, and serum potassium measurements.

Urinary aldosterone is increased on normal-salt diet (not detectable on all days); cannot be reduced by high-sodium intake and DOCA administration. 24-hour urinary aldosterone is best initial screening procedure (normal salt intake, no drugs).

Plasma renin is markedly decreased (normal or increased in secondary aldosteronism). It cannot be stimulated by use of salt restriction and upright posture to deplete plasma volume.

Hypokalemia (usually <3.0 mEq/L) is alleviated by administration of spironolactone* and by sodium restriction but not by potassium replacement therapy. May be normal in cases of shorter duration before classic clinical picture develops.

Saline infusion causes significant fall in serum potassium and in corrected potassium clearance. This hypokalemia induced by sodium loading is a reliable screening test.

Saline infusion (2 L normal saline in 4 hours) suppresses plasma aldosterone to <5 ng/100 ml in hypertensive patients without primary aldosteronism but not in patients with primary aldosteronism. (Plasma aldosterone level is first increased by having patient in upright position for 2 hours.) Since plasma aldosterone levels vary from moment to moment, a single specimen may not properly reflect adrenal secretion.

Urine is neutral or alkaline (pH >7.0) and not normally responsive to ammonium chloride load. Its large volume and low specific gravity are not responsive to vasopressin or water restriction (decreased tubular function, especially reabsorption of water). Proteinuria is intermittent or persistent. There is hyperkaluria even with low potassium intake. Sodium output is reduced.

There is absence of hyponatremia or slight hypernatremia, hypochloremia, and alkalosis (CO_2 content >25 mEq/L; blood pH tends to increase).

Glucose tolerance is decreased in $\leqq 50\%$ of patients.

Plasma cortisol and ACTH are normal.

Urine 17-KS and 17-OHKS are normal.

---

*Administration of spironolactone for 3 days increases serum potassium >1.2 mEq/L. It also increases urine sodium and decreases urine potassium. Negative potassium balance recurs in 5 days. It increases urinary aldosterone (this is variable in hypertensive and normal people).

Table 61. Laboratory Differentiation of Primary and Secondary Aldosteronism

Testing Procedure	Primary Aldosteronism	Secondary Aldosteronism
Etiology	Usually due to tumor (adenoma more frequent than carcinoma); may be due to bilateral hyperplasia	1. Edematous conditions (e.g., cirrhosis, nephrosis, congestive heart failure) 2. Hypertension (e.g., essential, malignant, renovascular renal artery stenosis) 3. Renal tubular dysfunction (e.g., renal tubular acidosis, Fanconi syndrome) 4. Hemorrhage
Blood electrolytes	Hypokalemia, usually with acidosis and hypernatremia	Depends on underlying condition
Plasma renin	Markedly D	N or I
Urinary 17-OHKS and 17-KS	Usually N; may be I in adrenal carcinoma	N
Urinary aldosterone	Markedly I	Markedly I
Aldosterone administration	Escapes from sodium retention after initial rise in serum sodium	Causes increased edema
Salt-loading	Does not suppress aldosterone secretion (as in normal person) and increases potassium excretion	
Low-sodium diet	Usually reduces potassium excretion	
Deoxycorticosterone administration	In adenoma, aldosterone level is *not* suppressed; in bilateral adrenal hyperplasia, aldosterone level *is* suppressed	

D = decreased; N = normal; I = increased.

Serum magnesium falls.

Total blood volume increases because of increased plasma volume.

Sodium level in sweat is low.

Salivary Na-K ratio <0.65 is consistent with diagnosis, but a higher ratio does not exclude it.

Measurement of aldosterone in blood from periphery and both adrenal veins confirms diagnosis by elevated level from side of lesion; opposite side has level close to that in peripheral blood. This also distinguishes unilateral adenoma from bilateral adenomas and hyperplasia and indicates location of lesion for surgeon.

Caused By

Single benign cortical adenoma (70% of patients)

Multiple benign cortical adenomas (15% of patients)

Bilateral cortical hyperplasia (9% of patients)

Normal size adrenal gland with normal architecture or focal nodular hyperplasia (6% of patients)

Rarely, adrenal carcinoma or heterotopic adrenal tissue

ALDOSTERONISM (SECONDARY)

Due To

Congestive heart failure

Cirrhosis with ascites (aldosterone 2000–3000 mg/day)

Nephrosis

Toxemia of pregnancy

Malignant hypertension

Low-sodium diet

Renin-producing renal tumor (see p. 451)

NORMOTENSIVE SECONDARY HYPERALDOSTERONISM (BARTTER'S SYNDROME)

Blood vessels are unable to respond normally to angiotensin; therefore there is no hypertension. To maintain blood pressure, juxtaglomerular apparatus secretes increased amounts of renin.

Increased urinary aldosterone with associated findings (e.g., hypokalemic alkalosis, inability to concentrate urine, proteinuria)

Increased plasma renin concentration

PSEUDOALDOSTERONISM DUE TO INGESTION OF LICORICE (AMMONIUM GLYCYRRHIZATE)

(excessive ingestion causes hypertension due to sodium retention)

Decreased serum potassium

Decreased aldosterone excretion in urine

Decreased plasma renin activity

Table 62. Laboratory Tests in Differential Diagnosis of Benign Pheochromocytoma and Neural Crest Tumors (Neuroblastoma, Ganglioneuroma)

Urinary Levels of	Pheochro-mocytoma	Neural Crest Tumor (neuroblastoma, ganglioneuroma)
Catecholamines	I	I
VMA	I	I
Metanephrines	I	I
Dopamine	N[a]	I
HVA	N[a]	I

I = increased; N = normal.

[a] I in malignant pheochromocytoma.

HYPOFUNCTION OF RENIN-ANGIOTENSIN-ALDOSTERONE SYSTEM
(differs from Addison's disease and congenital adrenal hyperplasia, which have deficiency of glucocorticoids as well as of mineralocorticoids)

Infrequent condition due to

   Rare congenital or acquired defect in aldosterone biosynthesis (renin normal or increased)

   Prolonged administration of heparin (very rare)

   Removal of unilateral aldosterone-secreting tumor (usually transient)

   Autonomic nervous system dysfunction; aldosterone deficiency causes impaired renal sodium conservation but without hyperkalemia

   Idiopathic hyporeninism

Hyperkalemia, urinary sodium loss, extracellular volume depletion corrected by administration of mineralocorticoids

Normal adrenal glucocorticoid response to ACTH stimulation test

Low 24-hour urinary excretion of aldosterone (normal = 3–32 μg/24 hours), with normal dietary intake of sodium and potassium; subnormal aldosterone response to sodium restriction

Mild hyperchloremic metabolic acidosis

Renal function frequently impaired (creatinine clearance rate may be 25–70 ml/minute

Laboratory findings of associated diseases (e.g., diabetes mellitus, gout, pyelonephritis)

Pseudohypoaldosteronism is a rare disease of children characterized by lack of renal tubular response to mineralocorticoid and presence of normal amount of aldosterone.

Table 63. Comparison of Pathologic Hypofunction of Renin-Angiotensin-Aldosterone System and Low-Renin Hypertension

Pathologic Hypofunction of Renin-Angiotensin-Aldosterone System	Low-Renin Hypertension
Hyperkalemia	Normal or low serum potassium
Urinary sodium loss	Sodium retention
Extracellular volume depletion	Increase in extracellular volume
Hypotension; may be normal	Persistent hypertension
Low renin-angiotensin-aldosterone activity	Low plasma renin activity with normal plasma and urinary levels of aldosterone

PHEOCHROMOCYTOMA
Blood and urine levels of norepinephrine and, to a lesser extent, epinephrine are increased, usually even when patient is asymptomatic and normotensive; rarely are increases found only following a paroxysm.

Urine VMA (vanillylmandelic acid, a catecholamine metabolite) excretion is considerably increased. This determination is simpler than for catecholamines and therefore is more commonly used. Beware of false increase due to foods (e.g., vanilla, fruits, especially bananas, coffee, tea) and drugs (e.g., vasopressor agents) ingested within 72 hours before the test (see p. 138). Beware of nonspecific techniques for VMA assay that fail to detect 30% of cases of pheochromocytoma.

Hyperglycemia and glycosuria are found in 50% of patients during an attack.

Glucose tolerance test frequently shows a diabetic type of curve.

Elevated BMR ($> +20\%$) occurs in $\cong 50\%$ of these patients, but other thyroid function tests are normal.

Urine changes are secondary to sustained hypertension.

$\leqq 15\%$ *of pheochromocytomas are malignant; 15% are extraadrenal; 10% are multiple.* Family inheritance in 10–20% of patients. Extensive surgical exploration may be required. Rarely, this syndrome is due to hyperplasia of the adrenal medulla.

"Incidental" pheochromocytomas have been discovered.

Five percent of patients with pheochromocytoma have normal blood pressure most or all of the time.

NEUROBLASTOMA, GANGLIONEUROMA, GANGLIOBLASTOMA

Urinary levels of catecholamines (norepinephrine, normetanephrine, dopamine, VMA, and HVA [homovanillic acid]) are increased.

Excretion of epinephrine is not increased.

Not all methods include dopamine in measurement of total catecholamines.

Not all patients have increased urinary levels of catecholamines, VMA, and HVA.

If only 1 of these substances is measured, only $\cong 75\%$ of cases are diagnosed.

If VMA and HVA or VMA and total catecholamines are measured, 95–100% of cases are diagnosed.

These tests are also useful for differentiating Ewing's tumor and metastatic neuroblastoma of bone and to show response to therapy (surgery, irradiation, or chemotherapy), which should bring return to normal in 1–4 months. Continued elevation indicates need for further treatment.

ADDISON'S DISEASE
(chronic adrenal insufficiency)

Serum potassium is increased.

Serum sodium and chloride are decreased.

Sodium-potassium ratio is $<30 : 1$.

Table 64. Laboratory Differentiation of Primary and Secondary Adrenal Insufficiency

Determination	Primary Adrenal Insufficiency	Adrenal Insufficiency Secondary to Hypopituitarism
After ACTH stimulation (see pp. 397–398)		
Urinary 17-OHKS and 17-KS levels	No responsive increase	Marked "staircase" response
Eosinophil count (decreases 80–90% daily in normal person)	Decreased < 20%	Decrease depends on degree of insufficiency
Blood ACTH level	Increased	Decreased

Blood volume is decreased; hematocrit level is increased (because of water loss).

BUN may be moderately increased.

Fasting hypoglycemia is present, with a flat oral glucose tolerance curve and insulin hypersensitivity. IV GTT shows a normal peak followed by severe prolonged hypoglycemia.

Neutropenia and relative lymphocytosis are common.

Eosinophilia is present (300/cu mm). (*A total eosinophil count of <50 is evidence against severe adrenocortical hypofunction.*)

Normocytic anemia is slight or moderate but difficult to estimate because of decreased blood volume.

Increased blood ACTH (200–1600 pg/ml) with wide variation between morning and evening levels in primary adrenal hypofunction but decreased or absent ACTH in pituitary hypoadrenalism. Increased ACTH level is quickly suppressed by replacement therapy.

Blood cortisol level is markedly decreased (< 5 μg/100 ml) and fails to rise to more than twice this level 1 hour after injection of ACTH. This is a reliable easy screening test to establish primary adrenocortical insufficiency.

Urine 17-OHKS are absent or markedly decreased.

Urine 17-KS are markedly decreased.

Urine 17-KGS are markedly decreased.

See Table 64 (above) for blood ACTH levels and response to ACTH stimulation of eosinophil count and of urinary steroids.

The Robinson-Power-Kepler water tolerance test (used as a screening procedure for Addison's disease) and the Cutler-Power-Wilder sodium chloride deprivation test have been replaced by the ACTH stimulation tests, which are more direct and more useful and avoid the risk of crisis that may be precipitated by the other two tests.

WATERHOUSE-FRIDERICHSEN SYNDROME

This is an acute adrenal insufficiency with degenerative changes in adrenal cortex; patient often dies before progression to cortical hemorrhage.

Dehydration occurs.

Azotemia is due to dehydration and shock affecting renal function.

Serum sodium and chloride are decreased and potassium is increased in some patients.

Hypoglycemia occurs regularly.

Direct eosinophil count is >50/cu mm (<50/cu mm in other kinds of shock).

Blood cortisol is markedly decreased (<5 μg/100 ml).

LABORATORY TESTS FOR EVALUATION OF FUNCTION OF OVARY

Estrogens
Increased in
    Granulosa cell tumor of ovary
    Theca-cell tumor of ovary
    Luteoma of ovary
    Pregnancy
Decreased in
    Primary hypofunction of ovary
    Secondary hypofunction of ovary

Pregnanediol
Increased in
    Luteal cysts of ovary
    Arrhenoblastoma of ovary
Decreased in
    Amenorrhea
    Threatened abortion (some patients)
    Fetal death
    Toxemia of pregnancy

Pituitary Gonadotropins
Increased in
    Primary hypogonadism
    Menopause
Decreased in
    Secondary hypogonadism

17-Ketosteroids
Increased in
    Virilizing ovarian tumors (e.g., adrenal rest tumor, granulosa cell tumor, hilar cell tumor, Brenner tumor, and, most frequently, arrhenoblastoma); increased in 50% of patients and normal in 50% of patients
Decreased in
    Primary ovarian agenesis

OVARIAN TUMORS

Feminizing Ovarian Tumors (e.g., granulosa cell tumor, thecoma, luteoma)
Pap smear of vagina and endometrial biopsy show high estrogen

effect and no progestational activity; no signs of ovulation during reproductive phase.
Urinary FSH is decreased (inhibited by increased estrogen).
Urine 17-KS and 17-OHKS are normal.
Pregnanediol is absent.

Masculinizing Ovarian Tumors
(e.g., arrhenoblastoma, hilar cell tumors, adrenal rest tumors)
Pap smear of vagina shows decreased estrogen effect.
Endometrial biopsy shows moderate atrophy of endometrium.
Urine FSH (gonadotropins) are low.
Urine 17-KS are normal or may be slightly increased in arrhenoblastoma. They may be markedly increased in adrenal tumors of ovary ("masculinovoblastoma"). They may be moderately increased in Leydig cell tumors.

> *In arrhenoblastoma there may be an increase of androsterone, testosterone, etc., excreted in urine even though the 17-KS are not much increased.*

> *In adrenal cell tumors of ovary, laboratory findings may be the same as in hyperfunction of adrenal cortex with Cushing's syndrome, etc.*

BMR is normal.

In some cases there are no endocrine effects from these tumors.
Some cases of arrhenoblastoma with masculinization also show evidence of increased estrogen formation.

Struma Ovarii
About 5–10% of cases are hormone-producing. Classic findings of hyperthyroidism may occur. These tumors take up radioactive iodine. *(Simple follicle cysts may also take up radioactive iodine.)*

Primary Chorionepithelioma of Ovary
Urinary chorionic gonadotropins are markedly increased.
Estrogen and progesterone secretion may be much increased.

Nonfunctioning Ovarian Tumors
Only effect may be hypogonadism due to replacement of functioning ovarian parenchyma.

PRECOCIOUS PUBERTY IN GIRLS

Due To
Diseases of central nervous system (usually floor of the third ventricle) with involvement of the posterior hypothalamus (e.g., tuberculous meningitis, epidemic encephalitis, other inflammations, tumors, tuberous sclerosis [more frequent in boys])
Polyostotic fibrosis dysplasia (Albright's syndrome)

Ovarian tumors (e.g., teratomatous choriocarcinomas, granulosa cell tumors, thecacell tumors, luteomas)

Adrenal adenoma or carcinoma, which may secrete estrogen and be associated with feminization without virilization in rare cases.

Iatrogenic cause or accidental ingestion or inunction of estrogens.

Laboratory Findings

Pap smear of vagina indicates estrogen effect.

Pituitary gonadotropin is usually low, with ovarian and adrenal lesions.

Increased 17-KS and estrogen excretion (above normal adult level) occur, with feminizing adrenal tumors.

Chorionic gonadotropin titers are increased in choriocarcinoma. (*Not all choriocarcinomas produce gonadotropin.*)

STEIN-LEVENTHAL SYNDROME (POLYCYSTIC OVARIAN DISEASE)

Serum luteinizing hormone (LH) is increased in approximately ≅60% of patients in association with normal or low follicule-stimulating hormone (FSH) level. Abnormally high LH/FSH ratio is more consistently abnormal than is either measurement alone.

Plasma testosterone is increased ≦200 μg/100 ml (>200 μg/100 ml usually indicates an androgen-producing tumor).

Plasma androstenedione is increased.

Approximately 85% of these patients have one or more abnormalities of serum LH/FSH ratio, testosterone, or androstenedione. Hyperandrogenism does not differentiate condition from congenital adrenal hyperplasia.

Urinary 17-KS are somewhat increased (higher values occur in congenital virilizing adrenal hyperplasia and hyperadrenalism due to Cushing's syndrome). Dexamethasone administration for 5 days causes partial suppression in cases of ovarian origin, but complete suppression suggests adrenal origin. Administration of gonadotropin increases urinary 17-KS.

Wedge biopsy of ovary may be required for confirmation of diagnosis.

Plasma cortisol, urinary 17-OHKS and 17-KGS are normal.

Because of erratic daily fluctuations of LH and androgens, daily plasma specimens for 3–5 days may be necessary.

"CONSTITUTIONAL" HIRSUTISM IN WOMEN

With normal menses and fertility, urine 17-KS are normal.

With amenorrhea, hypomenorrhea, or oligomenorrhea, urine 17-KS may be slightly increased.

LABORATORY TESTS IN DIFFERENTIAL DIAGNOSIS OF PATIENTS WITH HIRSUTISM AND DIMINISHED MENSES

Urine 17-Hydroxyketosteroids

Normal

    Constitutional hirsutism

Stein-Leventhal syndrome
Mild adrenogenital syndrome
Masculinizing tumor of ovary
Increased
Cushing's syndrome

Urine 17-Ketosteroids
Normal
Constitutional hirsutism
Stein-Leventhal syndrome
Masculinizing tumor of ovary
Cushing's syndrome
Slight increase
Constitutional hirsutism
Stein-Leventhal syndrome
Mild adrenogenital syndrome
Cushing's syndrome
Marked increase
Masculinizing tumor of adrenal gland
Adrenogenital syndrome

Urine 17-Ketosteroids Decreased by Daily Prednisone
Poor response
Constitutional hirsutism
Stein-Leventhal syndrome
Masculinizing tumor of ovary
Good response
Adrenogenital syndrome

Urine 17-Ketosteroids Further Decreased by Daily Stilbestrol and Prednisone
No response
Constitutional hirsutism
Masculinizing tumor of ovary
Adrenogenital syndrome
Response
Stein-Leventhal syndrome (testosterone level also decreases)

SECONDARY AMENORRHEA
If increased LH and normal FSH
Polycystic ovarian disease (Stein-Leventhal syndrome)
Early pregnancy
Ectopic gonadotropin production by neoplasm (e.g., lung, gastrointestinal tract)
If increased LH and increased FSH
Ovarian failure
If decreased LH and decreased FSH
Pituitary or hypothalamic impairment
Clomiphene citrate should be administered for 5–10 days; if gonadotropin level rises or menses return, cause is probably hypothalamic
Administer hypothalamic luteinizing hormone–releasing factor (LRF); normal or exaggerated response in hypothalamic

amenorrhea (cause in 80% of patients); smaller or no response in pituitary tumor or dysfunction

TURNER'S SYNDROME (OVARIAN DYSGENESIS)

Barr bodies are negative (male) in 80% of patients.

Chromosomal pattern—45 chromosomes (monosomy X with XO; or if XX, one X is abnormal; or XO mosaic)

Because of the frequency with which 45 X cells are admixed with 46 XX cells, it is impossible to exclude the diagnosis (i.e., 45 X karyotype) by either buccal smear or chromosome analysis alone.

Biopsy of ovary shows connective tissue stroma with rare follicular structure.

Vaginal smear and endometrial biopsy are atrophic.

17-KS and 17-OHKS are normal.

ACTH is normal.

FSH is increased.

BMR, PBI, T-3, etc., are usually normal.

About 50% of patients with primary amenorrhea have Turner's syndrome or sometimes testicular feminization.

TURNER'S SYNDROME IN THE MALE

Biopsy of testicle reveals dysgenetic tubules with few or no germ cells.

Chromosomal pattern—46 chromosomes (XY pattern with very defective Y that is equivalent to XO)

MENOPAUSE (FEMALE CLIMACTERIC)

Urinary gonadotropin is increased.

Urinary estrogens are decreased.

Urinary 17-KS are decreased.

Plasma gonadotropin is increased.

Table 65. Laboratory Differentiation of Primary and Secondary (to Pituitary Defect) Hypogonadism

Determination	Primary Hypogonadism	Hypogonadism Secondary to Pituitary Defect
Level of FSH and gonadotropin in urine	High	Low
After administration of gonadotropins 17-KS excretion	Does not increase	Increases
Clinical evidence of hypogonadism	Does not subside	Subsides with Increased sperm count Increased estrogenic effect in woman's Pap smear

SECONDARY OVARIAN INSUFFICIENCY
Urinary gonadotropin is decreased or absent.

GALACTORRHEA-AMENORRHEA SYNDROMES
Chiari-Frommel syndrome—postpartum occurrence
Argonz-del Castillo syndrome—spontaneous occurrence
Forbes-Albright syndrome—demonstrable pituitary tumor
"Postpill" syndrome following use of birth control pills; may also occur following use of other drugs (e.g., reserpine, phenothiazines)

Increased serum prolactin (normal level <20 ng/ml)
Serum levels of LH and progesterone decreased to values seen during follicular phase rather than luteal phase of menstrual cycle (serum progesterone, value <1.0 ng/ml during follicular phase and >2.0 ng/ml only in postovulatory luteal phase of the normal menstrual cycle)
Endogenous gonadotrophins normal or low compared to increased levels in normal postpartum nursing mothers
Normal serum thyroxine and RAIU
Normal metyrapone test for pituitary adrenal reserve

Administer luteinizing hormone–releasing factor (LRF) and then measure serum LH at 15-minute intervals for 2 hours.
In pituitary adenoma patient's levels of serum LH do not exceed 30 mIU/ml and curve is flat.
In Chiari-Frommel and postpill syndromes average peak levels are >80 mIU/100 ml with a higher curve.
In premature ovarian failure the curve is very high, with peak level approaching 500 mIU/100 ml.

Syndrome due to pituitary adenoma tends to produce a much higher serum prolactin level (usually much >200 ng/ml), and this level decreases <50% in response to water-loading test as compared to other syndromes listed above, in which the serum prolactin levels are not so markedly elevated and are reduced >50% (and often undetectable) in response to water-loading test.

LABORATORY TESTS FOR EVALUATION OF FUNCTION OF TESTICLE

Chorionic Gonadotropins in Urine
Increased in
Choriocarcinoma
Seminoma

Serum AFP
Serum alpha-fetoprotein (AFP) levels >40 ng/ml are found in 75% of patients with teratocarcinoma.
90% of patients with testicular tumors are positive for AFP or urinary chorionic gonadotropin, or both; these are valuable for gauging efficacy of chemotherapy. 30% of patients receiving in-

tensive chemotherapy apparently have a complete clinical remission; AFP levels may remain elevated although lower than pretreatment levels.

Serum AFP is not increased in pure seminoma without teratomatous component.

Pituitary Gonadotropins in Urine
Increased in
Primary hypogonadism
Decreased in
Secondary hypogonadism

17-Ketosteroids in Urine
(indicative of adrenal rather than testicular status)
Increased in
Interstitial cell tumor
Decreased in
Primary hypogonadism
Secondary hypogonadism

Plasma Testosterone
Decreased in
Primary hypogonadism
Secondary hypogonadism

Semen Analysis
Sterile males usually show
Volume of <3 ml
<20 million sperm/ml
<25% motility

Biopsy of Testicle
Evidence of atrophy in sterility study
Diagnosis of tumor

Normal spermatogenesis associated with normal endocrine findings in patient with aspermia and infertility suggests a mechanical obstruction to sperm transport that may be correctable.

Chromosome Analysis
Turner's syndrome (gonadal dysgenesis)—usually negative for Barr bodies
Klinefelter's syndrome—positive for Barr bodies
Pseudohermaphroditism—chromosomal sex corresponding to gonadal sex

GERMINAL APLASIA
Buccal smears are normal (negative for Barr bodies).
Chromosomal pattern is normal.
Urinary gonadotropin is normal.

Urinary pituitary gonadotropin is increased.

17-KS are decreased.

There is azoospermia.

Biopsy of testicle shows that Sertoli's and Leydig's cells are intact and germinal cells are absent.

KLINEFELTER'S SYNDROME

Buccal smears are positive for Barr bodies.

Biopsy of testicle shows atrophy, with hyalinized tubules lined only by Sertoli's cells, clumped Leydig's cells, and failure of spermatogenesis.

There is azoospermia.

Abnormal chromosomal pattern. XY males have an extra X; usually XXY; may have additional X (e.g., XXYY, XXXY, XXXXY).

Testosterone levels are usually decreased.

Urinary gonadotropin level is elevated.

LABORATORY STUDIES FOR AMBIGUOUS GENITALIA IN CHILDHOOD AND INFANCY

Determine sex chromatin pattern in buccal smears and urinary 17-KS excretion; biopsy of gonads may be indicated.

If buccal smear pattern positive (e.g., XX, XXY) and urinary 17-KS are normal, diagnosis may be

> Female pseudohermaphroditism, nonadrenal type
> True hermaphroditism
> Klinefelter's syndrome

If buccal smear pattern is positive and urinary 17-KS are increased, diagnosis may be

> Female pseudohermaphroditism (congenital adrenogenital or iatrogenic)
> True hermaphroditism
> Arrhenoblastoma, mother or fetus (rarely)

If buccal smear pattern negative (e.g., XY, XO) and urinary 17-KS are normal, diagnosis may be

> Turner's syndrome
> Abdominal testes in male
> Feminizing testes (undescended)
> True hermaphroditism
> Absence of testes
> Male pseudohermaphroditism due to deficient testes

If buccal smear pattern is negative and urinary 17-KS are increased, diagnosis may be

> Male pseudohermaphroditism due to congenital lipoid adrenal hyperplasia (rarely)

MALE CLIMACTERIC

There is decreased testosterone level in blood (<300 ng/ml) and urine (<100 μg/24 hours).

Urinary gonadotropin level is elevated. (Gonadotropin is decreased when low testosterone level is due to pituitary tumor, gout, or diabetes.)

EVALUATION OF PLACENTAL-FETAL FUNCTION
(to monitor high-risk pregnancy)

Maternal Serum
Heat-stable alkaline phosphatase (56°C for 30 minutes) progressively increases as pregnancy approaches term. If >50% of alkaline phosphatase is heat stable, placenta size is compatible with mature fetus. Decline after 34th week of gestation has been suggested as an indication for delivery.

Human placental lactogen (HPL) increases to level of 6–9 μg/24 hours as pregnancy approaches term. Fetal danger is indicated at <4.0 μg (e.g., severe hypertension, idiopathic placental insufficiency). Serial determinations are more useful than a single value. Abnormally high levels in diabetic patients correlate with proliferative retinopathy. If value is low, estriol in 24-hour urine or L/S ratio in amniotic fluid should be measured.

Maternal Urine
Estriol level is ideally measured every 48 hours as pregnancy approaches term to provide the most accurate information about fetal well-being.

> Normal is >25 mg/24 hours.
> Abnormal is <12 mg/24 hours or a fall of 50% from previous determination: it indicates the need to terminate pregnancy.
>> 8–12 mg/24 hours is compatible with attempt at vaginal delivery.
>> <8 mg/24 hours suggests need for abdominal delivery.
>> >12 mg/24 hours after 34th week—fetal or neonatal mortality is rare.
>> 4–12 mg/24 hours at time of delivery—live birth likely but difficulties in neonatal period and small percentage of neonatal deaths are expected.
>> <4 mg/24 hours—stillbirth is more likely and possibly many difficulties may be expected in neonatal period.

Abnormal estriol level warns of impaired intrauterine environment and indicates when fetus would be helped by termination of pregnancy. L/S ratio separates infants susceptible to RDS from those with mature lungs, thus indicating relative risk of inducing delivery.

Human chorionic gonadotropin (HCG) may be elevated in overt diabetes mellitus and erythroblastosis fetalis but is not useful for detecting fetal distress. Falling values in early pregnancy indicate threatened or missed abortion and rising values indicate hydatidiform mole.

Pregnanediol level parallels estriol level but does not give additional information and is not widely used. May remain normal after fetal death. Fall in pregnanediol associated with a late rise in HCG may precede premature labor and intrauterine fetal death.

Development of radioimmunoassay techniques is making possible determinations of HPL, HCG, and even estriol using serum rather than 24-hour urine samples.

ACROMEGALY AND GIGANTISM
(usually due to eosinophilic adenoma of pituitary)
Serum growth hormone (measured by radioimmunoassay; still limited availability) *(Avoid stress before and during venipuncture because stress stimulates secretion of growth hormone.)*

Fasting level above 5 ng/ml in men is diagnostic of acromegaly; not diagnostic in women because of wide fluctuations in levels in acromegalic range.

Most patients of both sexes show a fall of <50% during glucose tolerance test, whereas normal subjects show almost complete suppression of growth hormone (or to <5 ng/ml) by induced hyperglycemia.

Glucose tolerance is impaired in most patients. Mild diabetes mellitus that is insulin-resistant is found in <15% of patients.

Secretory activity of tumor is indicated when

Serum phosphorus is increased.

Serum alkaline phosphatase may be increased.

BMR is increased. *(PBI and RAIU are normal.)*

Urine calcium is increased.

Urine hydroxypyroline is increased.

Biopsy of costochondral junction evidences active bone growth.

Serum growth hormone level is increased (immunologic assay method is not generally available).

IV ACTH administration may cause excessive increase in urine 17-KS but normal 17-OHKS excretion.

Adrenal virilism and increased urine 17-KS are common in women.

Urine 17-KS, 17-KGS, and pituitary gonadotropins are usually normal or may be slightly changed but not diagnostically useful.

Rare associated endocrinopathies are hyperthyroidism, hyperparathyroidism, pheochromocytoma, insulinoma.

CBC and ESR are normal.

In inactive cases, all secondary laboratory findings may be normal.

In late stage, panhypopituitarism may develop.

PITUITARY GROWTH HORMONE DEFICIENCY
There may be isolated deficiency with dwarfism or associated with TSH deficiency, with ACTH deficiency, or with TSH and ACTH deficiencies.

Serum growth hormone levels are decreased (measured by radioimmunoassay <1.0 ng/ml) with no response 4 hours after oral glucose load and serum growth hormone level increases to >10 ng/ml after IV insulin (0.1 unit/kg) is administered.

Decreased fasting blood sugar (<50 mg/100 ml) is frequent; responds to growth hormone therapy.

Unresponsiveness to insulin-induced hypoglycemia (blood sugar at 90 minutes is >15 mg/100 ml below the fasting level) occurs in ≅50% of patients with isolated deficiency of growth hormone but almost all with combined ACTH and growth hormone deficiencies.

Serum phosphorus and alkaline phosphatase are decreased in prepubertal child but normal in adult-onset cases.

TSH deficiency (see Hypothyroidism, pp. 379, 383 and Table 55, p. 383)

ACTH deficiency (see tests of adrenal function and adrenal-pituitary function, pp. 397–399)

Gonadotropins are decreased or absent from urine in postpubertal patients (but increased levels occur in primary hypogonadism).

May Be Due To
Pituitary
    Congenital hypoplasia or absence, atrophy, fibrosis, cystic changes with calcification, etc.
Hypothalamus
    Progressive degenerative changes, which may cause multiple deficiency or isolated growth hormone deficiency types
Familial and genetic types
    Isolated growth hormone deficiency or multiple deficiency types

HYPOPITUITARISM

Due To
Pituitary necrosis secondary to postpartum hemorrhage (Sheehan's syndrome)
Craniopharyngioma, chromophobe adenoma, eosinophilic adenoma
Meningioma
Metastatic tumor (especially breast)
Granulomatous lesion (e.g., sarcoidosis, Hand-Schüller-Christian syndrome)

See sections on secondary insufficiency of gonads, thyroid, adrenals. All of these may be involved or only one (usually gonadal first).
See Diabetes Insipidus, p. 422.

ANOREXIA NERVOSA
BMR may be low.
PBI is usually normal.
Urine 17-KS and 17-OHKS may be low; in panhypopituitarism (Simmond's disease) these are practically absent.
Metyrapone administration shows limited pituitary ACTH reserve in ≅ 50% of patients; the rest show a normal response. Panhypopituitarism patients are unresponsive. This is a most useful procedure for distinguishing anorexia nervosa from panhypopituitarism.
Insulin tolerance test is the same as in panhypopituitarism.

DISEASES OF HYPOTHALAMUS

Due To
Neoplasms (primary or metastatic cancer, craniopharyngioma) (most frequent cause)

Inflammation (e.g., tuberculosis, encephalitis)
Trauma (e.g., basal skull fractures, gunshot wounds)
Intracranial xanthomatosis
Other

Manifestations
Sexual abnormalities are the most frequent manifestations of hypothalamic disease.
    Precocious puberty
    Hypogonadism (frequently as part of Fröhlich's syndrome)
Diabetes insipidus is a frequent but not an early manifestation of hypothalamic disease.

FRÖHLICH'S SYNDROME (ADIPOSOGENITAL DYSTROPHY)
Usually this is a transient functional disorder of the hypothalamus.
No deficiency of ACTH, TSH, or growth hormone is seen.
If there is a thyroid or adrenal hypofunction, an organic lesion, especially craniopharyngioma, should be suspected.

PRECOCIOUS PUBERTY IN BOYS
Precocious puberty occurs occasionally in boys with hepatoblastoma.
Urine contains chorionic gonadotropin-like substance.
There is secondary Leydig's cell hyperplasia.

See Pineal Tumors (below) and Diseases of Hypothalamus (above).

PINEAL TUMORS
Boys—precocious puberty in 30% of patients.
Girls—delayed pubescence

Diabetes insipidus occurs occasionally.

"ESSENTIAL" HYPERNATREMIA
This condition is due to a hypothalamic lesion (e.g., infiltration of histiocytes, neoplasm) that causes impaired osmotic regulation but intact volume regulation of antidiuretic hormone secretion.
Serum sodium shows sustained but fluctuating elevations, corrected by administration of antidiuretic hormone but not corrected by fluid administration.
Serum osmolality is increased.
Serum creatinine, BUN, and creatinine clearance are normal.
There is spontaneous excretion of random specimens of urine that may be very concentrated or very dilute and opposite to plasma osmolality.

DIABETES INSIPIDUS
Urine
    Low specific gravity (usually ≤ 1.004) is found.
    Large volume (4–15 liters/24 hours) is characteristic.
    Urine does not become concentrated when fluids are withheld.
    There is no response to hypertonic NaCl IV (normal person shows decrease in urine volume during and after infusion).

Vasopressin (Pitressin) injection decreases urine flow (does not cause decrease in nephrogenic diabetes insipidus), and specific gravity becomes normal.

Antidiuretic Response (increase in urine osmolality equal to, or more than, plasma osmolality with urine-serum ratio $\geqq 1.0$) *To Stimuli Listed Below*	*Hypophyseal Diabetes Insipidus (vasopressin deficiency)*	*Nephrogenic Diabetes Insipidus (renal insensitivity to vasopressin)*	*Primary Polydipsia*
Dehydration for 8–12 hours	No response	No response	Response
Nicotine (smoke 2 cigarettes) during water diuresis	No response	No response	Response
3% NaCl given IV (10 ml/kg in 30 minutes) during water diuresis	No response	No response	Response
Administer vasopressin (25–50 mU IV or 2.5–5.0 U IM)	Response	No response	Response
Plasma vasopressin level in response to dehydration, nicotine, and 3% NaCl (see above)	Low to absent	Elevated	Elevated

INAPPROPRIATE SECRETION OF ANTIDIURETIC HORMONE

Decreased serum sodium and chloride
Normal serum potassium, CO_2, and BUN
Decreased serum osmolality
Increased urine osmolality
Increased ratio of urine osmolality-serum osmolality
Increased urine sodium
Responds to water restriction but not to administration of isotonic or even hypertonic saline
May be associated with
    Acute intermittent porphyria
    Brain tumor (primary or metastatic)
    Pneumonia
    Pulmonary tuberculosis
    Tuberculous meningitis
    Systemic neoplasm
    Other

NONENDOCRINE NEOPLASMS CAUSING ENDOCRINE SYNDROMES

Tumors secrete polypeptides that have hormonal activity.
Cushing's syndrome* due to
    Bronchogenic carcinoma and carcinoid
    Thymoma

*Cushing's syndrome due to these neoplasms cannot be distinguished from Cushing's syndrome due to excessive pituitary secretion of ACTH by use of dexamethasone suppression test or metyrapone test.

Hepatoma
Carcinoma of ovary
Also carcinoma of thyroid, pancreas, etc.
Hypoglycemia. Patients show variable sensitivity to tolbutamide.
Not associated with decreased serum phosphorus as in
insulin-induced hypoglycemia.
Bronchogenic carcinoma
Carcinoma of adrenal cortex (6% of patients)
Hepatoma (23% of patients)
Fibrosarcoma (most frequently)
Thyrotoxicosis. Signs and symptoms are rare, but PBI, RAIU,
etc., are increased.
Tumors of GI tract, hematopoietic, pulmonary, etc.
Trophoblastic tumors in women
Choriocarcinoma of testis
Precocious puberty in boys
Hepatoma
Hypercalcemia simulating hyperparathyroidism*
Renal carcinoma
Squamous cell carcinoma of upper respiratory tract
Carcinoma of breast (occurs in 15% of patients with bone
metastases)
Malignant lymphoma, etc.

See also Carcinoid Syndrome (below), Precocious Puberty in Girls
(pp. 412–413), Precocious Puberty in Boys (p. 422), Secondary
Polycythemia (p. 313), Inappropriate Secretion of Antidiuretic
Hormone (p. 423).

CARCINOID SYNDROME
The syndrome occurs in patients with malignant carcinoids (argen-
taffinomas).
Urinary level of 5-hydroxyindolacetic acid (5-HIAA) (a metabolite
of serotonin) is increased, usually when tumor is far advanced
(i.e., large liver metastases), but may not be increased despite
massive metastases. Useful in confirming diagnosis in only 5–7%
of patients with a carcinoid tumor.
Blood serotonin may be increased (>0.4 μg/ml).
VMA and catecholamines in urine are at normal levels.
Laboratory findings due to other aspects of carcinoid syndrome are
noted (e.g., pulmonary valvular stenosis, tricuspid valvular insufficiency, heart failure, liver metastases, electrolyte disturbances).

*Serum calcium level is $\leqq 21$ mg/100 ml; less marked increase with renal
tumors. Serum phosphorus is decreased in $> 50\%$ of patients. Alkaline
phosphatase is frequently increased but not difficult to evaluate because of
liver metastases. Serum proteins are not consistently abnormal. Urine calcium and phosphorus and renal tubular reabsorption of phosphate are not
useful in differential diagnosis.

MULTIPLE ENDOCRINE ADENOMAS (MEA SYNDROME)

	Wermer's Syndrome (MEA I)	*Sipple's Syndrome (MEA II)*
Characteristic neoplasms	Pituitary adenoma Islet cell adenoma or carcinoma Parathyroid adenoma or hyperplasia	Medullary thyroid carcinoma Pheochromocytoma Parathyroid adenoma or hyperplasia Mucosal neuroma
Associated neoplasms	Adrenal cortical adenoma Renal cortical adenoma Thyroid carcinoma or hyperplasia Carcinoid Lipoma Gastric polyp Mediastinal endocrine neoplasm Gastrinoma (see p. 395)	

GENITOURINARY DISEASES

RENAL GLYCOSURIA
(glycosuria when serum glucose is <180 mg/100 ml)
Due to proximal tubular damage
    Fanconi syndrome
    Heavy-metal poisoning
    Nephrotic phase of glomerulonephritis
Due to increased glomerular filtration rate without tubular damage
    Pregnancy
Oral and IV glucose tolerance tests normal
Ketosis absent

RENAL DISEASES THAT MAY BE FOUND WITHOUT PROTEINURIA
Congenital abnormalities
Renal artery stenosis
Obstruction of GU tract
Pyelonephritis
Stone
Tumor
Polycystic kidneys
Hypokalemic nephropathy
Hypercalcemic nephropathy
Prerenal azotemia

PROTEINURIA PREDOMINANTLY GLOBULIN RATHER THAN ALBUMIN
Multiple myeloma
Macroglobulinemia
Primary amyloidosis
Adult Fanconi syndrome (some patients)

ORTHOSTATIC PROTEINURIA
First morning urine before arising shows high specific gravity but
    no protein.
Urine after arising may contain protein ≦3gm/L but usually
    <1gm/day.
Urine microscopy is normal.
Orthostatic proteinuria is usually considered benign, but some pa-
    tients show pathologic changes on renal biopsy and ultimately
    manifest chronic renal disease.

SOME GLOMERULAR CAUSES OF PROTEINURIA
Immune complexes (e.g., nephritis of SLE, poststreptococcal
    glomerulonephritis, membranous glomerulonephritis)
Antiglomerular basement membrane antibodies (e.g., Goodpas-
    ture's syndrome)
Deposition of abnormal material (e.g., amyloidosis, diabetes mel-
    litus)
Pyelonephritis

Table 66. Urinary Findings in Various Diseases

Disease	Volume	Specific Gravity	Protein[a]	RBCs[b]	WBCs and Epithelial Cells[b]	Casts[c,d]	Comment
Normal	600–2500	1.003–1.030	0 (0.05 gm)	0–occ. (0–0.130)	0–0.65	0–occ. (2000/24 hrs)	
Acute febrile states	D	I	Trace to +			Few	
Orthostatic proteinuria	N	N	I (up 1 gm)	N (0–0.130)	0–3	V; H & G	Normal when recumbent; abnormalities after upright posture
Glomerulonephritis							
Acute	D	I	2–4+ (0.5–5)	1–4+ (1–1000)	1–400	2–4+; H & G; *RBC, epithelial, mixed RBC & epithelial*	Gross hematuria or "smoky" urine
Latent			(0.1–2)	(1–100)	1–20	*RBC*, H & G	
Nephrosis ("nephrotic stage")	D	I	4+ (4–40)	0–few (0.5–50)	20–1000	*Epithelial, fatty,* waxy; H & G	Fat-laden epithelial cells, anisotropic fat in epithelial cells and casts
Terminal	I or D	D; fixed	1–2+ (2–7)	Trace–1+ (0.5–10)	1–50	1–3+ *Broad, waxy,* H & G, epithelial	

427

Table 66 (Continued)

Disease	Volume	Specific Gravity	Protein[a]	RBCs[b]	WBCs and Epithelial Cells[b]	Casts[c,d]	Comment
Pyelonephritis							
Acute	N	N	0–2+ (0.5–2)	Few (0–1)	20–2000	WBC, H & G bacteria	Bacteria, many WBCs in clumps
Chronic	N or D	N or D	2–4+ (0–5)	Few (0–1)	0.5–50	Same as acute; often few or none	Same as acute; findings may be intermittent
Renal tuberculosis			(0.1–3)	(1–20)	1–50	WBC, H & G	Tubercle bacilli
Disseminated lupus erythematosus	V	N or D	1–4+ (0.5–20)	1–4+ (1–100)	1–100	1–4+ RBC, fatty, waxy; H & G	
Toxemia of pregnancy	D	I	3–4+ (0.5–10)	0–1+ (0–1)	1–5	3–4+ H & G	
Malignant hypertension	V	D; fixed	1–2+ (1–10)	Trace–1+ (1–100)	1–200	1–2+ H & G, RBC, fatty	Increasing uremia with minimal or marked proteinuria and hematuria
Benign hypertension	N or I	N or D	0–1+	0–trace (1–5)		0–1+ H & G	
Congestive heart failure	D	I	1–2+	0–1+		1+ H & G	

Intercapillary glomerulosclerosis (Kimmelstiel-Wilson syndrome)			1-4+ (2-20)	(0-1)	1-30	Epithelial, fatty H & G	Frequently associated: pyelonephritis and nephrosclerosis
Lower nephron nephrosis							
Acute	D	I		1-4+	1-4+	RBC; H & G, epithelial	
Diuretic	I		0.5-10.0	(0-1)	1-100	Broad, waxy, epithelial, H & G	

D = decreased; I = increased; occ. = occasionally; N = normal; V = variable; H & G = hyaline and granular casts.

[a]Protein = quantitative values in ( ) given as gm/24 hours.

[b]= quantitative values given as cells $\times 10^6$/24 hours.

[c]Cast requires examination of fresh or preserved urine and acid pH.

[d]Italics denote most important or diagnostic finding.

Vascular disease (e.g., hypertension, congestive heart failure)
Congenital (e.g., Alport's syndrome of progressive interstitial ne-
phritis and progressive nerve deafness)
Unknown etiology (e.g., lipoid nephrosis)
Physiologic (e.g., orthostatic, exercise, fever)

SOME TUBULAR CAUSES OF PROTEINURIA*
Fanconi's syndrome
Renal tubular acidosis
Medullary cystic disease
Pyelonephritis
Cystinosis
Wilson's disease
Oculocerebral renal syndrome
Renal transplantation
Sarcoidosis
Cadmium toxicity
Balkan nephropathy

RENAL TUBULAR ACIDOSIS IN ADULTS

Proximal Tubule Due To
Multiple myeloma with Bence Jones proteinuria
Wilson's disease; other heavy-metal intoxication
Drugs—toxic effects (e.g., due to sulfonamides, degraded tetracy-
cline, amphotericin B)
Rejection of renal transplant
Fanconi syndrome (not due to other causes)

Caused by defect in bicarbonate reabsorption
    Low plasma bicarbonate concentration
    Alkaline urine that becomes acid if extracellular bicarbonate
      level is decreased below the patient's maximum reabsorp-
      tive limit
    Normal urine pH in the absence of bicarbonate in the urine

Distal Tubule Due To
Increased serum globulins (especially gamma) (e.g., SLE, Sjög-
ren's syndrome, Hodgkin's disease, sarcoidosis, chronic active
hepatitis, cryoglobulinemia)
Potassium depletion nephropathy
Pyelonephritis
Medullary sponge kidney
Ureterosigmoidostomy
Primary (may be hereditary)
Hereditary insensitivity to antidiuretic hormone (vasopressin)
Various renal diseases (e.g., obstructive uropathy, hypercalcemia,
potassium-losing disorders, medullary cystic disease, polyar-
teritis nodosa, amyloidosis, Sjögren's syndrome)

Caused by inability of tubular cell to secrete enough H^+
    Hyperchloremic acidosis, hypokalemia, low plasma bicarbo-
    nate concentration

*Proteinuria refers to protein excretion of >150 mg/day.

Alkaline urine that persists at any level of plasma bicarbonate

Absence of other tubular defects

Laboratory findings due to complications (e.g., nephrocalcinosis, nephrolithiasis, interstitial nephritis)

ACUTE RENAL FAILURE

Early Stage

Urine is scant in volume (often <50 ml/day) for ≦2 weeks; anuria for >24 hours is unusual. Urine usually bloody (because RBCs and protein are present, specific gravity may be high). Urine sodium concentration is usually >50 mEq/L.

WBC is increased even without infection.

BUN rises ≦20 mg/100 ml/day in transfusion reaction. It rises ≦50 mg/100 ml/day in overwhelming infection or severe crushing injuries. Serum creatinine is increased.

Hypocalcemia may occur.

Disproportionately increased serum phosphorus and creatinine indicates tissue necrosis.

Serum amylase and lipase may be increased without evidence of pancreatitis.

Metabolic acidosis is present.

Second Week

Urine becomes clear several days after onset of acute renal failure, and there is a small daily increase in volume. Daily volume of 400 ml indicates onset of tubular recovery. Daily volume of 1000 ml occurs in several days or ≦2 weeks. RBCs and large hematin casts are present. Protein is slight or absent.

Azotemia increases. BUN continues to rise for several days after onset of diuresis.

Metabolic acidosis increases.

Serum potassium is increased (because of tissue injury, failure of urinary excretion, acidosis, dehydration, etc.) EKG changes are always found when serum potassium is >9 mEq/L but are rarely found when it is <7 mEq/L.

Serum sodium is often decreased, with increased extracellular fluid volume.

Anemia usually appears during second week.

Bleeding tendency is frequent, with decreased platelets, abnormal prothrombin consumption, etc.

Diuretic Stage

Large urinary potassium excretion may cause decreased serum potassium level.

Urine sodium concentration is 50–75 mEq/L.

Serum sodium and chloride may increase because of dehydration from large diuresis if replacement of water is inadequate.

Hypercalcemia may occur in some patients with muscle damage.

Azotemia disappears 1–3 weeks after onset of diuresis.

Later Findings

Anemia may persist for weeks or months.

Pyelonephritis may first occur during this stage.

Renal blood flow and glomerular filtration rate do not usually become completely normal.

Recovery from renal cortical necrosis complicating pregnancy may be followed by renal calcification, contracted kidneys, and death from malignant hypertension in 1–2 years.

If there is complete anuria for >48 hours, suspect urinary tract obstruction, bilateral renal vascular thrombi or emboli, cortical necrosis, or acute glomerulonephritis.

Suspect cortical necrosis if proteinuria is >3–4 gm/L, BUN does not fall, and diuresis does not occur.

Suspect urinary tract obstruction if recurrent oliguria and increasing azotemia occur during period of diuresis.

Due To

Renal parenchymal damage (usually tubular injury)
  Poisoning (e.g., carbon tetrachloride, toluene, phosphorus, mercury bichloride)
  Intravascular hemolysis
  Necrotizing pyelonephritis
  Polyarteritis nodosa
  Hypersensitivity reaction (e.g., penicillin)
  Other
Prerenal—decreased renal blood flow with ischemia ("lower nephron nephrosis")
  Shock due to various causes
  Renal vascular occlusion
  Other
Postrenal—renal outflow obstruction
  Precipitation of sulfonamides
  Mechanical obstruction (cancer, calculi, ligation, etc.)
  Other
Often, combined mechanisms (e.g., crushing injury with myoglobinemia plus shock, shock plus intravascular hemolysis from transfusion reaction or bacteremia or infusion of distilled water during prostatectomy)

Indications for Artificial Dialysis in Acute Renal Failure

Uncontrollable hyperkalemia

Increasing acidosis in which congestive heart failure contraindicates sodium administration

Simplified treatment of oliguria in presence of severe infection, tissue damage, etc.

CHRONIC RENAL INSUFFICIENCY

BUN and serum creatinine are increased and renal function tests are impaired (see pp. 93–97).

Loss of renal concentrating ability (nocturia, polyuria, polydipsia) is an early manifestation of progressive renal functional impairment. Specific gravity is usually same as that of glomerular filtrate.

Hypotonic urine unresponsive to vasopressin may occur in

Table 67. Laboratory Differentiation of Prerenal Azotemia and Acute Renal Failure[a]

Measurement	Prerenal Azotemia	Acute Renal Failure
Urine creatinine–serum creatinine ratio (the most important criterion for differentiation)	>14:1	<14:1
Urine urea–BUN ratio	>14:1	<14:1
Urine sodium concentration	<10 mEq/L	>20 mEq/L
$\dfrac{\text{Creatinine urine: serum ratio}}{\text{Urine sodium concentration}}$	<1	>3
Urine osmolality	100 mOsm >Serum osmolality	< Serum osmolality
Urine sediment	Normal	Casts, RBCs

[a]These laboratory findings are difficult or impossible to interpret if mannitol or diuretics have been administered.

    Obstructive uropathy
    Chronic pyelonephritis
    Nephrocalcinosis
    Amyloidosis
    Familial nephrogenic diabetes insipidus
Serum sodium is decreased (because of tubular damage with loss in urine, vomiting, diarrhea, diet restriction, etc.). The decrease is indicated by increased urine sodium levels (>5–10 mEq sodium/L). It may occur in any renal disease, especially when polyuria is marked, but is more common with obstructive uropathy, chronic pyelonephritis, and interstitial nephritis than with chronic glomerulonephritis.
Serum potassium is increased (on account of dietary sodium restriction and increased potassium ingestion, acidosis, oliguria, tissue breakdown). Decreased serum potassium with increased loss in urine (>15–20 mEq/L) occurs in primary aldosteronism. It may occur in malignant hypertension, tubular acidosis, Fanconi syndrome, nephrocalcinosis, diuresis during recovery from tubular necrosis.
Acidosis (due to renal failure to secrete acid as NH_4^+ and to reabsorb filtered bicarbonate) is present.
Serum calcium is decreased (because of decreased serum albumin, increased serum phosphorus, decreased calcium absorption in intestine, etc.). Tetany is rare. Secondary parathyroid hyperplasia may occur, but hypercalcemia is not found.
Serum phosphorus increases when creatinine clearance falls to $\cong 25$ ml/minute.

Serum alkaline phosphatase may be normal or may be increased with renal osteodystrophy.

Serum magnesium increases when glomerular filtration rate falls to < 30 ml/minute.

Increase in serum uric acid is usually < 10 mg/100 ml. Secondary gout is rare. If clinical gout and family history of gout are present or if serum uric acid level is > 10 mg/100 ml, rule out primary gout nephropathy.

Blood organic acids, phenols, indoles, certain amino acids, etc., are increased.

Normochromic normocytic anemia is usually proportionate to the degree of azotemia.

Bleeding tendency is evident. There may be decreased platelets, increased capillary fragility, abnormal TGT and prothrombin consumption (possible platelet defect), normal bleeding and clotting time.

Gastrointestinal hemorrhage from ulcers anywhere in GI tract may be severe.

Laboratory findings due to uremic pericarditis, pleuritis, and pancreatitis are noted. (BUN is usually > 100 mg/100 ml.)

Laboratory findings due to uremic meningitis are noted ($\cong 50\%$ of these patients have increased CSF protein or leukocytes; protein may be reduced by hemodialysis; pleocytosis is not related to degree of azotemia).

Serum albumin and total protein are decreased. *When there is edema without hypoproteinemia or heart failure, rule out acute glomerulonephritis, toxemia of pregnancy, excess fluid intake in oliguria during acute tubular necrosis or terminal renal failure.*

Due To (see appropriate separate sections)
Primary renal disease
    Vascular lesions
        Nephrosclerosis, benign or malignant
        Renal artery stenosis or thrombosis
        Renal vein thrombosis
        Acute ischemic tubular necrosis, renal cortical necrosis
    Glomerular lesions—glomerulonephritis
    Tubular or interstitial lesions
        Infectious—chronic pyelonephritis, tuberculosis
        Other
            Fanconi syndrome and renal tubular acidosis
            Heavy-metal poisoning
            Analgesic abuse
            Irradiation nephritis
            Chronic interstitial nephritis
    Congenital
        Polycystic disease
        Congenital hypoplastic kidneys
Systemic diseases involving the kidney
    Collagen diseases
        SLE
        Polyarteritis nodosa
        Scleroderma

Subacute bacterial endocarditis
Goodpasture's syndrome
Allergic purpura, etc.
Metabolic diseases
Diabetes mellitus
Gout
Amyloidosis
Hypercalcemic nephropathy
Hypokalemic nephropathy
Urinary tract obstruction
Neoplasms (e.g., carcinoma of cervix)
Stones
Retroperitoneal fibrosis
Prostatic enlargement
Urethral stricture
Congenital urethral or bladder defects
Other
Multiple myeloma
Sickle cell anemia
Hemoglobinurias (e.g., paroxysmal nocturnal)

POSTSTREPTOCOCCAL ACUTE GLOMERULONEPHRITIS IN CHILDREN

Evidence of infection with Group A beta-hemolytic *Streptococcus* by
Culture of throat
Serologic findings indicative of recent streptococcal infection
Antistreptolysin O titers (ASOT) of >250 Todd units (increased in 80% of patients)

Table 68. Classification of Acute Glomerulonephritis[a]

Type	Traits	Prognosis
Diffuse proliferative and exudative	Characteristic of poststreptococcal nephritis in children	Most cases heal
Diffuse extracapillary	"Rapidly progressive glomerulonephritis"; may be associated with Goodpasture's syndrome, Henoch-Schönlein purpura, or periarteritis nodosa	Prognosis usually grave
Focal	May occur in systemic disease (e.g., SLE, periarteritis nodosa, Henoch-Schönlein purpura)	May progress to diffuse type

[a]Chronic (sclerosing) glomerulonephritis may be the end stage for any of the acute forms.

Antihyaluronidase
Antistreptokinase
Antidesoxyribonuclease-beta
Antidiphosphopyridine-nucleotidase
Antinicotinamide-adeninedenucleotidase, etc.

Urine

Hematuria—gross or only microscopic. Microscopic hematuria may occur during the initial febrile upper respiratory infection (URI) and then reappear with nephritis in 1–2 weeks. It lasts 2–12 months; usual duration is 2 months.

RBC casts show glomerular origin of hematuria.

WBC casts and WBCs show inflammatory nature of lesion.

Granular and epithelial cell casts are present.

Fatty casts and lipid droplets occur several weeks later; not related to hyperlipemia.

Proteinuria is usually <2 gm/day (but may be $\leqq 6$–8 gm/day). May disappear while RBC casts and RBCs still occur.

Oliguria is frequent.

Azotemia is found in $\cong 50\%$ of patients.

Glomerular filtration rate usually shows greater decrease than renal blood flow; therefore filtration factor is decreased.

PSP excretion is normal in cases of mild to moderate severity; increases with progression of disease.

ESR is increased.

Leukocytosis is present, with increased polynuclear neutrophils.

There is mild anemia, especially when edema is present (may be due to hemodilution, bone marrow depression, or increased destruction of RBCs).

Serum proteins are normal or there is nonspecific decrease of albumin and increase of alpha$_2$ and sometimes of beta and gamma globulins.

Serum cholesterol may be increased.

Serum complement falls 24 hours before onset of hematuria and rises to normal when hematuria subsides.

Antihuman kidney antibodies are present in serum in 50% of patients.

Decreased urinary aldosterone occurs in the presence of edema.

Renal biopsy shows characteristic findings with electron microscopy and immunofluorescence.

Azotemia with high urine specific gravity and normal PSP excretion usually means acute glomerulonephritis.

Clinical Course

Patients usually recover in 2–4 weeks; 10% die within a few months. A second attack is unusual after repeated urinalysis is normal. Marked proteinuria for >4 months suggests poor prognosis.

Acute nephritis in Schönlein-Henoch anaphylactoid purpura has a poorer initial prognosis and more often becomes chronic.

Acute glomerulonephritis in adults causes death or becomes chronic in 25–50% of patients. There may be a long latent period with only proteinuria and abnormal microscopical urinary findings.

RAPIDLY PROGRESSIVE NONSTREPTOCOCCAL GLOMERULONEPHRITIS

Preceded by nonstreptococcal respiratory or gastrointestinal viral illness in many patients.

No cultural or serologic (e.g., ASOT) evidence of recent streptococcus infection.

Oliguria with urine volume often <400 ml/day.

Hematuria is often gross.

RBCs, WBCs, and casts are present in urine.

Proteinuria is usually >3 gm/day.

Azotemia is usually marked, with BUN >80 mg/100 ml and serum creatinine >10 mg/100 ml (in poststreptococcal type, BUN is usually 30–100 mg/100 ml and serum creatinine 1.5–4 mg/100 ml).

Scrum complement levels are normal.

Renal biopsy and immunofluorescent antibody findings.

Prognosis is poorer than in poststreptococcal glomerulonephritis.

MEMBRANOPROLIFERATIVE GLOMERULONEPHRITIS

Marked proteinuria and nephrotic type of syndrome is found in 70% of patients.

Normal serum C_4 but prolonged or permanent depression of beta$_1$-complement (C_3) is found in 60–80% of patients; clinical course is not related to serum complement levels.

Clinical course may be clinically active, or there may be periods of remission; 50% have chronic renal insufficiency in 10 years.

Renal biopsy and immunofluorescent antibody findings.

NEPHROTIC SYNDROME

Characterized By

Marked proteinuria—usually >4.5 gm/day; usually exclusively albuminuria in children with lipoid nephrosis, but in glomerulonephritis high- and low-molecular weight proteins are present.

Decreased serum albumin—usually <2.5 gm/100 ml—and total protein

Increased serum cholesterol (free and esters)—usually >350 mg/100 ml. (Low or normal serum cholesterol occurs with poor nutrition and suggests poor prognosis.)

Increased serum phospholipids, neutral fats, triglycerides, low-density beta-lipoproteins, and total lipids

Serum alpha$_2$ and beta globulins are markedly increased and gamma globulin is decreased, alpha$_1$ is normal or decreased. If gamma globulin is increased, rule out systemic disease (e.g., SLE).

Urine containing doubly refractive fat bodies as seen by polarizing microscopy; many granular and epithelial cell casts

Hematuria—may be present in 50% of patients but is usually minimal and not part of syndrome

Azotemia—may be present but not part of syndrome

Changes secondary to proteinuria and hypoalbuminemia (e.g., de-

Table 69. Comparison of Some Serologic Tests in Different Types of Glomerulonephritis

Type of Glomerulonephritis	Culture for Group A Streptococcus	ASOT	Serum Beta$_1$-C (C$_3$)	Serum C$_4$	Anti-DNA
Poststreptococcal	+	+	D	D	–
Membranoproliferative	–	–	D or N	N	–
Nephritis of SLE	–	–	D	D	+
Rapidly progressive nonstreptococcal	–	–	N	N	–

+ = positive; – = negative; D = decreased; N = normal.

creased PBI, decreased serum calcium, decreased serum
ceruloplasmin, increased fibrinogen)
Increased ESR due to increased fibrinogen
Changes due to primary disease (see below)
Increased susceptibility to infection (most frequently peritonitis)
during periods of edema
Serum beta$_1$-C complement is normal in idiopathic lipoid nephrosis
but decreased when there is underlying glomerulonephritis.

Etiology
Renal
    Glomerulonephritis (>50% of patients)
    Lipoid nephrosis (10% in adult patients; 80% in children)
Systemic
    SLE (20% of patients)
    Amyloidosis
    Myeloma
    Diabetic glomerulosclerosis (15% of patients)
Venous obstruction
    Renal vein thrombosis
    Obstruction of inferior vena cava (thrombosis, tumor)
    Constrictive pericarditis
    Tricuspid stenosis
    Congestive heart failure
Infections (e.g., subacute bacterial endocarditis)
Allergic (e.g., serum sickness)
Toxic (e.g., heavy metal, drugs)

CHRONIC GLOMERULONEPHRITIS

Various Clinical Courses
Early death after marked proteinuria, hematuria, oliguria, progressive increasing uremia, anemia
Intermittent or continuous or incidental proteinuria, hematuria
with slight or absent azotemia, and normal renal function tests
(may develop into late renal failure or may subside)
Exacerbation of chronic nephritis (with accentuation of proteinuria, hematuria, and decreased renal function) shortly following streptococcal upper respiratory infection.
Nephrotic syndrome (see preceding section)

*Compared to pyelonephritis, chronic glomerulonephritis shows
lipid droplets and epithelial and RBC casts in urine, more
marked proteinuria (>2–3 gm/day), poorer prognosis for equivalent amount of azotemia.*

NEPHROSCLEROSIS
"Benign" nephrosclerosis ("essential hypertension")
    Urine contains little or no protein or microscopic abnor-
    malities.
    10% of patients develop marked renal insufficiency.
"Accelerated" nephrosclerosis ("malignant hypertension")
    Syndrome may occur in the course of "benign" nephro-

sclerosis, glomerulonephritis, unilateral renal artery occlusion, or any cause of hypertension.

Increasing uremia is associated with minimal or marked proteinuria and hematuria.

RENAL CALCULI
(autopsy incidence = 1.12%; cause of death = 0.38%)

Calcium oxalate alone or with phosphate is the constituent of kidney stones in 65% of patients in the United States.

35% of patients have increased urinary calcium, i.e., >250 mg/24 hours in females and >300 mg/24 hours in males (50–75% of hyperparathyroidism patients have renal calculi).

20–30% of patients have

Bone diseases—destructive (e.g., metastatic tumor) or osteoporosis (e.g., immobilization, Paget's disease, Cushing's syndrome)

Milk-alkali (Burnett's) syndrome

Hypervitaminosis D

Sarcoidosis

Renal tubular acidosis (Type I)

Hyperthyroidism

Other

50–60% of patients have

Idiopathic hypercalciuria—usually bilateral and occurring in males. Does not respond to cortisone; becomes normal with very low calcium intake. Normal serum calcium. Serum parathormone is most often increased.

Oxalate is the constituent of renal calculi in 65% of all patients, but hyperoxaluria is a relatively rare cause of these calculi and is due to

Increased ingestion of oxalate or precursor

Primary hyperoxaluria, Types I and II. Secondary pyelonephritis may cause death at an early age.

Methoxyflurane anesthesia

Hyperoxaluria secondary to ileal disease, which causes hyperabsorption of dietary oxalate

Magnesium ammonium phosphate is the constituent of renal calculi in 15% of patients. It occurs almost exclusively in patients with recurrent urinary tract infections by urea-splitting organisms, particularly *Proteus* species, and in patients with persistently alkaline urine.

Cystine stones form when urine contains >300 mg/day of cystine in congenital familial cystinuria. Urine shows cystine crystals. Cyanide-nitroprusside test is positive.

Uric acid is present in calculi in 10% of patients.

Gout. 25% of patients with primary gout and 40% of patients with marrow-proliferative disorders have calculi.

Urine is more acid than normal (e.g., patients with chronic diarrhea, ileostomy).

>50% of patients with urinary calculi have normal serum and urine uric acid levels.

Xanthine is present in children with inborn error of metabolism.

Hereditary glycinuria is a rare familial disorder associated with renal calculi.

Microscopic hematuria is found in 80% of patients.
In renal colic, hematuria and proteinuria are present, and there is an increased WBC due to associated infection.

OBSTRUCTIVE UROPATHY
(unilateral or bilateral; partial or complete)
Partial obstruction of both kidneys may cause increasing azotemia with normal or increased urinary output (due to decreased renal concentrating ability).
Partial obstruction may cause inexplicable wide variations in BUN and urine volume in patients with azotemia. PSP excretion is less in first 15-minute period than in any later period. There is considerable PSP excretion after the 2-hour test period.
In unilateral obstruction, BUN usually remains normal unless underlying renal disease is present.
Laboratory findings due to superimposed infection or underlying disease are noted.
Laboratory findings due to underlying disease
  Obstruction of bladder (e.g., benign prostatic hypertrophy, carcinoma of prostate or bladder, urethral stricture, neurogenic bladder dysfunction [multiple sclerosis, diabetic neuropathy])
  Obstruction of both ureters (e.g., infiltrating neoplasm [especially of uterine cervix], bilateral calculi, congenital anomalies, retroperitoneal fibrosis)

If ureter is obstructed >4 months, functional recovery is unlikely. When obstruction is relieved, most functional recovery takes place in 2–3 weeks; then there is continued improvement for several months.

PYELONEPHRITIS
Bacteriuria (see p. 128). Colony count of >100,000/ml of urine (properly collected) indicates active infection. If the count is 10,000 to 100,000/ml, it should be repeated. Bacteria seen on gram stain of uncentrifuged urine indicates bacteriuria.
A culture should be performed for identification of the specific organism and determination of antibiotic sensitivity.
Microscopical examination of urine sediment. WBC casts are very suggestive of pyelonephritis. Glitter cells may be seen.
Pyuria is present in only 50% of patients with chronic urinary tract infection and asymptomatic bacteriuria. Bacteriuria and pyuria are often intermittent; in the chronic atrophic stage of pyelonephritis, they are often absent.
Urine concentrating ability is decreased relatively early in chronic infection compared to other renal diseases.
Albuminuria is usually <2 gm/24 hours (≦2+ qualitative) and therefore helps to differentiate pyelonephritis from glomerular disease, in which albuminuria is usually >2 gm/24 hours. Al-

Table 70. Characteristic Features in Differential Diagnosis of Hypercalciuria[a]

Measurement	Primary Hyperparathyroidism	Absorptive Hypercalciuria	Renal Hypercalciuria	Normocalciuric Nephrolithiasis
Serum calcium	I	N	N	N
Urine calcium				
Fasting	I	N	I	N
After calcium load	I	I	I	N or I
Urine cyclic AMP				
Fasting	I in 30%	N	Usually I	N
After calcium load	I in 82%	N	N	N
Serum parathormone	I	N	I	N

N = normal; I = increased.

[a]See reference given as source for normal values and test procedures.

Source: C.Y.C. Pak et al., A simple test for the diagnosis of absorptive, resorptive and renal hypercalciurias. *N. Engl. J. Med.* 292:497, 1975.

buminuria may be undetectable in a very dilute urine associated with fixed specific gravity.

There is a decrease in 24-hour creatinine clearance before a rise in BUN and blood creatinine takes place.

Hyperchloremic acidosis (due to impaired renal acid excretion and bicarbonate reabsorption) occurs more often in chronic pyelonephritis than in glomerulonephritis.

Renal blood flow and glomerular filtration show parallel decrease proportional to progress of renal disease. Comparison of function in right and left kidneys shows more disparity in pyelonephritis than in diffuse renal disease (e.g., nephrosclerosis, glomerulonephritis).

Fluctuation in renal insufficiency (e.g., due to recurrent infection, dehydration) with considerable recovery is more marked and frequent in pyelonephritis than in other renal diseases.

Laboratory findings of associated diseases, e.g., diabetes mellitus, urinary tract obstruction (stone, tumor, etc.), neurogenic bladder dysfunction, are present.

Laboratory findings due to sequelae (e.g., papillary necrosis, bacteremia) are present.

When urine cultures are persistently negative in the presence of other evidence of pyelonephritis, specific search should be made for tubercle bacilli (e.g., culture, guinea pig inoculation).

"Cured" patient should be followed with routine periodic urinalysis and colony count for at least 2 years because asymptomatic recurrence of bacteriuria is common.

PAPILLARY NECROSIS OF KIDNEY
Findings of associated diseases
    Diabetes mellitus
    Urinary tract infection
    Chronic overuse of phenacetin
Sudden diminution in renal function; occasionally oliguria or anuria with acute renal failure
Hematuria

RENAL ABSCESS
(due to metastatic infection not related to previous renal disease)
Urine
    Trace of albumin
    Few RBCs (may have transient gross hematuria at onset)
    No WBCs
    Very many gram-positive cocci in stained sediment
WBC high (may be >30,000/cu mm)

Complications
Sudden rupture into renal pelvis—urine suddenly cloudy and contains very many WBCs and bacteria
Renal carbuncle formation
Rupture into perirenal space
Secondary pyelonephritis

PERINEPHRIC ABSCESS

Laboratory findings due to underlying or primary diseases (see above)

> Hematogenous from distant foci (e.g., furuncles, infected tonsils) usually due to staphylococci and occasionally streptococci
>
> Direct extension from kidney infection (e.g., pyelonephritis, pyonephrosis) due to gram-negative rods and occasionally tubercle bacilli
>
> Infected perirenal hematoma (e.g., due to trauma, tumor, polyarteritis nodosa) due to various organisms

Urine changes due to underlying disease

> Urine may be normal and sterile. (*Do acid-fast smear and culture for tubercle bacilli.*)

Increased polynuclear leukocytes

Increased ESR

Positive blood culture (some patients)

RENAL TUBERCULOSIS

Should be ruled out when there is unexplained albuminuria, pyuria, microhematuria, but cultures for pyogenic bacteria are negative, especially in presence of TB elsewhere

Urine culture for TB

Guinea pig inoculation

See Table 66, pp. 427–429.
See Tuberculosis, pp. 473–474, for general findings.

HORSESHOE KIDNEYS

Laboratory findings due to complications

> Renal calculi
>
> Pyelonephritis
>
> Hematuria

POLYCYSTIC KIDNEYS

Polyuria is common.

Hematuria may be gross and episodic or an incidental microscopical finding.

Proteinuria may be an incidental finding of routine analysis.

Renal calculi may be associated.

Superimposed pyelonephritis is frequent.

Death occurs within 5 years after BUN rises to 50 mg/100 ml.

Death usually occurs in early infancy, or in middle age when superimposed nephrosclerosis of aging or pyelonephritis has exhausted renal reserve.

Cerebral hemorrhage causes death in 10% of patients; intracranial berry aneurysms are frequently associated.

MEDULLARY CYSTIC DISEASE

Anemia is often severe and out of proportion to degree of renal failure.

Polyuria

Salt-losing syndrome

Death from renal insufficiency (may take many years)

Urinalysis shows minimal or no proteinuria; presence of RBCs, WBCs, casts, or bacteria is rare. Specific gravity may be decreased.

Serum alkaline phosphatase may be increased when bone changes occur.

SPONGE KIDNEY
Findings due to complications
    Hematuria
    Infection
    Renal calculi within cysts
Disease asymptomatic, not progressive

HEREDITARY NEPHRITIS
May be classified into two types
    Angiokeratoma corporis diffusum (familial condition of abnormal glycolipid deposition in glomerular epithelial cells, nervous system, heart, etc.)
        Proteinuria begins in second decade.
        Urine may contain lipid globules and foam cells.
        Uremia occurs by fourth or fifth decade.
    Familial autosomal dominant disease associated with nerve deafness and lens defects. Renal disease is progressive.
        Hematuria, gross or microscopic, is common; more marked after occurrence of unrelated infection. Other laboratory findings are the same as in other types of nephritis.

ARTERIAL INFARCTION OF KIDNEY
Microscopic or gross hematuria is usual.
BUN is normal unless other renal disease is present.
In some cases, urine shows no albumin or abnormal sediment at time of analysis.
WBC, SGOT, SGPT are increased if area of infarction is large; peak by second day; return to normal by fifth day.
Serum and urine LDH may be increased markedly.
CRP and serum LDH peak on third day; return to normal by tenth day.
Changes in serum enzyme levels, WBC, CRP, ESR are similar in time changes to those in myocardial infarction.
Plasma renin activity may rise on second day, peak about 11th day, and remain elevated for more than a month.

RENAL VEIN THROMBOSIS
Hematuria
Proteinuria
Oliguria and uremic death if bilateral
WBC increased
Anemia common
Possibly, low platelet count
Laboratory findings due to underlying causative condition (e.g.,

hypernephroma, metastatic cancer, trauma, polyarteritis, papillary necrosis, amyloidosis)

See Nephrotic Syndrome, p. 437.

RENAL ARTERIOVENOUS FISTULA
Hematuria
Laboratory findings due to congestive heart failure and hypertension

RENAL CHANGES IN BACTERIAL ENDOCARDITIS
There are three types of pathologic changes: diffuse subacute glomerulonephritis, focal embolic glomerulonephritis, microscopic or gross infarcts of kidney.
Laboratory findings due to bacterial endocarditis are noted (see p. 175).
Albuminuria is almost invariably present, even when no renal lesions are found.
Hematuria (usually microscopic, sometimes gross) is usual at some stage of the disease, but repeated examinations may be required.
Renal insufficiency is frequent (15% of cases during active stage; 40% of fatal cases).
  BUN is increased—usually 25–75 mg/100 ml.
  Renal concentrating ability is decreased.

KIDNEY DISORDERS IN GOUT
Kidney stones occur in 15% of patients with gout; may occur in absence of arthritis.
Early renal damage is indicated by decreased renal concentrating ability, mild proteinuria, and decreased PSP excretion.
Later renal damage is shown by slowly progressive azotemia with slight albuminuria and slight or no abnormalities of urine sediment.
Arteriolar nephrosclerosis and pyelonephritis are usually associated.
Renal disease causes death in $\leq$50% of patients with gout.

KIMMELSTIEL-WILSON SYNDROME (DIABETIC INTERCAPILLARY GLOMERULOSCLEROSIS)
The disease usually occurs after associated diabetes mellitus has been present >10 years; it is not related to control of diabetes. Occasionally it is associated only with prediabetes.
Proteinuria is usual (may be earliest clinical clue) and may be marked (often more than 5 gm/day). Nephrotic syndrome is often associated.
Urine shows many hyaline and granular casts and double refractile fat bodies. Hematuria is rare.
Serum protein is decreased.
Azotemia develops gradually after several years of proteinuria.
Biopsy of kidney is diagnostic.
Laboratory findings are those due to frequently associated infections of the urinary tract.

See sections on diabetes mellitus, acidosis, papillary necrosis, urinary tract infection, diabetic neuropathy.

RENAL DISEASE IN POLYARTERITIS NODOSA

Renal involvement occurs in 75% of patients.

Azotemia is often absent or only mild and slowly progressive.

Albuminuria is always present.

Hematuria (gross or microscopic) is very common. Fat bodies are frequently present in urine sediment.

There may be findings of acute glomerulonephritis with remission or early death from renal failure.

Always rule out polyarteritis in any case of glomerulonephritis, renal failure, or hypertension that shows unexplained eosinophilia, increased WBC, or laboratory evidence of involvement of other organ systems.

NEPHRITIS OF SYSTEMIC LUPUS ERYTHEMATOSUS (SLE)

Renal involvement occurs in two-thirds of patients with SLE.

Nephritis of SLE may occur as acute, latent, or chronic glomerulonephritis, nephrosis, or asymptomatic albuminuria.

Urine findings are as in chronic active glomerulonephritis.

Azotemia or marked proteinuria usually indicates death in 1–3 years.

Signs of SLE (e.g., positive LE test) may disappear during active nephritis, nephrosis, or uremia.

RENAL DISEASE IN SCLERODERMA

Renal involvement occurs in two-thirds of patients; one-third die of renal failure.

Proteinuria may be minimal and is usually <2 gm/day; this may be the only finding for a long time.

Azotemia usually signals death within a few months.

Terminal oligura or anuria may occur.

TOXEMIA OF PREGNANCY

Proteinuria varies from a trace to very marked ($\leqq$800 mg/100 ml, equivalent to 15–20 gm/day). >15 mg/100 ml may indicate early toxemia.

RBCs and RBC casts are not abundant; hyaline and granular casts are present.

BUN, renal concentrating ability, and PSP excretion are normal unless the disease is severe or there is a prior renal lesion. (*BUN usually decreases during normal pregnancy because of increase in glomerular filtration rate.*)

Serum uric acid is increased (decreased renal clearance of urate) in 70% of patients in absence of treatment with thiazides, which can produce hyperuricemia independent of any disease.

Serum total protein and albumin commonly are markedly decreased.

There may be multiple clotting deficiencies in severe cases.

Biopsy of kidney can establish diagnosis; rules out primary renal disease or hypertensive vascular disease.

GFR and renal plasma flow are 10–30% less than in normal pregnancy but may appear normal, increased, or decreased compared to rates in nonpregnant women. (Normally GFR increases gradually to a maximum of 40% more than nonpregnant level by 32nd week, then decreases slightly until term. Renal plasma flow is not so markedly increased. Therefore the filtration fraction—GFR-RPF ratio:—increases slightly.)

Tubular reabsorption of sodium, water, urea, and uric acid is increased (perhaps on account of decreased GFR). Sodium excretion is decreased $\geqq 35\%$.

Beware of associated or underlying conditions–hydatidiform mole, twin pregnancy, prior renal disease.

KIDNEY IN MULTIPLE MYELOMA

Renal function is impaired in >50% of patients: usually there is loss of renal concentrating ability and azotemia.

Proteinuria is very frequent and is due to albumin and globulins in urine; Bence Jones proteinuria may be intermittent.

There is severe anemia out of proportion to azotemia.

Occasional changes due to altered renal tubular function are present.

> Renal glycosuria, aminoaciduria, decreased serum uric acid, renal potassium wasting
> Renal loss of phosphate with decreased serum phosphorus and increased alkaline phosphatase
> Nephrogenic diabetes insipidus
> Oliguria or anuria with acute renal failure precipitated by dehydration

Changes due to associated amyloidosis are found (see pp. 520–521).

Changes due to associated hypercalcemia are found.

See Multiple Myeloma, pp. 322–323.

PRIMARY OR SECONDARY AMYLOIDOSIS OF KIDNEY

Persistent proteinuria that varies from mild, with or without hematuria, to severe, with nephrotic syndrome.

Vasopressin-resistant polyuria is present if the medulla alone is involved (rare).

See Amyloidosis, pp. 520–521.

SICKLE CELL NEPHROPATHY

Gross and microscopic hematuria is common.

Early decrease of renal concentrating ability is evident even with normal BUN, glomerular filtration rate, and renal plasma flow; it occurs in sickle cell trait as well as the disease, but progressive nephropathy occurs only with the disease. The decrease is temporarily reversed in children by transfusion but not in adults.

RENAL DISEASE IN ALLERGIC (HENOCH-SCHÖNLEIN) PURPURA

Urine is abnormal in 25–50% of patients, but renal biopsy is abnormal in most (usually a focal proliferative glomerulonephritis).

Clinical picture varies from minimal urinary abnormalities to severe, rapidly progressive nephritis that is indistinguishable from glomerulonephritis. Nephrotic syndrome may occur. Chronic course, with remissions and exacerbations and permanent renal damage, may occur.

Serum complement is normal.

HEMOLYTIC-UREMIC SYNDROME

Usually occurs in a child less than age 2 who develops urinary findings of acute glomerulonephritis after several days of gastroenteritis.

Severe hemolytic anemia is present at onset or within a few days; hemoglobin is often <6 gm/100 ml. Burr RBCs are always seen in peripheral blood smear.

Platelet count is usually decreased.

WBC is normal.

Coombs' test is negative.

Serum complement is normal.

Laboratory findings indicate progressive renal disease or recovery.

Azotemia, with BUN frequently >100 mg/100 ml.

HEPATORENAL SYNDROME

Oliguria

Azotemia

Decreased sodium in serum and urine

High specific gravity of urine

Decreased renal blood flow and glomerular filtration rate

HYPERCALCEMIC NEPHROPATHY

Diffuse nephrocalcinosis is the result of prolonged increase in serum and urine calcium (due to hyperparathyroidism, sarcoidosis, vitamin D intoxication, multiple myeloma, carcinomatosis, milk-alkali syndrome, etc.).

Urine is normal or contains RBCs, WBCs, WBC casts; proteinuria is usually slight or absent.

Early findings are decreased renal concentrating ability and polyuria.

Later findings are decreased glomerular filtration rate, decreased renal blood flow, azotemia.

Renal insufficiency is insidious and slowly progressive; it may sometimes be reversed by correcting hypercalcemia.

See various primary causative diseases.

IRRADIATION NEPHRITIS

Exposure (one or both kidneys) to >2300 rads for 6 weeks or less.

Latent period is >6 months.
Slight proteinuria is present.
Hematuria and oliguria are absent.
Refractory anemia is present.
Progressive uremia is found; may be reversible later.
Renal biopsy.

LABORATORY CRITERIA FOR KIDNEY TRANSPLANTATION
Donor: Three successive urinalyses and cultures must be negative.
Donor and recipient must show
  ABO and Rh blood group compatibility
  Leukoagglutinin compatibility
  Platelet agglutinin compatibility

ANALGESIC NEPHROPATHY
See Phenacetin—Chronic Excessive Ingestion, p. 526.

LABORATORY FINDINGS OF KIDNEY TRANSPLANT REJECTION
Total urine output is decreased.
Proteinuria is increased.
Cellular or granular casts appear.
Urine osmolality is decreased.
Blood urea nitrogen rises.
Hyperchloremic renal tubular acidosis may be an early sign of rejection or indicate smoldering rejection activity.
Renal clearance values decrease.
Sodium iodohippurate ^{131}I renogram is altered.
Biopsy of kidney shows a characteristic microscopic appearance.

LEUKOPLAKIA OF RENAL PELVIS
Cell block of urine shows keratin or keratinized squamous cells.

CARCINOMA OF RENAL PELVIS AND URETER
Hematuria is present.
Renal calculi are associated.
Urinary tract infection is associated.
Cytologic examination of urinary sediment for malignant cells is necessary.

HYPERNEPHROMA OF KIDNEY
Even in the absence of the classic loin pain, flank mass, and hematuria, hypernephroma should be ruled out in the presence of these *unexplained* laboratory findings
  Abnormal liver function tests (in absence of metastases to liver) found in 40% of these patients, e.g., increased serum alkaline phosphatase, thymol turbidity, prolonged prothrombin time, retention of BSP, altered serum protein values (decreased albumin, increased alpha$_2$ globulin)
  Hypercalcemia
  Polycythemia
  Leukemoid reaction
  Refractory anemia and increased ESR

Amyloidosis
Cushing's syndrome
Salt-losing syndrome

For laboratory assistance in diagnosis
Exfoliative cytology of urine for tumor cells
Test for increased urine LDH level
Radioisotope scan of kidney

Needle biopsy is not recommended.

RENIN-PRODUCING RENAL TUMORS
(hemangiopericytomas of juxtaglomerular apparatus; Wilms' tumor; rarely lung cancer)
Plasma renin activity is increased, with levels significantly higher in renal vein from affected side.
Plasma renin activity responds to changes in posture but not to changes in sodium intake.
Plasma renin activity maintains circadian rhythm despite marked elevation.
Secondary aldosteronism is evident, with hypokalemia, etc. (see pp. 406, 407).
Laboratory changes (and hypertension) are reversed by removal of tumor.

BENIGN PROSTATIC HYPERTROPHY
Laboratory findings are those due to urinary tract obstruction and secondary infection.

PROSTATITIS
Most frequently due to
Streptococcus faecalis
Staphylococcus albus
Escherichia coli
Proteus mirabilis
Pseudomonas
Klebsiella
The acute form usually shows laboratory findings of infected urine (WBCs in centrifuged sediment of last portion of voided specimen; positive culture).
In the chronic form, prostatic fluid usually shows >10–15 WBCs (pus cells). Cultures are frequently positive (see bacteria listed above).
Laboratory findings due to associated or complicating conditions (e.g., epididymitis) may be present.

POSTVASECTOMY STATUS
Sperm count may fall to low levels after 3 or 4 ejaculations and then rise abruptly before falling again.
Ten ejaculations may be required before sperm count reaches 0.
Three consecutive azoospermic specimens are recommended before dispensing with contraception.
Reanastomosis of the vas deferens may occur.

NONSPECIFIC URETHRITIS
Diagnosis is made by exclusion, using laboratory methods.

Gram stain of urethral exudate shows polynuclear leukocytes without bacteria. Urethral culture is negative. These test results are presumptive evidence for diagnosis of nonspecific urethritis.

Fresh preparations and cultures are negative for *Trichomonas* and *Candida*.

The presumptive agent is *Chlamydia* (obligate intracellular bacteria that are cultured like viruses), which can be isolated in >40% of men and 30% of women with nonspecific urethritis.

Laboratory findings of complications
> Prostatitis (20% of patients)
> Epididymitis (3% of patients)
> Urethral stricture (<5% of patients)
> Reiter's syndrome (2% of patients)

This is the most frequent venereal disease.

See Gonococcal Infections, pp. 459–460.

CARCINOMA OF PROSTATE
Increased serum acid phosphatase indicates local extension or distant metastases. It is increased in 80% of patients with bone metastases, 20% of patients with extension into periprostatic soft tissue but without bone involvement, 5% of patients with carcinoma confined to gland. Occasionally it remains low despite active metastases. Increased serum acid phosphatase shows pronounced fall in activity within 3–4 days after castration or within 2 weeks after estrogen therapy is begun; may return to normal or remain slightly elevated; failure to fall corresponds to the failure of clinical response that occurs in 10% of the patients. Most patients with invasive carcinoma show a significant increase in serum acid phosphatase after massage or palpation; this rarely occurs in patients with normal prostate, benign prostatic hypertrophy, or in situ carcinoma, or in patients with prostate carcinoma who are receiving hormone treatment.

Alkaline phosphatase is increased in 90% of patients with bone metastases. Increases with favorable response to estrogen therapy or castration and reaches peak in 3 months, then declines. Recurrence of bone metastases causes new rise in alkaline phosphatase.

Anemia is present.

Carcinoma cells may appear in bone marrow aspirates.

Fibrinolysins are found in 12% of patients with metastatic prostatic cancer; occur only with extensive metastases and are usually associated with hemorrhagic manifestations; they show fibrinogen deficiency and prolonged prothrombin time.

Urinary tract infection and hematuria occur late.

Needle biopsy of suspicious nodules in prostate is called for.

Cytologic examination of prostatic fluid is not generally useful.

CARCINOMA OF BLADDER
Hematuria is present.

Biopsy of tumor should be taken.

Cytologic examination of urine for tumor cells is useful. (It may be of most value in screening dye workers in chemical industry.)

Urinary LDH level may be particularly useful in screening studies to discover asymptomatic patients with neoplasm of GU tract.

Laboratory findings due to complications will stem from infection or from obstruction of ureter.

Laboratory findings due to preexisting conditions (e.g., schistosomiasis, stone, or infection)

RETROPERITONEAL FIBROSIS

ESR is increased.

Leukocytosis is present.

Occasionally eosinophilia occurs.

Serum protein and A/G ratio are normal; if the person is chronically ill, total protein may be decreased.

Gamma globulins may be increased.

Anemia is present.

Laboratory findings due to ureteral obstruction are made.

The condition may be primary, due to angiomatous lymphoid hamartoma, or secondary to administration of methysergide.

VULVOVAGINITIS

Due To

Bacteria, especially gonococcus (see p. 459); also *Hemophilus vaginalis* (gram stain of smear, culture)

Fungi, especially *Candida albicans*, diagnosed by culture on Nickerson's or Sabouraud's medium and also by identification on Papanicolaou smears

Trichomonas, diagnosed by hanging drop preparation; often seen in routine urinalysis on microscopical examination

Local cause is most common (e.g., poor hygiene, pinworms, scabies, foreign body).

In nongonorrheal cases, smear shows more epithelial cells and fewer WBCs compared to gonorrhea. Gram stain may show many or few bacteria, which are often mixed (i.e., gram-positive and gram-negative; cocci and bacilli).

CARCINOMA OF UTERUS

Carcinoma of the Corpus

Cytologic examination (Pap smear) is positive in $\cong 70\%$ of patients; a false negative result occurs in 30% of patients. Therefore a negative Pap smear does not rule out carcinoma.

Pap smear from aspiration of endometrial cavity is positive in 95% of patients. Endometrial biopsy may be helpful, but a negative result does not rule out carcinoma.

Diagnostic curettage is the only way to rule out carcinoma of the endometrium.

Carcinoma of the Cervix

Pap smear for routine screening in the general population may be positive for carcinoma of the cervix in $\cong 6$ of every 1000 women

(prevalence); only 7% of these lesions are invasive. The prevalence rate is greatest in certain groups:
  Women ages 21–35 years, with peak in 31st to 35th year
  Black and Puerto Rican women
  Women who use birth control pills rather than diaphragm for
      contraception
  Women with early onset or long duration of sexual activity

Vaginal pool Pap smear has an accuracy rate of ≅80% in detecting carcinoma of the cervix. Smears from a combination of vaginal pool, exocervical, and endocervical scrapings have an accuracy rate of 95%.
After an initial abnormal smear, the follow-up smear taken in the next few weeks or months may not always be abnormal; there is no clear explanation for this finding. Biopsy shows important lesions of the cervix in some of these patients. Therefore an abnormal initial smear requires further investigation of the cervix regardless of subsequent cytologic reports.

Late Cases
Laboratory findings due to obstruction of ureters with pyelonephritis, azotemia, etc., may be present.
General effects of cancer are found.

RUPTURED TUBAL PREGNANCY
Increased WBC usually returns to normal in 24 hours. Persistent increase may indicate recurrent bleeding. 50% of patients have normal WBC; 75% of the patients have WBC <15,000/cu mm. Persistent WBC >20,000/cu mm may indicate pelvic inflammatory disease.
Anemia is present but often precedes the tubal pregnancy in impoverished populations. Progressive anemia may indicate continuing bleeding into hematoma. Absorption of blood from hematoma may cause increased serum bilirubin.
Pregnancy tests are positive in ≅50% of patients.

ALTERED LABORATORY TESTS DURING PREGNANCY
Hemoglobin decreases slightly to as low as 10 gm/100 ml, with corresponding decrease of hematocrit.
RBC is decreased ≤10–15% because of increased plasma volume.
Blood volume is increased ≤45%, and plasma volume is decreased by 25–55% by 32d week.
WBC is increased during late pregnancy and labor.
Increased ESR is due to increased fibrinogen.
Serum iron is decreased and TIBC is increased during last half of pregnancy.
Serum albumin is decreased ≅1 gm/100 ml during last 2 trimesters.
Serum alpha$_1$ globulin is markedly increased in last 2 trimesters.
Serum alpha$_2$ globulin is increased in last 2 trimesters.
Serum beta globulin is slightly increased in second trimester.
Serum gamma globulin may decrease slightly in last trimester.

Blood fibrinogen is moderately increased by fourth month; increased one-third by term.

Serum ceruloplasmin, copper, transferrin, and alpha$_1$ antitrypsin are increased in last trimester.

Serum glucose is occasionally decreased.

Glucose tolerance is decreased during last trimester.

Glomerular filtration rate (GFR) and renal plasma flow are increased.

Blood urea nitrogen and creatinine decrease $\cong 25\%$, especially during first 2 trimesters.

BUN of 18 mg/100 ml and creatinine of 1.2 mg/100 ml are definitely abnormal in pregnancy although normal in nonpregnant women.

Serum cholesterol increases after 8th week to maximum by 30th week.

Serum PBI is increased throughout pregnancy.

Serum T-3 uptake is decreased and T-4 is increased. Free thyroxine factor (T-3 × T-4) is normal. TBG is increased. BMR is moderately increased, especially in last trimester.

In late pregnancy, Factor XI is decreased and Factors II, VII, VIII, IX, and X are increased.

Serum CPK may be decreased during 8th to 20th week (maximum at 12th week). CPK is frequently definitely increased during last few weeks. Serum LDH is occasionally slightly increased.

At parturition there is a significant increase in serum of CPK with a smaller increase of LDH and SGOT. Levels become normal in 2–5 days.

In toxemia of pregnancy, serum SGOT and SGPT are increased; more marked increases occur with greater severity of toxemia.

Serum alkaline phosphatase is increased (2–3 times) and serum ICD is increased in third trimester. In toxemia, rise in serum alkaline phosphatase is greater. Alkaline phosphatase falls with intrauterine fetal death.

Serum leucine aminopeptidase (LAP) may be moderately increased throughout pregnancy.

Abnormal BSP retention occurs during last month.

Occasionally cold agglutinins may be positive and osmotic fragility increased.

Urine volume may increase $\leqq 25\%$ in last trimester.

Proteinuria is common ($\cong 20\%$ of patients).

Glycosuria is common with decreased glucose tolerance.

Lactosuria should not be confused with glucose in urine.

Urine porphyrins may be increased.

Urinary gonadotropins (HCG) are increased (see "Pregnancy Test," p. 120).

Urine estrogens increase from 6 months to term ($\leqq 100$ μg/24 hours).

Urine 17-ketosteroids rise to upper limit of normal at term.

Plasma renin is increased.

Serum aldosterone is increased.

Gastric HCl and pepsin may be decreased.

ALTERED LABORATORY TESTS DURING MENSTRUATION
Platelet count is decreased by 50–70%; returns to normal by fourth day.
Hemoglobin is unchanged.
Fibrinogen is increased.
Serum cholesterol may increase just before menstruation.
Serum PBI may decrease slightly after menstruation.
Urine volume, sodium, and chloride decrease premenstrually and increase postmenstrually (diuresis).
Urine protein may increase during premenstrual phase.
Urine porphyrins increase.
Urine estrogens decrease to lowest level 2–3 days after onset.

INFECTIOUS DISEASES

PNEUMOCOCCAL INFECTIONS

Pneumonia

Increased WBC (usually 12,000–25,000/cu mm) with shift to the left; normal or low WBC in overwhelming infection, in aged patients, or with other causative organisms (e.g., Friedländer's bacillus)

Blood culture positive for pneumococci in 25% of untreated patients during first 3–4 days

Gram stain of sputum—many polynuclear leukocytes, many gram-positive cocci in pairs and singly; direct pneumococcus typing using Neufeld capsular swelling method rarely done now

Pleural effusion in ≅5% of patients

Laboratory findings due to complications (endocarditis, meningitis, peritonitis, arthritis, empyema, etc.)

Endocarditis

See pp. 175–176.

Meningitis

See pp. 250, 251.

Laboratory findings due to associated or underlying conditions—pneumococcal pneumonia, endocarditis, otitis, sinusitis, multiple myeloma

Peritonitis

Positive blood culture

Increased WBC

Ascitic fluid—identification of organisms by gram stain and culture

See section on laboratory findings in body fluids, p. 145.

STREPTOCOCCAL INFECTIONS

(uncommon under age 2)

Group A streptococci showing beta hemolysis

  Upper respiratory infection

  Scarlet fever

WBC is usually increased (14,000/cu mm) early. It becomes normal by end of first week. (*If still increased, look for complication, e.g., otitis.*) Increased eosinophils appear during convalescence, especially with scarlet fever.

Urine may show transient slight albumin, RBCs, casts, without sequelae.

ASO titer (see pp. 122–123)

See sections on rheumatic fever and acute glomerulonephritis, pp. 173–174, 435–436.

Acute glomerulonephritis follows streptococcal infection after latent period of 1–2 weeks; preceding infection may be

> *pharyngeal or of the skin. Latent period prior to onset of acute rheumatic fever is 2–4 weeks; preceding infection is pharyngeal but rarely of the skin.*

Group A streptococci are the most frequent type of streptococci causing
>   Otitis media, mastoiditis, sinusitis, meningitis, cerebral sinus thrombosis
>   Pneumonia, empyema, pericarditis
>   Bacteremia, suppurative arthritis
>   Puerperal sepsis
>   Lymphangitis, lymphadenitis, erysipelas, cellulitis
>   Impetigo (in older children, is often mixed infection with staphylococci that overgrow the culture plate)
>
>   WBC is markedly increased ($\leqq$20,000–30,000/cu mm).
>   Streptococci appear in smears and cultures from appropriate sites.
>   Blood culture may be positive.

Streptococcus viridans (alpha-hemolytic streptococci) causes
>   Subacute bacterial endocarditis (see pp. 175–176)

Streptococcus faecalis (enterococcus; Group D streptococci) causes
>   Bacterial endocarditis
>   Urinary tract infection

Anaerobic streptococci
>   Associated with coliform bacilli, clostridia, *Bacteroides*
>   Compound fractures and soft-tissue wounds
>   Puerperal and postabortion sepsis
>   Visceral abscesses (e.g., lung, liver, brain)
>   Associated with *Staphylococcus aureus*
>   Gangrenous postoperative abdominal incision
>   Without associated bacteria
>   Burrowing skin and subcutaneous infection

STAPHYLOCOCCAL INFECTIONS

Pneumonia—often secondary to measles, influenza, mucoviscidosis, debilitating diseases such as leukemia and collagen diseases or to prolonged treatment with broad-spectrum antibiotics
>   WBC is increased (usually >15,000/cu mm).
>   Sputum contains very many leukocytes with intracellular gram-positive cocci.
>   Bacteremia occurs in <20% of patients.

Acute osteomyelitis—due to hematogenous dissemination
>   Bacteremia occurs in >50% of early cases.
>   WBC is increased.
>   Anemia develops.
>   Secondary amyloidosis occurs in long-standing chronic osteomyelitis.

Endocarditis—occurs in valves without preceding rheumatic disease and showing little or no previous damage; causes rapid severe damage to valve, producing acute clinical course of mechanical heart failure (rupture of chordae tendineae, perforation of valve, valvular insufficiency) plus results of acute severe infection

Metastatic abscesses occur in various organs.

Anemia develops rapidly.

WBC is increased (12,000–20,000/cu mm); occasionally is normal or decreased.

From 1 to 13% of cases of bacterial endocarditis are due to coagulase-negative Staphylococcus albus; *bacterial endocarditis due to* Staphylococcus albus *is found following cardiac surgery in one-third and without preceding surgery in two-thirds of patients.*

WBC is increased.

Bacteremia is common.

Food poisoning—due to enterotoxin

Culture of staphylococci from suspected food (especially custard and milk products and meats)

Necrotizing enterocolitis of infancy as seen in Hirschsprung's disease

Impetigo—especially in infants between ages 3 weeks and 6 months

Meningitis (see pp. 250, 251)

MENINGOCOCCAL INFECTIONS
Meningococcemia

Meningitis (see pp. 250, 251)

Waterhouse-Friderichsen syndrome (see pp. 410–411)

Increased WBC (12,000–40,000/cu mm)

Gram-stained smears of body fluids

Tissue fluid from skin lesions

Buffy coat of blood

Cerebrospinal fluid *(Pyogenic meningitis in which bacteria cannot be found in smear is more likely to be due to meningoccus than to other bacteria.)*

Nasopharynx

Culture (use chocolate agar incubated in 10% CO_2)—blood, spinal fluid, skin lesions, nasopharynx, other sites of infection

Urine—may show albumin, RBCs; occasional glycosuria

Cerebrospinal fluid (see Table 29, pp. 240–244)

Markedly increased WBC (2500–10,000/cu mm), almost all polynuclear leukocytes

Increased protein (50–1500 mg/100 ml)

Decreased glucose (0–45 mg/100 ml)

Positive smear and culture

Laboratory findings due to complications (e.g., disseminated intravascular coagulation, pp. 337–339) and sequelae (e.g., subdural effusion)

GONOCOCCAL INFECTIONS
Genital infection

Gram stain of smear from involved site, especially urethra, prostatic secretions, cervix, pelvic inflammatory disease.

(Smear may become negative within hours of antibiotic therapy.)

Bacterial culture *(use special media such as Thayer-Martin)* should always be taken at the same time (before beginning antibiotic therapy). In ≅2% of male patients, gram stain of urethral exudate is negative when a simultaneous culture of the same material is positive.

Fluorescent antibody test on smear of suspected material

Beware of concomitant inapparent venereal infection that may be suppressed but not adequately treated by antibiotic therapy of gonorrhea.

Proctitis

Gram-stained smears are not sufficiently reliable.

Bacterial culture on special media (e.g., Thayer-Martin) is required for confirmation.

Rectal biopsy shows mild and nonspecific inflammation. In a few cases, gram stain of tissue section may reveal small numbers of gram-negative intracellular diplococci after prolonged examination.

Rectal gonorrhea accompanies genital gonorrhea in 20–50% of women and is found without genital gonorrhea in 6–10% of infected women. Therefore rectal cultures for gonococcus should be taken in all suspected cases of gonorrhea.

Arthritis

Synovial fluid (see Table 34, pp. 274–275)

Variable; may contain few leukocytes or be purulent

Gonococci identified in about one-third of patients

Gonococcal complement-fixation test for differential diagnosis of other types of arthritis. Not a reliable test in urethritis but may rarely be helpful in arthritis, prostatitis, and epididymitis. Becomes positive at least 2–6 weeks after onset of infection, remains positive for 3 months after cure. If test is negative, it should be repeated; two negative tests help to rule out gonococcus infection. False positive test may occur after gonococcus vaccine has been used. Test is of limited value and is seldom used.

Associated nonbacterial ophthalmitis in ≦20% of patients

Rarely, other sites

Ophthalmitis of newborn

Acute bacterial endocarditis (toxic hepatitis common) (see pp. 175–176). *(Gonococcus is the most common bacteria infecting tricuspid or pulmonic valves.)*

Bacteremia—resembles meningococcemia

Peritonitis and perihepatitis following spread from pelvic inflammatory disease

INFECTIONS WITH COLIFORM BACTERIA
(*Escherichia coli*, *Enterobacter-Klebsiella* group, paracolon group)

Bacteremia

Secondary to infection elsewhere; occasionally due to transfusion of contaminated blood

Secondary to debilitated condition in 20% of patients (e.g., malignant lymphoma, irradiation or anticancer drugs, steroid therapy, cirrhosis, diabetes mellitus)

Gram-negative shock occurs in 25% of patients.
> Azotemia
> Increased serum potassium
> Decreased serum sodium
> Metabolic acidosis
> Increased SGOT (decreased hepatic perfusion)
> Increased serum amylase (decreased renal perfusion)
> Other findings due to shock
>> Shock is most frequently from urinary tract, gastrointestinal tract, uterus, lung—in that order.
> *Escherichia coli* is the most frequent organism; it causes the lowest mortality (45%) and the lowest incidence of shock. *Pseudomonas aeruginosa* has the highest mortality (85%). *Klebsiella-Enterobacter,* paracolon bacilli, and *Proteus mirabilis* are intermediate, with 70% mortality.

Urinary tract infection (75% of cases due to *E. coli*)

Infections of intestinal tract and biliary tree (e.g., appendicitis, cholecystitis)

Wound infections, abscesses, etc.

Sepsis neonatorum (bacterial infection during the first 30 days of life with primary involvement of blood and, frequently, meninges)
> Positive blood culture. *Escherichia coli* and *Klebsiella-Enterobacter* cause ≅75% of cases. Group B and Group D streptococci and *Listeria monocytogenes* cause most of the other cases. May also be caused by a large variety of other bacteria. *Incidence of contaminated blood cultures is high in newborns. Negative blood culture does not rule out this condition; should take cultures from umbilical stump, skin lesions, mucous membranes, urine.*
> Positive culture of cerebrospinal fluid occurs frequently. *There may be no WBC increase early in the course of the disease.*
> WBC is variable; leukopenia is often associated with a high mortality.
> Anemia and decreased platelets may occur.
> Laboratory findings due to involvement of other organs (e.g., kidney, with albumin, cells, or casts increased in urine; liver, with increased direct or indirect bilirubin).

Gastroenteritis in young children and infants—identification of specific enteropathogenic strains by fluorescent antibody technique

Pneumonia—1% of primary bacterial pneumonias due to *Klebsiella* (Friedländer's bacilli), especially in alcoholics
> WBC is often normal or decreased.
> Sputum is very tenacious; is brown or red. Smear shows en-

capsulated gram-negative bacilli. *(Gram stain of sputum in lobar pneumonia allows prompt diagnosis of this organism and appropriate therapy.)* Bacterial culture confirms diagnosis.
Laboratory findings due to complications (lung abscess, empyema) are present.

Rarely chronic lung infection due to Friedländer's bacilli simulates tuberculosis.

PROTEUS INFECTIONS
Proteus infections usually follow other bacterial infections.
Indolent skin ulcers (decubital, varicose ulcers)
Burns
Otitis media, mastoiditis
Urinary tract infection
Bacteremia

Characteristic spreading growth on culture plate may obscure associated bacteria since Proteus *infection frequently is part of mixed infection; antibiotic sensitivity testing may not be possible.*

PSEUDOMONAS INFECTIONS
Pseudomonas infections occur in various sites.

Due To
Replacement of normal bacterial flora or initial pathogen because of antibiotic therapy (e.g., urinary tract, ear, lung)
Burns
Debilitated condition of patient (e.g., premature infants, the aged, patients with leukemia)

Decreased WBC during bacteremia in patients with leukemia or burns is more frequently due to Pseudomonas *than to other gram-negative rods.*

BACTEROIDES INFECTION
This is usually a component of mixed infection with coliform bacteria, aerobic and anaerobic streptococci or staphylococci.
Local suppuration or systemic infection is secondary to disease of the female genital tract, intestinal tract, or tonsillar region.
Laboratory findings due to complications (e.g., thrombophlebitis, endocarditis, metastatic abscesses of lung, liver, brain, joint) are present.
Laboratory findings due to underlying conditions (e.g., recent surgery, cancer, arteriosclerosis, diabetes mellitus, alcoholism, prior antibiotic treatment, and steroid, immunosuppressive, or cytotoxic therapy) are present.

TYPHOID FEVER
(due to *Salmonella typhosa*)

WBC is decreased—4000–6000/cu mm during first 2 weeks, 3000–5000/cu mm during next 2 weeks; ≧10,000/cu mm suggests perforation or suppuration.

Decreased ESR is found.

Normocytic anemia is frequent; with bleeding, anemia becomes hypochromic and microcytic.

Blood cultures are positive during first 10 days of fever in 90% of patients and during relapse; <30% are positive after third week.

Stool cultures are positive after tenth day, with increasing frequency up to fourth or fifth week. Positive stool culture after 4 months indicates a carrier.

Urine culture is positive during second to third week in 25% of patients, even if blood culture is negative.

Widal reaction. H and O agglutinins appear in serum after 7–10 days, increase to peak in third to fifth week, then gradually fall for several weeks; there is no increase during relapse. O appears before H and is usually higher at first; during convalescence H titer becomes higher than O. Positive Widal test may occur on account of typhoid vaccination or previous typhoid infection; nonspecific febrile disease may cause this titer to increase (anamnestic reaction). Rising titer (especially of O) on serial determinations may be necessary for proper evaluation. Usual criteria for serologic diagnosis in unvaccinated patients is fourfold increase in O titer or O titer >1:50 or 1:100 in a single specimen or during first 2–3 weeks of illness. ≦5% of healthy unvaccinated individuals may have O titer of 1:50.

> Early treatment with chloramphenicol or ampicillin may cause titer to remain negative or low.
>
> Increase in O titer may reflect infection with any organism in the Group D salmonellae (e.g., *S. enteritidis, S. panama*) and not just *S. typhosa*.
>
> Because of differences in commercially manufactured antigens, there may be a twofold to fourfold difference in O titers on the same sample of serum tested with antigens of different manufacturers.
>
> H titer is very variable and may show nonspecific response to other infections; it is therefore of little value in diagnosis of typhoid fever.

Laboratory findings due to complications

> Increased serum LDH, alkaline phosphatase, and SGOT is frequent; increased CPK occurs in some patients
>
> Intestinal hemorrhage is occult in 20% of patients, gross in 10%; it occurs usually during second or third week. It is less frequent in treated patients.
>
> Intestinal perforation occurs in 3% of untreated patients.
>
> Relapse occurs in ≦20% of patients. Blood culture becomes positive again; Widal titers are unchanged.
>
> Secondary suppurative lesions (e.g., pneumonia, parotitis, furunculosis) are found.
>
> Abnormal liver function tests (e.g., serum bilirubin, SGOT) occur in ≅25% of patients as an incidental finding. Hepatitis is the chief clinical feature in ≅5% of patients.

INFECTIONS DUE TO OTHER *SALMONELLA* ORGANISMS

Enteritis
> Stool culture remains positive for 1–4 weeks, occasionally longer.
> WBC is normal.

Paratyphoid fever—usually due to *Salmonella paratyphi A* or *B* or to *S. choleraesuis*
> Cultures of blood and stool and decreased WBC show same values as indicated in preceding section.

Bacteremia—especially due to *S. choleraesuis*
> Blood cultures are intermittently positive.
> Stool cultures are negative.
> WBC is normal. It increases ($\leqq 25,000$/cu mm) with development of focal lesions (e.g., pneumonia, meningitis, pyelonephritis, osteomyelitis).

Local infections
> Meningitis, especially in infants
> Local abscesses with or without preceding bacteremia or enteritis

One-third of patients are predisposed by underlying disease (e.g., malignant lymphoma, disseminated lupus erythematosus). Bacteremia and osteomyelitis are more common in patients with sickle hemoglobinopathy. Bacteremia is more common in patients with acute hemolytic *Bartonella* infection.

Agglutination tests on sera from acute and convalescent cases are often not useful unless present in high titer ($\geqq 1 : 560$) or rising titer is shown.

BACILLARY DYSENTERY
(due to *Shigella* species)

Stool culture is positive in >75% of patients.
> Rectal swab can also be used.

Microscopy of stool shows mucus, RBCs, and leukocytes.
Serologic tests are not useful.
WBC is normal.
Blood cultures are negative.
Laboratory findings due to complications
> Marked loss of fluid and electrolytes
> Intestinal bleeding
> Relapse (in 10% of untreated patients)
> Carrier state
> Acute arthritis—especially untreated disease due to *S. shigae* (culture of joint fluid negative)

CHOLERA
(due to *Vibrio comma*)

Stool culture is positive. One may also identify organism in stool using immunofluorescent techniques.
Laboratory findings due to marked loss of fluid and electrolytes
> Loss of sodium, chloride, and potassium
> Hypovolemic shock

Metabolic acidosis
Uremia

INFECTIONS WITH *VIBRIO FETUS*
Clinical types
> Occasional cases of subacute bacterial endocarditis, septic arthritis, meningoencephalitis, etc.; *seen especially in cases of thrombophlebitis of all limbs*

Culture of infected material from appropriate sites (incubate blood culture in $< 10\%$ CO_2)

Complement-fixation test positive during active phase.

HEMOPHILUS INFLUENZAE INFECTIONS
(due to *Hemophilus influenzae*)
Clinical types
> Upper respiratory infections
> Lower respiratory infections
> Otitis media
> Empyema
> Meningitis
> Pyarthrosis, single or multiple

Increased WBC (15,000–30,000/cu mm) and polynuclear leukocytes

Positive blood culture in $\cong 50\%$ of patients with meningitis

Infants less than age 1 commonly have empyema, bacteremia, and meningitis concomitantly; therefore CSF should always be examined in infants with empyema.

PERTUSSIS (WHOOPING COUGH)
(due to *Bordetella pertussis*)
Marked increase in WBC ($\leqq 100,000$/cu mm) and $\leqq 90\%$ mature lymphocytes

Negative blood cultures

Positive cultures from nasopharynx or cough plate

PARAPERTUSSIS
(due to *B. parapertussis*)
There are increased WBCs (usually 12,000–25,000/cu mm) and lymphocytes.

Isolation of organism by culture from nasopharynx or cough plate differentiates condition from pertussis.

CHANCROID
(due to *H. ducreyi*)
Biopsy of genital ulcer or regional lymph node is helpful.

Smear of genital ulcer or regional lymph node stained with Unna-Pappenheim method shows bacteria.

Smear of lesion for Donovan bodies is negative.

Dark-field examination of lesion for treponemae is negative.

Serologic tests for syphilis are negative.

Cultures of lymph node aspirate are more frequently positive than cultures from lesion. Culture is of limited practical value.

BRUCELLOSIS

Agglutination reaction becomes positive during second to third week of illness; 90% of patients have titers of $\geqq 1:320$. Rising titer is of diagnostic significance. False negative results are rare. False positive test results may occur with tularemia or cholera or with cholera vaccination or after brucellin skin test. In chronic localized brucellosis, titers may be negative or $\leqq 1:200$. They may remain positive long after infection has been cured.

Multiple blood cultures should be performed. (Brucella abortus *requires 10% CO_2 for culture.*) They are more likely to be positive with high agglutination titer.

Bone marrow culture is occasionally positive when blood culture is negative. It may show microscopic granulomas

Opsonophagocytic test and complement-fixation test are not generally useful.

WBC is usually $<10,000$/cu mm, with a relative lymphocytosis. Decreased WBC occurs in one-third of patients.

ESR is increased in $<25\%$ of patients and usually in nonlocalized type of brucellosis.

Anemia appears in $<10\%$ of patients and usually with localized type of disease.

Biopsy of tissue may show nonspecific granulomas suggesting a diagnosis of brucellosis. Tissue may be used for culture.

Liver function tests may be abnormal.

TULAREMIA
(due to *Pasteurella tularensis*)

Clinical types
  Typhoidal
  Ulceroglandular
  Glandular
  Pneumonic
    Rarely oculoglandular, gastrointestinal, endocardial, meningeal, osteomyelitic, etc.

Agglutination reaction becomes positive in second week of infection. Significant titer is $1:40$; usually it becomes $\geqq 1:320$ by third week. Peaks at 4–7 weeks ($\leqq 1:1000$), then gradually decreases during next year; appreciable titer persists for many years. May cross-react with *Brucella* agglutinins.

Culture and animal inoculation (positive with $\geqq 5$ organisms) of suspected material from appropriate site are performed. (Positive blood culture is rare; regional lymph node and mucocutaneous lesions are usually positive.)

WBC is usually normal.

ESR may be increased in severe typhoidal forms; it is normal in other types.

Biopsy of involved lymph node shows a characteristic histologic picture.

PLAGUE
(due to *Pasteurella pestis*)

Clinical types
  Bubonic

Primary septicemic

Pneumonic

Identify bacteria by smear, culture, fluorescent antibody technique, or animal inoculation of suspected material from appropriate site (e.g., lymph node aspirate, blood, sputum).

Serum hemagglutination antibodies are present.

WBC is increased (20,000–40,000/cu mm), with increased polynuclear leukocytes.

INFECTIONS WITH *PASTEURELLA MULTOCIDA*

Clinical types

Localized suppurative infections (e.g., osteomyelitis, cellulitis)

Bacteremia with endocarditis, meningitis, etc.

Respiratory tract infection

Gram stain and culture of bacteria from appropriate sites are performed (e.g., blood, skin, spinal fluid).

WBC is increased

GLANDERS
(due to *Malleomyces mallei*)

Clinical types

Acute fulminant

Chronic disseminated granulomas and abscesses in skin, respiratory tract, etc.

Culture or animal inoculation of infected material from appropriate sites is performed.

Agglutination and complement-fixation tests are positive in chronic disease.

WBC is variable.

MELIOIDOSIS
(due to *Pseudomonas pseudomallei*)

Clinical types

Acute febrile

Chronic febrile with abscesses in bone, skin, viscera

Infection is occasionally transmitted among narcotic addicts using needles in common.

Culture or animal inoculation of infected material from appropriate sites is performed (e.g., pus, urine, blood, sputum).

Agglutination test is positive in chronic disease; an occasional false positive test occurs.

WBC is normal or increased.

INFECTIONS WITH *MIMAE-HERELLEA*

Clinical types

Bacteremia, bacterial endocarditis, meningitis, pneumonia, etc.

Often associated with intravenous catheters or cutdowns

Bacteria are isolated from appropriate sites (e.g., blood, spinal fluid, sputum).

GRANULOMA INGUINALE
(due to Donovan body)
Wright-stained or Giemsa-stained smears of lesions show intracytoplasmic Donovan bodies in large mononuclear cells in acute
stage; they may be present in chronic stages.
Biopsy of lesion shows suggestive histologic pattern and is usually
positive for Donovan bodies in acute stage.
Serologic tests for syphilis are negative unless concomitant infection is present.
Dark-field examination for syphilis is negative.

LISTERIOSIS
(due to *Listeria monocytogenes*)
Especially in newborn from antepartum infection of mother
>Findings due to meningitis or disseminated abscesses of
>viscera are made.
>WBC is increased, and other evidence of infection is found.
>Gram stain of meconium shows gram-positive bacilli. *This
>should be done whenever mother is febrile before or at onset
>of labor.*

Infection of adult nonpregnant patients is associated with debilita-
tion (e.g., alcoholism, diabetes mellitus, adrenocorticoid therapy).
>Laboratory findings due to bacteremia, endocarditis, skin in-
>fection, etc., are present.

ANTHRAX
(due to anthrax bacillus)
Identification of gram-positive bacillus in material by gram stain,
culture, and animal inoculation from site of involvement (fluid
from cutaneous lesions; sputum and pleural fluid from patients
with pulmonary disease; stool or vomitus from patients with
intestinal disease; blood from patients with bacteremia)
WBC and ESR normal in mild cases; increased in severe cases
With meningeal involvement
>CSF bloody
>CSF smear and culture positive for bacilli

Precipitin antibodies with high or increasing titer sometimes useful
in pulmonary or intestinal disease

DIPHTHERIA
(due to *Corynebacterium diphtheriae*)
WBC is increased ($\leqq 15,000$/cu mm). If $>25,000$/cu mm are found,
there is probably a concomitant infection (e.g., hemolytic streptococcal).
Smear from involved area stained with methylene blue is positive
in $>75\%$ of patients.
Culture from involved area is positive within 12 hours on Loeffler's
medium (more slowly on blood agar). *If there has been prior
antibiotic therapy, culture may be negative or take several days
to grow.* Penicillin G eliminates *C. diphtheriae* within 12 hours;
without therapy organisms usually disappear after 2–4 weeks.
Fluorescent-antibody staining of material from involved area pro-

vides more rapid diagnosis, with a higher percentage of positive results.

Laboratory findings of peripheral neuritis (see pp. 257–258) are present in 10% of patients, usually during second to sixth week. Increased CSF protein may be of prolonged duration.

Laboratory findings of myocarditis (which occurs in ≦ two-thirds of patients) are present.

Albumin and casts are frequently present in urine; blood is rarely found.

Hemagglutination titer assays antitoxin titer of patient's serum. Fourfold increase in titer in acute and convalescent sera confirms diagnosis.

A moderate anemia is common.

Decreased serum glucose occurs frequently.

TETANUS
(due to *Clostridium tetani*)
WBC is normal.
Urine is normal.
CSF is normal.
Identification of organism in local wound is difficult and not usually helpful.

BOTULISM
(due to *Clostridium botulinum*)
CSF is normal.
Usual laboratory tests are not abnormal or useful.
Diagnosis is made by injecting suspected food intraperitoneally into mice, which will die in 24 hours unless protected with specific antiserum.

CLOSTRIDIAL GAS GANGRENE, CELLULITIS, AND PUERPERAL SEPSIS
(due to *Clostridium perfringens, C. septicum, C. novyi,* etc.)
WBC is increased (15,000 to >40,000/cu mm).
Platelets are decreased in 50% of patients.
In postabortion sepsis, sudden severe hemolytic anemia is common. Hemoglobinemia, hemoglobinuria, increased serum bilirubin, spherocytosis, increased osmotic and mechanical fragility, etc., may be associated.
Protein and casts are often present in urine.
Renal insufficiency may progress to uremia.
Smears of material from appropriate sites show gram-positive rods, but spores are not usually seen and other bacteria are often also present.
Anaerobic culture of material from appropriate site is positive.
Clostridia are frequent contaminants of wounds caused by other agents. Other bacteria may cause gas formation within tissues.

ANAEROBIC INFECTIONS
Frequently several anaerobic organisms are present simultaneously and are often associated with aerobic bacteria as well. If

cultures from suspicious sites are reported as negative, the culturing for anaerobic organisms has not been performed properly.

Mixed aerobic-anaerobic infections are often successfully treated by suppressing only the anerobes.

The most common anaerobic organisms cultured are *Bacteroides* and *Clostridia* species and streptococci.

The most commonly associated aerobic bacteria are the gram-negative enteric bacteria (*Escherichia coli, Klebsiella, Proteus, Pseudomonas,* enteroccoci).

Anaerobic organisms should be sought particularly in cultures from intra-abdominal infections (e.g., bowel perforations, acute appendicitis, biliary tract disease), obstetric and gynecologic infections (e.g., pelvic abscess, Bartholin gland abscess, postpartum, postabortion, posthysterectomy infections), chest infections (e.g., bronchiectasis, lung abscess, necrotizing pneumonia), urinary tract, soft tissue infections, <5% of endocarditis cases (especially streptococci), 10% of cases of bacteremia.

Bacteremia due to anaerobic organisms is characterized by high incidence of jaundice, septic thrombophlebitis, and metastatic abscesses; the gastrointestinal tract and the female pelvis are the usual portals of entry (in aerobic bacteremia, the urinary tract is the most common portal of entry).

LEPTOSPIROSIS
(most frequently due to *Leptospira icterohaemorrhagiae, L. canicola,* and *L. pomona*)

Normochromic anemia is present.

WBC may be normal or $\leq$40,000/cu mm in Weil's disease.

ESR is increased.

Urine is abnormal in 75% of patients: proteinuria, WBCs, RBCs, casts.

Liver function tests are abnormal in 50% of patients.
    Increased serum bilirubin
    Increased alkaline phosphatase
    Increased SGOT and SGPT, but average levels are not as high as in hepatitis

    Increased CPK in about one-third of patients during first week may help to differentiate condition from hepatitis.

    Reversed A/G ratio
    Abnormal flocculation tests

CSF is abnormal in cases with meningeal involvement ($\leq$ two-thirds of patients)
    Increased cells ($\leq$500/cu mm), chiefly mononuclear type
    Increased protein ($\leq$80 mg/100 ml)
    Glucose and chloride normal
    Organisms are not found in CSF.

Blood culture is positive during first 3 days of disease in $\leq$90% of patients.

Urine cultures may be positive only intermittently and are difficult because of contamination and low pH. They are rarely positive after the fourth week.

Of the serologic tests the hemolysis test is most useful. Agglutination, complement fixation, and hemolysis antibodies reach peaks in 4–7 weeks and may last for many years. An increasing titer is diagnostic. An individual titer of 1:300 is suggestive.

RELAPSING FEVER
(due to *Borrelia recurrentis, B. novyi, B. duttonii*)

Identification of organism by
　　Wright or Giemsa stain or dark-field microscopy of peripheral blood smear or buffy coat
　　Intraperitoneal injection of rats

Agglutination of *Proteus* OX-K

Biologic false positive serologic test for syphilis in ≦25% of patients

Increased WBC (10,000–15,000/cu mm)

Protein and mononuclear cells sometimes increased in CSF.

Laboratory findings due to complications (e.g., hemorrhage, rupture of spleen, secondary infection)

INFECTIONS WITH *STREPTOBACILLUS MONILIFORMIS* (RAT-BITE FEVER, HAVERHILL FEVER, ETC.)

Clinical types
　　Rat-bite fever
　　Febrile rash with multiple joint type of arthritis

Isolation of bacteria from appropriate sites (e.g., blood, pus, joint fluid) during acute febrile stage

Agglutination antibodies in serum during second to third week; rising titer significant

INFECTIONS WITH *BARTONELLA BACILLIFORMIS*

Oroya Fever

Sudden very marked anemia is found.

Blood smears may show gram-negative bacilli in ≦90% of RBCs (Giemsa stain); they are also present in monocytes. Bacteria are also present in phagocytes of reticuloendothelial system.

Blood culture is positive. *(Use special enriched media.)*

Beware of secondary Salmonella *infection.*

Verruga Peruana

Moderate anemia is found.

Blood smears and blood cultures are positive for bacilli.

SYPHILIS
(due to *Treponema pallidum*)

Primary Syphilis

Dark-field examination of genital lesion is made; if it is negative, regional lymph node aspirate may be used. *Examination will be negative if there has been recent therapy with penicillin or other treponemicidal drugs*. Can also use immunofluorescent staining of smears from lesion, a procedure that allows properly prepared specimens to be mailed to the laboratory.

Serologic test shows rising titer with or without positive dark-field examination. VDRL does not become positive until 7–10 days after appearance of chancre.

Biopsy of suspected lesion is done for histologic examination.

Secondary Syphilis
Dark-field examination of mucocutaneous lesions is positive.
Serologic tests are almost always positive in high titer.

Latent Syphilis
A positive serologic test is the only diagnostic method.

Congenital Syphilis
Dark-field examination of mucocutaneous lesions or scraping from moist umbilical cord is positive.

Serologic tests are positive and show rising or very high titer. *The serologic test may be positive because of maternal antibodies but without congenital syphilitic infection.* Rising infant's titer or titer higher than mother's establishes diagnosis of congenital syphilis. If mother has been adequately treated, infant's titer falls steadily to nonreactive level in 3 months. If mother acquires syphilis late in pregnancy, infant may be seronegative and clinically normal at birth and then manifest syphilis 1–2 months later.

Late Syphilis
CNS
    Meningitis
        ≤ 2000 lymphocytes/cu mm
        Positive serologic test in blood and spinal fluid
    Meningovascular disease
        Increased cell count
        Increased protein
        Positive serologic test in blood and spinal fluid
        Laboratory findings due to cerebrovascular thrombosis
    Tabes dorsalis
        Early—increased cell count and protein and positive serologic test in blood and spinal fluid (titer may be low)
        Late—$\cong 25\%$ of patients may have normal spinal fluid and negative serologic tests in blood and spinal fluid
    General paresis (spinal fluid always abnormal in untreated patients)
        Increased cells and protein
        Positive serologic test (titer usually high)
    CSF cell count should return to normal within 3 months after therapy; otherwise retreatment is indicated.
    Asymptomatic CNS lues
        May have negative blood and positive spinal fluid serologic test
        Increased cell count and protein is index of activity

Cardiovascular syphilis-VDRL—usually reactive but titer often low

Gummatous lesions-VDRL—almost always reactive, usually in high titer

Cardiovascular, liver, etc., involvement

Biopsy of skin, lymph node, larynx, testes, etc.

Adequately treated primary and secondary syphilis usually show falling titer and become serologically nonreactive in about 9 and 12 months, respectively; 2% of patients remain positive for several years. Therapy causes a negative reagin test in 75% of patients with early latent syphilis in 5 years, but less than 25% of patients with late syphilis become nonreactive although titers may fall steadily over a long period. In contrast to the VDRL the FTA-ABS remains reactive once it has become reactive, except for early primary syphilis, and cannot be used to confirm a cure.

If late syphilis of any type is suspected, always do FTA-ABS, even if VDRL is nonreactive.

One-third of patients with only weakly reactive VDRL are reactive with more sensitive test (e.g., TPI); weakly reactive VDRL should always be confirmed with FTA-ABS.

VDRL may be nonreactive in undiluted serum in presence of an actual high titer ("prozone" phenomenon) in 1% of patients with secondary syphilis.

See Serologic Tests for Syphilis, pp. 121–122.

YAWS (due to *Treponema pertenue*), PINTA (due to *T. carateum*), BEJEL (due to a treponema indistinguishable from *T. pallidum*)

Positive serologic tests for syphilis

Positive dark-field demonstration of a treponema in smears from appropriate lesions

TUBERCULOSIS

Acid-fast stained smears and cultures (and occasionally guinea pig inoculation) of concentrates of suspected material from involved sites (e.g., sputum, gastric fluid, effusions, urine, CSF, pus) should be performed on multiple specimens. If negative, guinea pig inoculation of this material may be needed.

WBC is usually normal. Granulocytic leukemoid reaction may occur in miliary disease. Active disseminated disease is suggested by more monocytes (10–20%) than lymphocytes (5–10%) in peripheral smear.

ESR is normal in localized disease; increased in disseminated or advanced disease. It is not used as index of activity.

Moderate anemia may be present in advanced disease.

Characteristic histologic pattern appears in random biopsy of lymph node, liver, bone marrow (especially in miliary dissemination), or other involved sites (e.g., bronchus, pleura).

Urine. Rule out renal tuberculosis in presence of hematuria (gross or microscopic) or pyuria with negative cultures for pyogenic bacteria.

Laboratory findings due to extrapulmonary tuberculosis
  Tuberculous meningitis
    CSF shows
      100–1000 WBC/cu mm (mostly lymphocytes)
      Increased protein (slight in early stages but continues to increase; >300 mg/100 ml associated with advanced disease; much higher levels when block of CSF occurs)
      Decreased glucose (<50% of blood glucose)
      Decreased chloride
      Increased tryptophan
      Acid-fast smear and culture from pellicle
    Serum sodium may be decreased (110–125 mEq/L) especially in aged; may also occur in overwhelming tuberculous infection.
  Tuberculous pleural effusion (see p. 145)
    Sputum is positive on culture in 25% of patients; pleural fluid is positive on culture in 25% of patients.
    Fluid is an exudate with increased protein (>3 gm/100 ml) and increased lymphocytes.
  Lymph nodes
    Culture is important to rule out infection due to other mycobacteria (atypical or anonymous).
Laboratory findings due to complications (see appropriate separate sections)
  Amyloidosis
  Addison's disease
  Other
Laboratory findings due to underlying diseases (e.g., diabetes mellitus, sickle cell anemia)

LEPROSY (HANSEN'S DISEASE)
(due to *Mycobacterium leprae*)
Mild anemia is found. Sulfone therapy frequently causes anemia, which indicates dosage change is needed.

Serum albumin is decreased, and serum globulin is increased.

ESR is increased.

Serum cholesterol is slightly decreased.

Serum calcium is slightly decreased.

False positive serologic test for syphilis occurs in ≦40% of patients.

Acid-fast bacilli are found in smear or tissue biopsy from nasal scrapings or lepromatous lesions. Acid-fast diphtheroids are not infrequently found in nasal septum smears or scrapings in normal persons, and *M. leprae* is not found here in two-thirds of early lepromatous cases. Therefore nasal smear may have very limited diagnostic value. Bacilli may show a typical granulation and fragmentation that precede the clinical improvement due to sulfone therapy. Larger, more nodular lesions are more likely to be positive. During lepra reactions, enormous numbers of bacilli may be present in skin lesions and may be found in peripheral blood smears. Bacilli are usually very difficult to find in skin lesions of tuberculoid leprosy.

Histologic pattern of the lesions is used for classification of type of leprosy.

Laboratory findings due to complications are noted.

Amyloidosis occurs in 40% of patients in the United States.

Other diseases (e.g., tuberculosis, malaria, parasitic infestation) may be present.

Sterility due to orchitis is very frequent.

SWIMMING-POOL DISEASE
(due to *Mycobacterium balnei*)

Histologic pattern of ulcerated skin lesions on extremities is that of nonspecific granuloma containing acid-fast bacilli.

Cultures from these lesions must be incubated at 31°C rather than 37°C.

ANTIBIOTIC TABLE

The summary of the selection of antibiotic drugs presented in Table 71 illustrates various approaches to the problems of treating infections rather than being an encyclopedic compendium of antibiotic sensitivity studies. The following points must be remembered when using this table.

Although in many cases an infection may be successfully treated without a culture, a sensitivity test should *always* be performed for the organism cultured in a particular case, since various strains of bacteria may have different antibiotic susceptibility. Tables published in the literature are useful general guides, but they may not be applicable to a specific case. Thus the antibiotic of choice may vary, depending on whether the infection is due to a community-acquired strain or to a hospital-acquired strain of bacteria. Some antibiotics may not be reliable; or they may cause toxic effects or provoke an allergic response.

Cultures should always be taken before antibiotic therapy has been administered. Repeat cultures should be taken if clinical response does not occur.

A smear for gram stain should always be taken at the same time as the culture; this is often a useful guide to the choice of antibiotics until the culture results are reported.

Causes of antibiotic treatment failure include

Improper laboratory techniques (e.g., taking the culture after beginning antibiotic treatment, using incorrect culture media, failing to use anaerobic methodology)

Mixed bacterial infections

Inadequate dosage of antibiotic

Interfering pathology (e.g., obstruction with lack of adequate drainage, immunologically compromised patient)

Since there are inherent delays in the publication of a book, the most current information is likely to be found in the periodical literature.

Table 71 should be used in conjunction with Table 15, pp. 147–151.

Table 71. Antibiotic Selection Guide for the More Common Infections

Organism	Infection Major	Infection Minor	Primary Choice[a]	Secondary Choice (if cannot use antibiotic of choice)[a]	Also Effective (usually no advantage over other choices)[a]
Gram-positive *Staphylococcus aureus*	Endocarditis Bacteremia Pneumonia Osteomyelitis		Nafcillin Oxacillin Methicillin Penicillin G (if sensitive)	Cephalosporins Clindamycin Vancomycin	
		Minor soft tissue	Dicloxacillin Cloxacillin Oxacillin Penicillin G (if sensitive)	Cephalosporins Clindamycin Erythromycin	
Streptococcus (Diplococcus) pneumoniae	Pneumonia with bacteremia		Penicillin G	Cephalosporins Chloramphenicol	Clindamycin Ampicillin
	Meningitis		Penicillin G	Chloramphenicol	Ampicillin
		Pneumonia Otitis	Penicillin G Penicillin V	Erythromycin	Ampicillin

Organism	Clinical condition			
Group A streptococci (beta-hemolytic)	Osteomyelitis Burns Sepsis Neonatal sepsis (Group B)	Penicillin G	Cephalosporins Clindamycin	Ampicillin
	Pharyngitis Otitis Impetigo	Benzathine penicillin G	Penicillin G Erythromycin Cephalosporins Clindamycin	Oxacillin Ampicillin Amoxicillin
	Prophylaxis of rheumatic fever	Penicillin G	Sulfadiazine	Erythromycin
Streptococcus viridans (alpha-hemolytic, including anaerobic streptococci)	Endocarditis Brain abscess	Penicillin G	Cephalosporins, or vancomycin + streptomycin, or kanamycin, or gentamicin	Ampicillin Chloramphenicol
Group D streptococci (enterococci)	Endocarditis Bacteremia	Penicillin G + streptomycin, or kanamycin, or gentamicin	Vancomycin + streptomycin, or kanamycin, or gentamicin	Ampicillin + streptomycin, or kanamycin, or gentamicin
	Urinary tract infection	Ampicillin	Tetracycline Trimethoprimsulfa Nitrofurantoin Nalidixic acid	Amoxicillin

(Continued)

477

Table 71 (Continued)

| Organism | Infection | | Primary Choice[a] | Secondary Choice (if cannot use antibiotic of choice)[a] | Also Effective (usually no advantage over other choices)[a] |
	Major	Minor			
Gram-positive *Corynebacterium diphtheriae*	Diphtheria		Erythromycin	Penicillin G	
Mycoplasma pneumoniae		Pneumonia Bronchitis	Erythromycin	Tetracycline	
Actinomyces israelii	Actinomycosis		Penicillin G	Tetracycline	Erythromycin Clindamycin
Treponema pallidum	Syphilis		Penicillin G	Tetracycline Erythromycin	
Gram-negative *Neisseria gonorrhoeae*	Bacteremia		Penicillin G	Cephalosporins Tetracyclines	
		Gonorrhea	Penicillin G + probenecid	Ampicillin + probenecid Amoxicillin + probenecid Tetracycline Spectinomycin	

Organism	Infection	Drug of first choice	Alternative drugs	
Neisseria meningitidis	Bacteremia	Penicillin G	Cephalosporins	Ampicillin
	Meningitis	Penicillin G	Chloramphenicol Cephalosporins Sulfa (frequently resistant) Tetracycline (frequently resistant)	Ampicillin
	Carrier state	Rifampin	Minocycline Sulfa (frequently resistant)	
Haemophilus influenzae	Meningitis Pneumonia Epiglottitis	Ampicillin + chloramphenicol (until proved sensitive to ampicillin)	Chloramphenicol	
	Otitis	Ampicillin Amoxicillin Penicillin + sulfa	Tetracycline Sulfa Erythromycin + sulfa	
Bordetella pertussis	Whooping cough	Erythromycin		

(Continued)

Table 71 (Continued)

Organism	Infection — Major	Infection — Minor	Primary Choice[a]	Secondary Choice (if cannot use antibiotic of choice)[a]	Also Effective (usually no advantage over other choices)[a]
Escherichia coli	Neonatal sepsis Bacteremia		Ampicillin Gentamicin for hospital-acquired infection	Kanamycin Cephalosporins Tetracyclines	Chloramphenicol Carbenicillin Tobramycin
		GU tract infection	Ampicillin	Sulfa	Amoxicillin
		Enteropathogenic diarrhea	Colistin	Nitrofurantoin Nalidixic acid Trimethoprimsulfa Cephalosporins	
Klebsiella	Bacteremia		Gentamicin	Kanamycin Cephalosporins Tetracyclines Chloramphenicol	Tobramycin Polymyxin B Colistimethate
		GU tract infection	Cephalosporins	Tetracyclines Trimethoprimsulfa Nitrofurantoin	
Pseudomonas	Sepsis Burns GU tract infection		Carbenicillin + tobramycin or gentamicin		Polymyxin B Colistimethate

Organism				
Enterobacter	GU tract infection	Carbenicillin indanyl Gentamicin		
	Bacteremia	Gentamicin	Kanamycin Carbenicillin Tetracyclines	Polymyxin B Colistimethate Tobramycin
Proteus mirabilis	GU tract infection	Trimethoprimsulfa	Carbenicillin indanyl Nitrofurantoin Tetracyclines	
	Bacteremia	Ampicillin	Kanamycin Gentamicin Cephalosporins Chloramphenicol	Carbenicillin Tobramycin
	GU tract infection	Ampicillin	Cephalosporins Nitrofurantoin Nalidixic acid	Amoxicillin Carbenicillin indanyl
Bacteroides	Bacteremia Abscess	Clindamycin	Penicillin G (except *B. fragilis*) Ampicillin (except *B. fragilis*) Carbenicillin Tetracyclines Chloramphenicol	

(Continued)

Table 71 (Continued)

Organism	Infection		Primary Choice[a]	Secondary Choice (if cannot use antibiotic of choice)[a]	Also Effective (usually no advantage over other choices)[a]
	Major	Minor			
Serratia	Bacteremia		Gentamicin + carbenicillin	Kanamycin Carbenicillin Chloramphenicol Trimethoprimsulfa	
Salmonella	Bacteremia		Ampicillin (if susceptible) Chloramphenicol	Amoxicillin Trimethoprimsulfa	
		Gastroenteritis	None unless there is invasion of tissues or blood or high risk patient (e.g., infant less than age 2 months, sickle cell disease)		
Shigella		Gastroenteritis	Trimethoprimsulfa	Ampicillin Tetracyclines	

[a]When more than one antibiotic appears in a box, only one is to be administered at a time unless combination is denoted by a plus sign.

Source: S. A. Plotkin, Current guide to antibiotic selection. *Consultant*, Dec., 1976.

RICKETTSIAL DISEASES

Weil-Felix reaction (see Table 72, p. 484)

Conplement-fixation or agglutination tests are positive in most cases when group-specific and type-specific rickettsial antigens are used. These tests permit differentiation of various rickettsial diseases. No test is available for trench fever. Rising titer during convalescence is the most important criterion. Early antibiotic therapy may delay appearance of antibodies for an additional 1–4 weeks, and titers may not be as high as when treatment is begun later. Low titers of complement-fixing antibodies may persist for years.

Guinea pig inoculation—scrotal reaction following intraperitoneal injection of blood into male guinea pig

Marked in Rocky Mountain spotted fever and endemic typhus

Moderate in boutonneuse fever

Slight in epidemic typhus and Brill-Zinsser disease

Negative in scrub typhus, Q fever, trench fever, and rickettsial pox

Test is not often used at present.

Microscopic examination of organisms following animal inoculation; test is not often used.

In less severe cases, blood findings are not distinctive.

In *severe cases,* the following changes are found:

Early in disease WBC is decreased and lymphocytes are increased (usually 4000–6000/cu mm; as low as 1200/cu mm in early scrub typhus). Later WBC increases to 10,000–15,000/cu mm with shift to the left and toxic granulation. If count is higher, rule out secondary bacterial infection or hemorrhage.

Mild normochromic normocytic anemia (as low as Hg = 9 gm/100 ml) appears around tenth day.

ESR is increased.

Total protein and serum albumin are decreased.

BUN may be increased (prerenal).

Serum chloride may be decreased.

Urine shows slight increase in albumin; granular casts.

CSF is normal despite symptoms of meningitis.

Blood cultures for bacteria are negative (to rule out other tickborne diseases, e.g., tularemia).

Laboratory findings due to specific organ involvement (e.g., pneumonitis, hepatitis) or due to complications (e.g., secondary bacterial infection, hemorrhage) are present.

Acute glomerulonephritis occurs in 78% of patients with epidemic typhus, 50% of patients with Rocky Mountain spotted fever, and 30% of patients with scrub typhus.

VIRAL PNEUMONIA DUE TO EATON AGENT (MYCOPLASMA PNEUMONIAE)

WBC is slightly increased (in 25% of patients) or is normal.

ESR is increased in 65% of patients.

Increased cold hemagglutination occurs late in course in 50% of patients ($\leqq$90% in severe illness); becomes positive at about seventh day, rises to peak at 4 weeks, then declines rapidly and

Table 72. Weil-Felix Reaction[a]

Disease	Rickettsia	Proteus OX-19	Proteus OX-2	Proteus OX-K	Comments
Spotted fevers					
Rocky Mountain spotted fever	R. rickettsii	1–4+	1–4+	0	
Boutonneuse fever	R. conorii	1–4+	2–3+	0	OX-19 frequently positive only in low titer
Other spotted fevers	Eg., R. australis, R. siberica	1–4+	2–3+	0	
Rickettsialpox	R. akari	0	0	0	
Typhus group					
Endemic (murine) typhus	R. mooseri	3–4+	Usually 0 or 1+	0	
Epidemic typhus	R. prowazekii	3–4+	Usually 0 or 1+	0	
Brill-Zinsser disease (recrudescent latent epidemic typhus)	R. prowazekii	Usually negative, or positive only in very low titer	0	0	
Scrub typhus	R. tsutsugamushi	0	0	3+	OX-K appears late in second week. Positive in ≅50% of patients
Q fever	R. burnetii	0	0	0	Usually pneumonitis. Hepatitis in ⅓ of severe cases. Occasional cases of subacute endocarditis
Trench fever	R. quintana	0	0	0	Can be grown on blood agar

[a]Weil-Felix reaction: Rise in titer by comparison of acute and later serum samples is most useful diagnostic procedure. Agglutinins appear in 5–8 days, reach peak in 1 month, then decrease to negative by 5–6 months. Reaction will not detect Q fever and rickettsialpox and is usually negative in Brill-Zinsser disease. May not differentiate epidemic and endemic typhus and spotted fever. Thus, is not useful for *early* diagnosis.

usually is negative by 4 months. May sometimes be present in other conditions (see p. 125).

Increased streptococcal MG agglutination occurs in 25% of patients; higher titer in more severe illness.

Serologic tests

Show fourfold increase in titer in complement-fixation and, less frequently, hemagglutination tests. Complement-fixation titer is the most useful serologic test; increase begins in 7–9 days; peak at 3–4 weeks may last for 4–6 months, then gradual fall for 2–3 years; if only a convalescent serum is available, a titer of >1 : 64 is highly suggestive of diagnosis of *Mycoplasma pneumoniae* infection.

Fluorescent antibody test is useful.

Isolation of organism by special techniques on broth media.

UPPER RESPIRATORY VIRAL INFECTION

Due to respiratory syncytial virus

ESR and WBC may be increased in children.

Pharyngeal smears may reveal many epithelial cells that contain cytoplasmic inclusion bodies.

Rise in titer of complement-fixing and neutralizing antibodies occurs during convalescence. Since complement-fixing antibodies soon disappear but neutralizing antibodies persist longer, the former should be used if reinfection is suspected.

Only virus isolation or rise in antibody titer during convalescence allows specific diagnosis.

Due to adenovirus (may cause at least six clinical syndromes involving pharynx, conjunctiva, and pneumonitis)

WBC is slightly decreased after about 7 days.

ESR is increased.

Complement-fixing and neutralizing antibodies appear after 1 week and peak in 2–3 weeks. Complement-fixing antibody decreases considerably in 2–3 months but neutralizing antibody may decrease only 2–3 times after 1–2 years. An increase in complement-fixing antibody titer during convalescence is presumptive evidence of infection but does not indicate the type of adenovirus.

Only virus isolation or rise in type-specific neutralizing antibody titer during convalescence allows specific diagnosis.

Due to rhinoviruses

WBC may be slightly increased.

ESR is increased in ≅35% of patients.

Serologic confirmation by rise in neutralizing antibody titer during convalescence or virus isolation allows specific diagnosis.

Complement-fixing antibody titer is not specific.

Due to parainfluenza virus

WBC is variable at first; later becomes normal or decreased.

INFLUENZA

WBC is usually normal (5000–10,000/cu mm) with relative lymphocytosis. Leukopenia occurs in 50% of the patients. WBC >15,000/cu mm suggests secondary bacterial infection.

Influenza virus antibody (hemagglutination inhibition, complement-fixation) titer shows fourfold increase in sera taken during
acute phase and 2–3 weeks later.

PARAINFLUENZA

Specific diagnosis requires recovery of virus in tissue-culture preparation.
Serologic tests include hemagglutination inhibition and tissue-
culture neutralization; complement-fixation serves only Types II
and III. Not useful for routine clinical studies.

TRACHOMA

Typical cytoplasmic inclusion bodies are in epithelial cells scraped
from conjunctiva of upper eyelid.
Secondary bacterial infection is common.

PSITTACOSIS

WBC may be normal or decreased in acute phase and increases
during convalescence.
ESR is increased or frequently is normal.
Cold agglutination is negative.
Albuminuria is common.
Sputum smear and culture shows normal flora.
Viral serologic tests. Positive complement-fixation test in early
stage is presumptive but is not conclusive because of cross-
reaction with lymphogranuloma venereum and false positive in
presence of some other infections (e.g., brucellosis, Q fever).
Rising complement-fixation titer is seen between acute-phase and
convalescent-phase sera.

COXSACKIEVIRUS AND ECHOVIRUS INFECTIONS
**(e.g., epidemic pleurodynia, "grippe," meningitis, myocarditis,
herpangina, etc.)**
Laboratory findings are not specific.
CSF
  Cell count is ≦500/cu mm, occasionally ≦2000/cu mm; pre-
  dominantly polynuclear leukocytes at first, then predomi-
  nantly lymphocytes.
  Protein may increase ≦100 mg/100 ml.
  Glucose is normal.
WBC varies but is usually normal.
Viral serologic tests show increasing titer of neutralizing or
complement-fixing antibodies between acute-phase and
convalescent-phase sera.

VIRAL GASTROENTEROCOLITIS
(especially echovirus)
Identified by exclusion by negative tests for other causes of the
symptoms (e.g., failure to find *Entamoeba histolytica, Shigella,
Salmonella*)

POLIOMYELITIS
CSF

Cell count is usually 25–500/cu mm; rarely is normal or ≦2000/cu mm. At first most are polynuclear leukocytes; after several days most are lymphocytes.

Protein may be normal at first; increased by second week (usually 50–200 mg/100 ml); normal by sixth week.

Glucose is usually normal.

GOT is always increased but does not correlate with serum GOT; reaches peak in 1 week and returns to normal by 4 weeks; level of GOT does not correlate with severity of paralysis.

CSF findings are not diagnostic but may occur in many CNS dieases due to viruses (e.g., Coxsackie, mumps, herpes), bacteria (e.g., pertussis, scarlet fever), other infections (e.g., leptospirosis, trichinosis, syphilis), CNS tumors, multiple sclerosis, etc.

Blood shows early moderate increase in WBC (≦15,000/cu mm) and polynuclear leukocytes; normal within 1 week.

Laboratory findings of associated lesions (e.g., myocarditis) or complications (e.g., secondary bacterial infection, stone formation in GU tract, alterations in water and electrolyte balance due to continuous artificial respiration) are present. Increased SGOT in 50% of patients is due to the associated hepatitis.

Viral serologic tests show fourfold increase in neutralizing antibody titer between acute-phase and convalescent-phase (after 3 weeks) sera, but titer has already reached peak at time of hospitalization in 50% of patients.

Virus may be cultured from stool up to early convalescence (done by the U.S. Public Health Service's Communicable Disease Center, Atlanta, Ga.).

LYMPHOCYTIC CHORIOMENINGITIS
WBC is slightly decreased at first; normal with onset of meningitis.

ESR is usually normal.

Thrombocytopenia develops during first week.

CSF
> Cell count is increased (100–3000 lymphocytes/cu mm, occasionally ≦30,000).
>
> Protein is normal or slightly increased.
>
> Glucose is usually normal.

Viral serologic tests show increasing titer between acute-phase and convalescent-phase sera in complement-fixing (after 2 weeks) and neutralizing (after 6–8 weeks) antibodies.

Viral isolation by animal inoculation is not routinely performed.

EASTERN AND WESTERN EQUINE ENCEPHALOMYELITIS
Marked decrease occurs in WBC with relative lymphocytosis.

CSF findings (see Table 29, pp. 240–244).

RABIES (HYDROPHOBIA)
WBC is increased (20,000–30,000/cu mm), with increased polynuclear leukocytes and large mononuclear cells.

Urine shows hyaline casts; reaction for albumin, sugar, and acetone may be positive.

CSF is usually normal or has a slight increase in protein and an increased number of mononuclear cells (usually <100/cu mm).

Brain of suspected animal shows Negri bodies (absent in >10% of animals with virus isolated from brain).

Fluorescent antibody examination of postmortem brain tissue is fast, accurate, and reliable.

Suspected animal dies within 7–10 days.

ENCEPHALOMYELITIS (VIRAL AND POSTINFECTIOUS)
CSF

> Early (first 2–3 days)
>> Cell count is usually increased (≦100/cu mm), mostly polynuclear leukocytes (higher total count and more polynuclear leukocytes in infants).
>> Protein is usually normal.
>> Glucose and choride are normal.
> Later (after third day)
>> Increased cell count is >90% lymphocytes.
>> Protein gradually increases after first week (≦100 mg/100 ml).
>> Glucose and chloride remain normal.

Viral serologic tests are for specific virus identification (fourfold increase from acute-phase sera to convalescent-phase sera in hemagglutination-inhibition, neutralization, or complement-fixation titers).

For additional laboratory tests see

> Cytomegalic inclusion disease (next section)
> Mumps (p. 489)
> Rabies (preceding section)
> Psittacosis (p. 486)
> Other

CYTOMEGALIC INCLUSION DISEASE
(limited to salivary gland involvement in 10% of infant autopsies; disseminated in 1–2% of childhood autopsies)

Intranuclear inclusions in epithelial cells in urine sediment and liver biopsy (more useful in infants than adults)

Hemolytic anemia with icterus and thrombocytopenic purpura in infants

Complement-fixation test on acute-phase and convalescent-phase sera

Evidence of damage to liver, kidney, brain

Laboratory findings due to predisposing or underlying conditions (e.g., malignant lymphoma, leukemia, refractory anemia, after renal transplant) or after receiving many transfusions of fresh blood; may be associated with *Pneumocystis carinii* pneumonia in adults

May cause a syndrome of heterophil-negative infectious mononucleosis in immunologically competent adults characterized by

> Normal or decreased WBC during first week followed by

increase to 15,000–20,000/cu mm with 60–80% lymphocytes, many of which are Downey cell type
Slightly increased ESR
Rise in cold agglutinin titer (same as in heterophil-positive
infectious mononucleosis)
Slight increase of SGOT and thymol turbidity; more marked
with clinical hepatitis in some cases
Rise in complement-fixing titer in 2–3 weeks to levels of
1 : 64–1 : 256
Same syndrome may follow immunosuppressive drug therapy
and multiple blood transfusions, as in open-heart surgery,
hemodialysis, etc.

MUMPS

Uncomplicated salivary adenitis
WBC and ESR are normal; WBC may be decreased, with
relative lymphocytosis.
Serum and urine amylase are increased during first week of
parotitis; therefore increase does not always indicate pancreatitis.
Serum lipase is normal.
Serologic tests
Serum neutralization test becomes positive by fifth day. It
is the most reliable and specific index of immunity but
also the most cumbersome and time-consuming.
Complement-fixation test becomes positive during second
week and remains elevated >6 weeks; paired sera
showing a fourfold increase in titer confirm recent infection. High titer suggests recent infection. Test correlates well with neutralization test.
Hemagglutination-inhibition reaction develops later and
persists longer (several months) than conplement-
fixation test. It is possibly useful for screening only at
high titers and is less sensitive and specific than neu-
tralization.
Complications of mumps
Orchitis (in 20% of postpubertal males but rare in children)
WBC is increased, with shift to the left. ESR is increased.
Sperm are decreased or absent after bilateral atrophy.
Ovaries are involved in 5% of adult females.
Pancreatitis (pp. 233–235) is much less frequent in children.
Serum amylase and lipase are increased. Patient may have
hyperglycemia and glycosuria.
Meningitis or meningoencephalitis (p. 251). Mumps causes
>10% of cases of aseptic meningitis. The disease may be
clinically identical with mild paralytic poliomyelitis. WBC is
usually normal. Serum amylase may be increased even if no
abdominal symptoms are present. CSF contains 0–2000
mononuclear cells.
Thyroiditis, myocarditis, arthritis, etc.

MEASLES (RUBEOLA)

WBC shows slight increase at onset, then falls to ≅5000/cu mm

490 III. Diseases of Organ Systems

with increased lymphocyte count. Increased WBC with shift to
the left suggests bacterial complication (e.g., otitis media,
pneumonia, appendicitis).

Mild thrombocytopenia in early stage.

Wright's stain of sputum or nasal scrapings show measles multinucleated giant-cells, especially during prodrome and early
rash.

Pap stain of urine sediment after appearance of rash shows intracellular inclusion bodies; more specific is fluorescent antibody
demonstration of measles antigen in urine sediment cells.

Viral serologic tests. Neutralizing antibody, complement-fixation,
and antihemagglutination tests become positive one week after
onset, evidencing infection.

Measles encephalitis. There is a marked increase in WBCs. CSF
may show slightly increased protein and $\leqq$500 mononuclear
cells/cu mm. $\leqq$ 10% of all measles patients have a significant
increase in cells in CSF.

Measles may cause remission in children with nephrosis.

RUBELLA (GERMAN MEASLES)

*It is important to identify exposure to rubella infection and suscep-
tibility status in pregnant women because infection in the first
trimester of pregnancy is associated with congenital abnormalities, abortion, or stillbirth in about 30% of patients; during
first month up to 80% of patients show this association.*

Viral serologic tests: hemagglutination inhibition (HAI),
complement-fixation, neutralization

Screening of pregnant women shows lack of susceptibility
(i.e., previous rubella infection) if HAI titer is >1:10–
1:20 or if complement-fixation test is positive.

Change in HAI titer from acute-phase to convalescent-phase
sera is the most useful technique to demonstrate a rise in
antibody titer.

With rubella rash, diagnosis is established if acute sample
titer is >1:10 or if convalescent-phase serum taken 7
days after rash shows a fourfold increase in titer.

If no rash develops in a patient exposed to rubella, a
convalescent-phase serum specimen taken 14–28 days
after exposure that shows a fourfold increase in titer
compared to the earlier sample indicates rubella infection.

Complement-fixation antibodies appear early (within 1 week
after rash); therefore acute-phase serum must be collected
promptly or the rise in titer may not be detected. They may
last for from 8 months $\leqq$some years. A positive test is useful to indicate recent infection or postinfection immunity.
Rate of false positive test is <2%.

Neutralization antibodies appear within 1–3 days after rash
and reach maximum in 2 weeks, and test may remain positive for >20 years; titer of $\geqq$1:8 indicates past infection
and therefore present immunity. A titer of 1:32 suggests

recent infection. In infants with congenital abnormalities, a high neutralization antibody titer establishes the diagnosis. Test is technically difficult to perform and requires 7–10 days.

WBC is inconstantly decreased before the rash; during the rash, lymphocytes are increased, and some of them may be abnormal.

Decreased platelet count within 1 week of onset of rash is frequent and may be marked.

Neonatal rubella may show laboratory findings of thrombocytopenia, hemolytic anemia, hepatitis, and encephalitis. The infant's antibody titer level parallels that of the mother. Diagnosis is confirmed if HAI titer persists after age 6 months in absence of postnatal infection. After age 3 when HAI titer has disappeared, rubella vaccine administration does not produce a rise in titer in patients with congenital rubella, but it does in normal children.

EXANTHEMA SUBITUM (ROSEOLA INFANTUM)
WBC is increased during fever, then decreased during rash, with relative lymphocytosis.

ERYTHEMA INFECTIOSUM (FIFTH DISEASE)
WBC is normal. Some patients have slight increase in eosinophils.

CHICKENPOX (VARICELLA)
Microscopic demonstration of very large epithelial giant cells with intranuclear inclusion in fluid or base of vesicle

Similar giant cells may occur in herpes simplex and herpes zoster.

WBC is normal; increased with secondary bacterial infection.

Serum electrophoresis may show decreased albumin with increased beta and gamma globulins.

SMALLPOX (VARIOLA)
Microscopic finding of cytoplasmic elementary bodies (Guarnieri bodies) in scrapings from base of skin lesions

Fluorescent antibody staining of virus from skin lesion

Viral serologic tests
> Increased titer of neutralizing antibody in acute-phase and convalescent-phase (2–3 weeks later) sera
> Rapid technique using vesicular fluid in hemagglutination, precipitation, or complement-fixation tests

WBC decreased during prodrome, increased during pustular rash

VACCINIA
(vaccine virus skin infection during vaccination against smallpox)
Guarnieri bodies (cytoplasmic inclusions) in skin lesions

Complications
> Progressive vaccinia. *Rule out malignant lymphoma, chronic lymphatic leukemia, neoplasms, hypogammaglobulinemia, and dysgammaglobulinemia.*
> Superimposed infection (e.g., tetanus)
> Postvaccinal encephalitis

HERPES SIMPLEX
WBC normal
Intranuclear inclusions in multinucleated giant cells in scrapi̇i̇
  skin lesions or vesicle fluid
Increased titer of complement-fixation and neutralizing antibdi
  is shown in convalescent-phase compared with acute-phas₂
  in primary infections; in recurrent infections a high titer ii
  sent in acute-phase sera.
Findings of encephalitis if this complication occurs
Causes 5% of cases of aseptic meningitis

HERPES ZOSTER (SHINGLES)
(reactivation of latent varicella virus)
Skin lesions may show intranuclear inclusions in degen
  epithelial cells or multinucleated giant cells.
40% of patients show increased cells ($\leqq$300 mononuclear/c
  in CSF.

LYMPHOGRANULOMA VENEREUM
WBC is normal or increased $\leqq$20,000/cu mm. There may b
  tive lymphocytosis or monocytosis.
ESR is increased.
Slight anemia may be present.
Serum globulin is increased with reversed A/G ratio during
  of activity.
Biologically false positive reaction for syphilis which be
  negative in a few weeks appears in 20% of patients. *If t*
  creases, beware of concomitant syphilitic infection.
Biopsy of regional lymph node shows stellate abscesses.
High complement-fixation titer (> 1:80) and increasing ti
  conversion of negative to positive indicate recent infection
  in titer evidences therapeutic success in acute stage. Per
  negative in the presence of disease is rare.

CAT-SCRATCH DISEASE
Microscopic examination of excised lymph node should be
Culture of involved lymph nodes is sterile.
ESR is usually increased.
WBC is usually normal but occasionally is increased $\leqq$13,
  mm; eosinophils may be increased.
Frei test is negative.
Skin test with cat-scratch antigen is positive.

YELLOW FEVER
Decreased WBC is most marked by sixth day, associate
  decreased leukocytes and lymphocytes.
Proteinuria occurs in severe cases.
Laboratory findings are those due to GI hemorrhage, wHv
  frequent; there may be associated oliguria and anuria.
Liver function tests are abnormal, but serum bilirubin i i
  slightly increased.
Biopsy of liver is taken for histologic examination.

Serum is positive by mouse intracerebral inoculation ≦ the fifth day; serum during convalescence protects mice.

DENGUE
WBC decreased (2000–5000/cu mm) with toxic granulation of leukocytes in early stage; often increased during convalescence
Children commonly have decreased platelets.

VIRAL EPIDEMIC HEMORRHAGIC FEVER
WBC is increased, with shift to the left.
Platelet count is decreased (< 100,000/cu mm) in 50% of patients.
Laboratory findings due to renal damage
> Proteinuria
> Oliguria with azotemia and hemoconcentration and abnormal electrolyte concentrations

Return of normal tubular function may take 4–6 weeks.

Other viral hemorrhagic fevers (e.g., Philippine, Thailand, Singapore, Argentinian, Bolivian, Crimean, Omsk, Kyasanur Forest) show much less severe renal damage and WBC is normal (Philippine, Thailand) or decreased.

COLORADO TICK FEVER
WBC is decreased (2000–4000/cu mm). The number of polynuclear leukocytes is decreased, but with shift to the left.
Viral serologic tests show an increase in complement-fixation and neutralizing antibodies in sera taken during acute and convalescent phases.
Blood should be inoculated into suckling mice.

PHLEBOTOMUS FEVER (SANDFLY FEVER)
Decreased WBC and lymphocytes with shift to the left of polynuclear leukocytes are most marked when fever ends.
CSF is normal.
Liver function tests are normal.
Urine is normal.

CRYPTOCOCCOSIS
(due to *Cryptococcus neoformans*)
Serologic tests
> Latex slide agglutination on serum and spinal fluid detects specific cryptococcal *antigen*. Use for screening of suspected cryptococcosis, since it is more sensitive than India ink smears of spinal fluid. Serum or cerebrospinal fluid is positive in most cases; when negative, agglutination test may be positive.
> Use whole yeast cell agglutination test for presence of *antibodies* in serum and cerebrospinal fluid. It is positive only in early CNS disease or no CNS involvement, may become positive only after institution of therapy. Rising titer may be a favorable prognostic sign.

Culture of cerebrospinal fluid for *Cryptococcus neoformans* on Sabouraud's medium becomes positive in 1–2 weeks (positive in 97%) followed by mouse inoculation. One may also get a positive culture from blood (25%), urine (37%), stool (20%), sputum (19%), and bone marrow (13%).

India ink slide of cerebrospinal fluid is positive in ≅ 50% of patients.

Cerebrospinal fluid cell count is almost always increased ≦800 cells (more lymphocytes than leukocytes). Protein is increased in 90% (≦500 mg/100 ml). Sugar is moderately decreased in ≅55% of patients. Relapse is less frequent when increase in protein and cells is marked rather than moderate.

In biopsy material, mucicarmine stain is positive; it is also positive on intraperitoneal injection of white mice.

There is evidence of coexisting disease in ≅50% of patients (especially those with diabetes mellitus, Hodgkin's disease, prior steroid therapy, lymphosarcoma, leukemia).

COCCIDIOIDOMYCOSIS
(due to *Coccidioides immitis*)
Serologic tests

Precipitin antibodies appear early, decrease after the third week, are uncommon after the fifth month. They occur at some stage of the disease in 75% of patients and usually indicate early infection. In primary infection, they are the only demonstrable antibodies in 40% of patients. If tests are negative, repeat 3 times at intervals of 1–2 weeks. *Beware of occasional cross-reaction with primary histoplasmosis and cutaneous blastomycosis.*

Complement-fixing antibodies appear later (positive in 10% of patients in first week), and the number rises with increasing severity. Antibodies decrease after 4–8 months but may remain positive for years. The titer is useful for following the course of the disease; a titer greater than 1 : 16 suggests dissemination; a fall in titer suggests effective therapy. Less than one-third of cases are positive in the first month; most positive reactions occur between the fourth and fifth weeks. The antibodies are usually present in disseminated disease.

Latex particle agglutination test shows 6% false positive reactions. Chief value is for screening purposes for detection of precipitin antibodies. A positive result should be confirmed with complement-fixation and precipitin antibody tests. A negative test does not rule out coccidioidomycosis.

Agar immunodiffusion test parallels latex particle agglutination test but is somewhat less sensitive. Its chief value is for screening purposes.

Smear (wet preparation in 20% KOH) and culture are taken from sputum, gastric contents, cerebrospinal fluid, exudate, skin scrapings, etc., on Sabouraud's medium or intraperitoneal injection of mice.

Biopsy of skin lesions and affected lymph nodes is made.

Cerebrospinal fluid in meningitis shows 100–200 WBCs/cu mm (mostly mononuclear), increased protein, frequently decreased glucose. Paretic colloidal gold curve may occur. Complement-fixing antibodies are present in 75% of meningitis patients.

Eosinophilia is ≦35%; >10% in 25% of patients.

WBC (with shift to the left) and ESR are increased.

HISTOPLASMOSIS
(due to *Histoplasma capsulatum*)

Culture is made (may be difficult) of skin and mucosal lesions, sputum, gastric washings, blood, bone marrow (Sabouraud's medium at room temperature; blood agar at 37°C not specific). Blood and bone marrow cultures are positive in 50% of patients. Mouse inoculation, especially from sputum, may give a positive subculture from spleen on Sabouraud's medium in 1 month. A positive skin test can cause conversion of serologic titers within 1 week.

Complement-fixation titers are positive in 90% of chronic cases and in 50% of acute pulmonary cases. Positive titers persist for months or years if disease remains active. They appear during the third to sixth week. A low titer in known cases may indicate a poor prognosis. Titers may be negative in severe disease.

Latex agglutination titers become positive in 2–3 weeks and revert to negative in 5–8 months, even with persistent disease. There are few false positives. A titer of 1:32 or more indicates active or very recent disease.

Biopsy is made of skin and mucosal lesions, bone marrow, and reticuloendothelial system.

Anemia and leukopenia are nonspecific.

ACTINOMYCOSIS
(due to *Actinomyces israelii*)

Recognition of organism in material (e.g., sinus tracts, abscess cavities, empyema fluid; *may be found normally in sputum*) from sites of involvement (especially jaw, lung, cecum)

    Sulfur granules show radial gram-positive bacilli or filaments with central gram-negative zone.

    No growth is seen on Sabouraud's medium.

    Anaerobic growth on blood agar shows small colonies after 4–6 days.

    Animal inoculation is negative.

    Anaerobic culture methods (e.g., Brewer's thioglycollate medium) are positive.

Histologic examination is suggestive; the diagnosis may be confirmed if a "ray fungus" is seen.

Serologic tests are not useful.

WBC is normal or slightly increased (≦14,000/cu mm); high WBC indicates secondary infection.

ESR is usually increased.

Normocytic normochromic anemia is mild to moderate.

Table 73. Summary of Laboratory Findings in Fungus Infections

Disease	Causative Organism	Blood	Cerebrospinal Fluid	Stool	Urine	Nasopharynx, Throat	Sputum, Lung	Gastric Washings	Vagina, Cervix	Exudates, Lesions, Sinus Tracts, Etc.	Skin, Nails, Hair	Bone Marrow	Lymph Node	Fresh Unstained Material	Stained Material	Culture	Animal Inoculation	Complement-Fixation	Agglutination	Precipitin	Histologic Examination
														Source of Material					*Serologic Tests*			
														Microscopic Examination								*Diagnostic Methods*
Cryptococcosis	*Cryptococcus neoformans*	+	+	+	+		+				+	+			+	+	+		+		+
Coccidioidomycosis	*Coccidioides immitis*		+				+	+			+			+		+	+	+		+	+
Histoplasmosis	*Histoplasma capsulatum*	+					+	+			+	+	+			+	+	+		+	+
Actinomycosis	*Actinomyces israelii*						+			+					+	+					+

Disease	Organism
Nocardiosis	*Nocardia asteroides*
North American blastomycosis	*Blastomyces dermatitidis*
South American blastomycosis	*Paracoccidioides brasiliensis*
Moniliasis	*Candida albicans*
Aspergillosis	*Aspergillus fumigatus*, others
Geotrichosis	*Geotrichum candidum*
Chromoblastomycosis	*Phialophora pedrosi, compactum*, etc.
Sporotrichosis	*Sporotrichum schenckii*
Rhinosporidiosis	*Rhinosporidium seeberi*

NOCARDIOSIS
(**due to** *Nocardia asteroides*)
Clinical types
> Lung abscess; metastatic brain abscesses in one-third of patients.
> Maduromycosis

Recognition of organism
> Direct smear—gram-positive and acid-fast (*may be over-decolorized by Ziehl-Neelsen stain for tubercle bacilli*)
> Positive culture on Sabouraud's medium and blood agar (*Beware of inactivation by concentration technique for tubercle bacillus.*)
> Positive guinea pig inoculation

May be saprophytic in sputum or gastric juice.

Rule out underlying pulmonary alveolar proteinosis, Cushing's syndrome.

BLASTOMYCOSIS
(**North American blastomycosis due to** *Blastomyces dermatitidis;*
South American blastomycosis due to *Paracoccidioides brasiliensis*)
Clinical types
> South American—involvement of nasopharynx, lymph nodes, cecum
> North American—involvement of skin and lungs
> Later, visceral involvement may occur in both types.

Recognition of organism in material (e.g., pus, sputum, biopsied tissue)
> Wet smear preparation in 20% KOH
> Positive culture on Sabouraud's medium at room temperature and blood agar at 37°C; slow growth of *P. brasiliensis* on blood agar ≦1 month
> Negative animal inoculation

Complement-fixation test is positive in high titer with systemic infection. High titer is correlated with poor prognosis.
WBC and ESR are increased.
Serum globulin is slightly increased.
Mild normochromic anemia is present.
Alkaline phosphatase may be increased with bone lesions.

MONILIASIS
(**due to** *Candida albicans*)
Positive culture on Sabouraud's medium and on direct microscopic examination of suspected material

In vaginitis, rule out underlying diabetes mellitus.
In skin and nail involvement in children, rule out congenital hypoparathyroidism and Addison's disease.
In septicemia with endocarditis, rule out narcotic addiction.
In GI tract overgrowth, rule out chemotherapy suppression of normal bacterial flora.

In positive blood culture, which is rare, rule out serious underlying disease (e.g., malignant lymphoma), multiple therapeutic antibiotics, and plastic intravenous catheters.

ASPERGILLOSIS
(due to *Aspergillus fumigatus* and other species)
Recognition of organism in material (especially sputum) from sites of involvement (especially lung; also brain, sinuses, orbit, ear)
Positive culture on most media at room temperature or 35°C.

Organisms occur as saprophytes in sputum and mouth. Confirm by staining organisms in biopsy specimens.

Laboratory findings due to underlying or primary disease
Superimposed on lung cavities caused by tuberculosis, bronchiectasis, carcinoma
Underlying condition (e.g., malignant lymphoma, irradiation, steroid, or antibiotic therapy)

GEOTRICHOSIS
(due to *Geotrichum candidum*)
Recognition of organisms from material from sites of involvement (respiratory tract; possibly colon)
Positive culture on Sabouraud's medium (room temperature).
Organisms occur as saprophytes in pharynx and colon.
Microscopic visualization of organisms in biopsy material

CHROMOBLASTOMYCOSIS
(due to *Phialophora pedrosi, P. compactum,* etc.)
Recognition of organism from sites of involvement (usually skin; rarely brain abscess)
Wet smear preparation in 10% KOH
Positive culture on Sabouraud's medium (slow growth)
Biopsy of tissue

SPOROTRICHOSIS
(due to *Sporotrichum schenckii*)
Recognition of organism in skin, pus, or biopsy
Positive culture on Sabouraud's medium from unbroken pustule. Intraperitoneal mouse inoculation of these colonies or of fresh pus produces organism-containing lesions.
Direct microscopic examination is usually negative.
Serum agglutinins, precipitins, and complement-fixation (titer of $\geqq 1:16$) antibodies can be demonstrated in extracutaneous disease (e.g., pulmonary, disseminated).

RHINOSPORIDIOSIS
(due to *Rhinosporidium seeberi*)
Recognition of organism in biopsy material from polypoid lesions of nasopharynx or eye (*cannot be cultured*)

Table 74. Summary of Laboratory Findings in Protozoan Diseases

Disease	Causative Organism	Blood	Cerebrospinal Fluid	Stool	Urine	Vagina	Urethra	Exudates, Ulcers, Skin Lesions	Bone Marrow	Spleen	Lymph Node Aspirate	Fresh Unstained Material	Stained Material	Culture	Animal Inoculation	Xenodiagnosis	Serologic Tests	Complement-Fixation	Others	Histologic Examination	Anemia	WBC Decreased	Monocytosis	Serum Globulin Increased	Cerebrospinal Fluid Abnormalities	Renal Function Abnormalities	Liver Function Abnormalities	Skeletal Muscle Abnormalities	Cardiac Abnormalities	Other
Malaria	*Plasmodium* species	+							+				+						+		+	+	+	+	+	+	+			
Trypanosomiasis Acute sleeping sickness	*T. rhodesiense*	+	+						+		+		+	rare	+						+		+	+	+					
Chronic sleeping sickness	*T. gambiense*	+	+						+		+		+		+			+			+		+	+	+					
Chagas' disease	*T. cruzi*	+											+	+		+		+		a					+			+	+	

a

	L. donovani													
Leishmaniasis Kala-azar	L. donovani	+					+[a]	+[a]			+	+	+	+
American muco-cutaneous	L. braziliensis			+		+[a]	+	+				+		
Oriental sore	L. tropica			+		+[a]	+	+						
Toxoplasmosis	T. gondii	+			+			+	+[b]	+[c]	+	+		
Interstitial plasma cell pneumonia	Pneumocystis carinii							+	++	++				+[d]
Amebiasis	Entamoeba histolytica						+	+	++[e]					
Giardiasis	G. lamblia	+[f]					+	+						
Balantidiasis	B. coli	+					+	+						
Coccidiosis	Isospora hominis or belli	+					+	+						
Trichomoniasis	T. vaginalis	++	++		+									

[a] Liver, lymph node.
[b] Hemagglutination, Sabin-Feldman dye test.
[c] Lymph node, muscle.
[d] Special stains.
[e] Rectum.
[f] Also duodenal washings.

Serologic tests can be performed at the Center for Disease Control (Atlanta, Ga.) on specimens submitted through state health department laboratories that do not perform such tests.

MUCORMYCOSIS
(due to *Mucorales fungi*)
Clinical types
> Cranial (acute diffuse cerebrovascular disease and ophthal-moplegia in uncontrolled diabetes mellitus with acidosis)
> Pulmonary (findings due to pulmonary infarction)
> In abdominal blood vessels (findings due to hemorrhagic infarction of ileum or colon)

Mycologic cultures from brain and spinal fluid are negative; may be positive from infected nasal sinuses or turbinate.

Laboratory findings of underlying disease (e.g., diabetes mellitus with acidosis, leukemia, irradiation or cytotoxic drugs, uremic acidosis) are present.

Laboratory findings due to complications (e.g., visceral infarcts) are present.

MALARIA
(due to *Plasmodium vivax, P. malariae, P. falciparum, P. ovale*)
Identification of organism is made in thin or thick smears of peripheral blood or bone marrow.

Anemia (average 2.5 million RBCs/cu mm in chronic cases) is usually hypochromic; may be macrocytic in severe chronic disease. Reticulocyte count is increased.

Monocytes are increased in peripheral blood; there may be pigment in large mononuclear cells occasionally.

WBC is decreased.

There is increased serum indirect bilirubin and other evidence of hemolysis.

Bone marrow shows erythroid hyperplasia, RBCs containing organisms, and pigment in RE cells. Marrow hyperplasia may fail in chronic phase. Agranulocytosis and purpura may occur late.

Serum globulin is increased (especially euglobulin fraction); albumin decreased.

ESR is increased.

Biologic false positive test of syphilis is frequent.

Osmotic fragility of RBCs is normal.

Acute hemorrhagic nephritis due to *P. malariae*
> Albuminuria
> Hematuria

Blackwater fever (massive intravascular hemolysis) due to *P. falciparum*
> Severe acute hemolytic anemia (1–2 million RBCs/cu mm) with increased bilirubin, hemoglobinuria, etc.
> May be associated with acute tubular necrosis with hemoglobin casts, azotemia, oliguria to anuria, etc.
> Parasites absent from blood

Laboratory findings due to involvement of organs
> Liver—vary from congestion to fatty changes to malarial hepatitis or central necrosis; moderate increase in SGOT, SGPT, and alkaline phosphatase
> Pigment stones in gallbladder
> Cerebral malaria

Serologic tests (performed in special reference laboratories, e.g., at the Center for Disease Control, Atlanta, Ga.)
Indirect fluorescent antibody test shows high sensitivity and specificity and is useful for diagnostic purposes.
Indirect hemagglutination can detect antibody many years after infection and is useful for prevalence studies.

TRYPANOSOMIASIS
Sleeping sickness
Acute (Rhodesian) due to *Trypanosoma rhodesiense*
Chronic (Gambian) due to *T. gambiense*
Identification of organism in appropriate material (blood, bone marrow, lymph node aspirate, cerebrospinal fluid) by thick or thin smears or concentrations, animal inoculation, rarely culture
Anemia
Increased serum globulin producing increased ESR, positive flocculation tests, etc.
Increased monocytes in peripheral blood
Cerebrospinal fluid
Increased number of cells (mononuclear type)
Increased protein (use as index to severity of disease and to therapeutic response)
Complement-fixation test specific for *T. gambiense*
Chagas' disease (American trypanosomiasis) due to *T. cruzi*
Identification of organism
Blood concentration technique during acute stage
Biopsy of lymph node or liver (shows leishmanial forms)
Culture on blood broth at 28°C from lymph node aspirate
Xenodiagnosis (laboratory-bred bug fed on patient develops trypanosomes in gut in 2 weeks)
Complement-fixation test positive in 50% of acute cases; specific and positive in >90% of chronic cases. In the acute infection the indirect hemagglutination test is more reliable.
Laboratory findings due to organ involvement (e.g., heart, central nervous system, skeletal muscle)

LEISHMANIASIS
Kala-azar (due to *Leishmania donovani*)
Organism identified in stained smears from spleen, bone marrow, peripheral blood, liver biopsy, lymph node aspirate
Culture (incubate at 28°C) from same sources
Complement-fixation test usually positive but also positive in tuberculosis
Anemia
Leukopenia
Thrombocytopenia
Increased serum globulin with decreased albumin and reversed A/G ratio
Increased ESR, abnormal cephalin flocculation, etc., due to increased serum globulin
Frequent urine changes

Proteinuria
Hematuria
Laboratory findings due to amyloidosis in chronic cases
American mucocutaneous leishmaniasis (due to *L. braziliensis*)
Organisms identified by direct microscopy, culture, or histologic examination in scrapings from lesions
Anemia sometimes present
Oriental sore (cutaneous leishmaniasis) (due to *L. tropica*)
Organisms identified by direct microscopy and culture in scrapings from lesion

TOXOPLASMOSIS
(due to *Toxoplasma gondii*)
Recognition of organism in appropriate material (cerebrospinal fluid, lymph node, muscle)
Smears stained with Wright's or Giemsa stain
Mouse inoculation
Histologic examination of tissue (e.g., lymph node, muscle)
Serologic tests are sensitive and specific, except for false positive indirect fluorescent antibody tests in patients with antinuclear antibodies (see Table 75, p. 506). Most recent serologic test is IgM-fluorescent antibody, which appears early and may disappear or fall to low titer as early as 1 month; absence of IgM antibodies signifies that infection is not acute.
Adult patients
WBC varies from leukopenia to leukemoid reaction; atypical lymphocytes may be found.
Anemia is present.
Serum gamma globulins are increased.
Heterophil agglutination is negative, but hematologic picture may exactly mimic infectious mononucleosis; eosinophilia in 10–20% of patients.
Laboratory findings are those due to involvement of various organ systems.
Lymph node shows distinctive marked hyperplasia; organism may be identified in histologic section.
Central nervous system shows CSF changes and organism can be identified in smear of sediment.
Disseminated form is an important complication of the immunologically compromised patient (e.g., lymphoma, leukemia, immunosuppressive drugs).

PNEUMOCYSTIS PNEUMONIA
(due to *Pneumocystis carinii*)
There are no specific laboratory tests.
No culture techniques are available.
No serologic techniques are available.
Lung biopsy is necessary to make a definite diagnosis. The organism is rarely found in sputum or bronchial washings.
Organisms are found in postmortem histologic preparations.
The morphology of the lung lesions suggests the diagnosis.

Organism does not stain with routine H & E stains; requires special stains (e.g., Giemsa, Schiff).

Laboratory findings are those of associated diseases (especially cytomegalic inclusion disease, systemic bacterial infections, especially *Pseudomonas* or *Staphylococcus*) or of underlying diseases (malignant lymphoma, leukemia, tuberculosis, cryptococcosis, premature or debilitated infants, immunoglobulin defects), administration of cytotoxic drugs and corticosteriods. These findings are present in 25% of patients who die after renal transplant.

Leukopenia indicates a poor prognosis.

Serologic tests are not useful. Complement fixation is positive in <20% of patients, and indirect fluorescent antibody is positive in 30%.

AMEBIASIS
(due to *Entamoeba histolytica*)

Microscopic examination of stool for *E. histolytica*. (*Beware of interfering substances in feces, e.g., bismuth, kaolin, barium sulfate, soap or hypertonic-salt enema solutions, antacids and laxatives, sulfonamides, antibiotic and antiprotozoal and antihelmintic agents.) Abundant RBCs but minimal WBCs on microscopic examination of stool helps to differentiate condition from bacillary dysentery (see p. 464).*

Biopsy of rectum for *E. histolytica*

Serologic tests

    Indirect hemagglutination test is sensitive and specific; associated with current or previous infection. A negative test is unlikely if amebic infection (especially hepatic) is present. Significant positive titer is $\geq 1:128$.

    Complement-fixation test is usually positive only during active (especially hepatic) disease. Usually reverts to normal 6 months after cure. Significant positive titer is $\geq 1:16$.

    Agar-gel diffusion test parallels complement-fixation test.

    Height of titer above significant levels or changing titers are not clinically significant.

    Increased serum alkaline phosphatase is not diagnostic in children, in whom it is normally increased.

Liver abscess

    Liver scanning

    Leukocytosis

    Increased ESR

    Animal inoculation of liver biopsy

See Chap. 27, p. 222.

GIARDIASIS
(due to *Giardia lamblia*)

Recognition of organism is achieved in stools or duodenal washings stained with iodine. Chronic infection may cause malabsorption syndrome.

Table 75. Serologic Tests for Toxoplasmosis

Test	Titer Indicates Possible Recent Infection[a]	Titer Strongly Suggests Recent or Present Infection[b]	Time of Rise of Titer	Duration of Rise of Titer
Sabin-Feldman dye	256	4096	Earliest 10–28 days	Indefinite 20–30 years
Complement fixation	8	32	14–28 days	Short-lived 2–4 years
Indirect fluorescent antibody	256	4096	Earliest 10–28 days	Indefinite 20–30 years
Indirect hemagglutination	256	4096	14–28 days	Indefinite 20–30 years

[a]Titer present in ≦10% of apparently healthy persons. Therefore perform serial titers at weekly intervals.
[b]Titers present in <1% of apparently healthy persons.

Indirect fluorescent antibody test gives results comparable to Sabin-Feldman dye test but has greater laboratory ease of performance and safety.

Indirect hemagglutination and complement-fixation tests may be negative in congenital toxoplasmosis and therefore are not recommended in this condition.

Sabin-Feldman dye and indirect fluorescent antibody test titers are usually the same in the newborn and in the mother for the first 30 days of the infant's life. In diagnosis of congenital toxoplasmosis, these tests are useful when a persistently elevated or rising titer is found in the infant 2–3 months after birth.

Presence of antibodies before pregnancy probably assures protection against congenital toxoplasmosis in the child.

BALANTIDIASIS
(due to *Balantidium coli*)
Recognition of organisms in stool (*Intermittent appearance requires repeated examinations.*)

COCCIDIOSIS
(due to *Isospora hominis* or *I. belli*)
Recognition of organism in $ZnSO_4$-concentrated stool specimens

TRICHOMONIASIS
(due to *Trichomonas vaginalis*)
Recognition of organism in material from vagina (occasionally from male urethra)

> Hanging drop preparation of freshly examined vaginal fluid. Frequently found in routine urinalysis.
>
> Frequently found in routine Papanicolaou smears (the organism is often not identified but may be associated with characteristic concomitant cytologic changes).

ASCARIASIS
(due to *Ascaris lumbricoides*)
Stools contain ova.
Eosinophils are increased during symptomatic phase, especially pulmonary phase.

TRICHURIASIS
(due to whipworm—*Trichuris trichiura*)
Stools contain ova.
Increased eosinophils ($\leq 25\%$), leukocytosis, and microcytic hypochromic anemia may be present.

PINWORM INFECTION
(due to *Enterobius vermicularis*)
Ova and occasionally adults are found on Scotch tape swab of perianal region. *Swab should be taken on first arising early in morning.*
Stool is usually negative for ova and adults.
Eosinophil count is usually normal; may be slightly increased.

VISCERAL LARVA MIGRANS
(due to *Toxocara canis* or *T. cati*)
WBC is increased; increased eosinophils are vacuolated and contain fewer than normal granules.
Serum gamma globulin is often increased.
Indirect hemagglutination and bentonite flocculation tests may be insensitive and nonspecific.
Disease may cause Loeffler's syndrome.
Biopsy of liver showing granulomas containing larvae is best procedure for definite diagnosis.

Table 76. Identification of Parasites

Organism	Stool	Other Body Sites
Nematodes		
Ascaris lumbricoides	O, A	Rarely L in sputum early
Trichuris trichiura	O	
Enterobius vermicularis	Usually neg.; A after enema	Scotch tape, perianal region—O and A
Strongyloides stercoralis	L	Occasionally L in sputum and duodenal contents
Ancylostoma duodenale	O, rarely L	
Necator americanus	O, rarely L	
Trichinella spiralis	Occasionally A and/or L	
Wuchereria bancrofti, W. malayi	None	Microfilariae in blood
Loa loa	None	Microfilariae in blood; adult under conjunctiva
Onchocerca volvulus	None	Adult in subcutaneous nodules
Dracunculus medinensis	None	L in fluid from ulcer
Cestodes		
Taenia solium	G, O, S; A after treatment	
Taenia saginata	G, O, S	Scotch tape, perianal region—O
Hymenolepis nana, H. diminuta	O	
Diphyllobothrium latum	O	
Echinococcus multilocularis	Not found	Histologic examination of biopsy specimen
Trematodes		
Schistosoma mansoni, S. japonicum,	O	See pp. 511–512
S. haematobium	None	O in urine
Clonorchis sinensis	O	O in duodenal contents
Opisthorchis felineus	O	O in duodenal contents
Paragonimus westermani	O	O in sputum
Fasciola hepatica	O	
Fasciolopsis buski	O, occasionally A	

O = ova; A = adult; L = larvae; G = gravid segments; S = scolex.

TRICHOSTRONGYLOSIS
(due to *Trichostrongylus* species)
Stools contain ova. *Usually a concentration technique is required; worm may be mistaken for hookworm.*
There is an increase in WBC and eosinophils ($\leq 75\%$) when patient is symptomatic.

STRONGYLOIDIASIS
(due to *Strongyloides stercoralis*)
Stools contain larvae. Larvae may also be found in duodenal washings. Larvae appear in sputum with pulmonary involvement.
Leukocytosis is common.

Increase in eosinophils is almost always present, but the number usually decreases with chronicity. Leukopenia and absence of eosinophilia are poor prognostic signs.

Condition is especially common in orphanages and mental institutions.

HOOKWORM DISEASE
(due to *Necator americanus* or *Ancylostoma duodenale*)
WBC is normal or slightly increased, with 15–30% eosinophils; in early cases ≦75% eosinophils is present.

Anemia due to blood loss is hypochromic microcytic. When anemia is more severe, eosinophilia is less prominent.

Hypoproteinemia may occur with heavy infestation.

Stools contain hookworm ova. Stools are usually positive for occult blood. Charcot-Leyden crystals are present in >50% of patients.

Laboratory findings are those due to frequently associated diseases (e.g., malaria, beriberi)

TRICHINOSIS
(due to *Trichinella spiralis*)
Eosinophilia appears with values of ≦85% on differential count and 15,000/cu mm on absolute count. It occurs about 1 week after the eating of infected food and reaches maximum after third week. It usually subsides in 4–6 weeks but may last up to 6 months and occasionally for years. Occasionally it is absent; it is usually absent in fatal infections.

Stool may contain adults and larvae *only* during the first 1–2 weeks after infection (during the stage of enteritis and invasion).

Indentification of larvae is made in suspected meat by acid-pepsin digestion followed by microscopic examination.

Muscle biopsy may show the encysted larvae beginning 10 days after ingestion. Direct microscopic examination of compressed specimen is superior to routine histologic preparation.

Serologic tests become positive 1 week after onset of symptoms in only 20–30% of patients and reach a peak of 80–90% of patients by fourth to fifth week. Rise in titer in acute- and convalescent-phase sera is diagnostic. Titers may remain negative in overwhelming infection. False positive results may occur in polyarteritis nodosa, serum sickness, penicillin sensitivity, infectious mononucleosis, malignant lymphomas, and leukemia.

> *Trichinella* complement-fixation test becomes positive ≅2 weeks after occurrence of eosinophilia. It may remain positive for 6 months.
>
> Bentonite flocculation test may remain strongly positive for 6 months; less strongly positive for another 6 months; becomes negative in 2–3 years. It is the best single test for diagnosis.
>
> Precipitin tests are also used.

Decrease in serum total protein and albumin occurs in severe cases between 2 and 4 weeks and may last for years.

Increased (relative and absolute) gamma globulins parallel titer of

serologic tests and of thymol turbidity. The increase occurs be-
tween 5 and 8 weeks and may last 6 months or more.
ESR is normal or only slightly increased.
BSP is usually normal.
Decreased serum cholinesterase often lasts 6 months.
Some serum enzymes may be increased (e.g., aldolase).
Urine may show albuminuria with hyaline and granular casts in
severe cases.
Cerebrospinal fluid. With meningoencephalitis, CSF may be nor-
mal or up to 300 lymphocytes/cu mm with increased protein.

FILARIASIS
(due to *Wuchereria bancrofti* or *W. malayi*)
Microfilariae appear in peripheral blood smear (Wright's or Giemsa
stain) or wet preparation.
Eosinophils are increased.
Biopsy of lymph node may contain adult worms.
Complement-fixation test may not be reliable.
Chyluria may occur

LOAIASIS
(due to *Loa loa*)
Marked increase of eosinophils (50–80%) may occur.

TAPEWORM INFESTATION
Due to *Taenia saginata* (beef tapeworm)
> In stool, ova cannot be distinguished from those of *T. solium*.
>> Proglottids establish diagnosis. Stool examination is posi-
tive in 50–75% of patients.
> Scotch tape swab of perianal region is positive in ≦95% of
patients.
> Eosinophils may be slightly increased.
Due to *Taenia solium* (pork tapeworm)
> Stool and Scotch tape swab of perianal region are examined.
> Eosinophils may be slightly increased.
> Cerebrospinal fluid may show increased eosinophils with cys-
ticercal meningoencephalitis.
Due to *Hymenolepis nana* (dwarf tapeworm)
> Stool shows ova, occasionally proglottids, etc.
Due to *Diphyllobothrium latum* (fish tapeworm)
> Stool shows ova.
> Macrocytic anemia (see p. 286) occurs when worm is in prox-
imal small intestine.
> Increased eosinophils and leukocytes are found.
Due to *Echinococcus granulosus (multilocularis)*
> Cystic lesion appears, especially in liver (see Metastatic or
Infiltrative Disease of Liver, p. 222). 65% of cysts occur in
lung, and the remaining 10% of cysts are widely scattered.
> Identification of scolices and hooklets is made in cyst fluid and
histologic examination.
> Eosinophils are occasionally increased; the number rises
dramatically in cyst leaks.

Stool examination is not helpful

Serologic tests. High titers ($\geqq$1024), indirect hemagglutination, and bentonite flocculation (>5) usually indicate disease; low titers are equivocal and may be found with collagen disease or cirrhosis. The tests often cross-react with cysticercosis antibody. They are more sensitive in presence of liver cysts (85%) than lung cysts (<50%).

SCHISTOSOMIASIS
(due to *Schistosoma mansoni, S. japonicum, S. haematobium*)

Acute

Eosinophilia occurs; may be 20–60%.

ESR is increased.

Serum globulin is increased.

Cephalin flocculation is positive.

Chronic

Ova appear in stools.

Unstained rectal mucosa examined microscopically may show living or dead ova when stools are negative.

Serologic tests are particularly useful for chronic infections when stools contain no ova; they are not useful to assess chemotherapeutic cure.

Fluorescent antibody test requires additional standardization.

Cercarial slide flocculation test has some technical shortcomings and difficulties; some cross-reaction to other infestations.

Bentonite flocculation test is somewhat less sensitive than cercarial slide test; some cross-reaction to other infestations.

Complement-fixation test is the best serologic procedure (100% specific and 95% sensitive).

Circumoval precipitin test is particularly useful for testing spinal fluid since it is specific for involvement of central nervous system; intestinal involvement alone causes positive reaction with serum but negative reaction with spinal fluid.

Cercarienhullen reaction test is performed with living infectious cercariae and therefore is not useful as a routine procedure.

Indirect hemagglutination test is more often used for epidemiologic studies.

Rectal biopsy of mucosal fold may show parasites and granulomatous lesions.

Multiple granulomatous lesions appear in uterine cervix.

Changes appear that are secondary to clay pipestem fibrosis of liver with portal hypertension, esophageal varices, splenomegaly, etc. Liver function changes are quite minimal; increased serum bilirubin is rare, even with advanced cirrhosis; abnormal BSP is infrequent. Increased serum globulin is frequent. Serum alkaline phosphatase is elevated in 50% of adult patients but is not useful in children.

Changes secondary to pulmonary hypertension are seen.
Ova appear in urine sediment and in biopsy of vesical mucosa in infection with *S. haematobium*.

PARAGONIMIASIS
(due to *Paragonimus westermani*)
Eosinophilia is usual.
Ova appear in sputum, which may contain blood.

CLONORCHIASIS
(due to *Clonorchis sinensis*)
Ova appear in stool or duodenal contents.
Complement-fixation test may be positive.
Clonorchiasis may cause laboratory findings due to biliary obstruction or recurrent cholecystitis.

OPISTHORCHIASIS
(due to *Opisthorchis felineus*)
Ova appear in stool or duodenal contents.

FASCIOLIASIS
(due to *Fasciola hepatica*)
Ova appear in stool or duodenal contents.
Eosinophils are increased.
Liver function tests are abnormal.

FASCIOLOPSIASIS
(due to *Fasciolopsis buski*)
Ova appear in stool.

OPPORTUNISTIC INFECTIONS
Laboratory findings due to underlying diseases (e.g., malignant lymphoma and leukemia, diabetes mellitus, immunoglobulin defects, following renal transplant, uremia, hypoparathyroidism, hypoadrenalism)
Laboratory findings due to administration of drugs (antibiotics, corticosteroids, cytotoxic and immunosuppressive drugs)
Associated with other factors (e.g., plastic intravenous catheters, narcotic addiction)
Laboratory findings due to particular organism (see appropriate separate sections)
  Cryptococcus neoformans
  Candida albicans
  Aspergillus
  Mucorales fungi
  Staphylococcus aureus
  S. albus, Bacillus subtilis, B. cereus, and other saprophytes
  Enteric bacteria (*Pseudomonas aeruginosa, Escherichia coli, Klebsiella-Enterobacter, Proteus*)

INTRAUTERINE AND PERINATAL INFECTIONS

Causative Agents	*Incidence/ 1000 Live Births*
Protozoal	
Toxoplasmosis	0.05 (congenital)
Bacterial	2.5–3.5 (perinatal)
Syphilis	0.12–0.2 (congenital)
Listerosis	
Escherichia coli	
Proteus	
Klebsiella	
Streptococci	
Staphylococci	
Streptococcus faecalis	
Mycoplasma	
Viral	
Rubella	0.25–0.3 (congenital)
Cytomegalic inclusion disease	0.5–1.0 (congenital)
Variola-vaccinia	
Herpes simplex	
Varicella-zoster	
Hepatitis B	
Poliomyelitis	
Influenza	
Mumps	
Coxsackie B, echovirus	

Laboratory Diagnosis (see appropriate separate sections)

Total IgM level may be increased in cord blood or in early weeks of life.

Specific antibody in IgM fraction may be present.

Antibody persists after the normal time for disappearance of maternal antibody (e.g., in congenital rubella, after age 6 months maternally transmitted antibody should have disappeared and postnatal infection is uncommon).

Identification of agent should be made (e.g., culture, dark-field or fluorescent microscopy).

Table 77. Commonly Associated Pathogens in Patients with Immunosuppression (for Organ Transplantation or Treatment of Malignancies)

Immune Response Depressed	Underlying Condition	Commonly Associated Pathogens
Humoral	Lymphatic leukemia	Pneumococci
	Lymphosarcoma	*Haemophilus influenzae*
	Multiple myeloma	Streptococci
	Congenital hypogamma-globulinemias	*Pseudomonas aeruginosa*
	Nephrotic syndrome	*Pneumocystis carinii*
	Treatment with cytotoxic or antimetabolite drugs	
Cellular	Terminal cancers	Tubercle bacillus
	Hodgkin's disease	*Listeria*
	Sarcoidosis	*Candida* species
	Uremia	*Toxoplasma*
	Treatment with cytotoxic or antimetabolite drugs or corticosteroids	*Pneumocystis carinii*
Leukocyte bactericidal	Myelogenous leukemia	Staphylococci
	Chronic granulomatous disease	*Serratia*
		Pseudomonas species
	Acidosis	*Candida* species
	Burns	*Aspergillus*
	Treatment with cortico-steroids	*Nocardia*
	Granulocytopenia due to drugs	

Table 78. Some Human Diseases That May Be Transmitted by Animal Pets

		Dogs	Cats	Birds	Farm Animals	Poultry	Rodents	Reptiles	Monkeys
BACTERIAL	*Salmonella* infections	+	+	+	+	+	+	+	+
	Bacillary dysentery								+
	Pasteurella infections	+	+		+	+	+		
	Anthrax	+			+				
	Brucellosis	+	+		+	+	+		
	Tularemia	+	+				+		
	Leptospirosis	+		+	+		+		
	Tuberculosis	+	+		+				
VIRAL	Rabies	+	+		+				
	Cat-scratch disease		+						
	Psittacosis			+			+		
	Encephalomyelitis			+	+				
	Lymphocytic choriomeningitis	+					+		
FUNGAL	Ringworm	+	+		+		+		
PARASITIC	Roundworm infestation	+	+						
	Tapeworm infestation	+	+		+				
	Visceral larva migrans	+	+						
	Cutaneous larva migrans	+	+						
	Scabies	+	+						
	Toxoplasmosis	+	+						

35

MISCELLANEOUS DISEASES

SYSTEMIC LUPUS ERYTHEMATOSUS (SLE)
LE test is positive in $\geqq 75\%$ of patients but may be intermittent and require repeated examinations. Other antinuclear and anticytoplasmic antibodies are often present (see the discussions of the LE cell test and serologic tests for SLE, p. 124).

Moderate normochromic normocytic anemia is usual; it may be hemolytic, with positive Coombs' test in 5% of patients.

Decreased WBC with or without neutropenia is usual; increased WBC occurs with secondary infections.

SLE may present as "idiopathic" thrombocytopenic purpura.

Serum gamma globulin is increased in 50% of patients; a continuing rise may indicate poor prognosis. Alpha$_2$ globulin is increased; albumin, decreased. Immunoglobulins may be abnormal on immunoelectrophoresis. Cephalin flocculation and thymol turbidity may be positive.

ESR and CRP are increased.

Abnormal serum proteins frequently occur.

Biologically false positive (BFP) test for syphilis is very common—occurs in $\leqq 20\%$ of patients. *(This may be the first manifestation of SLE and may precede other features by many months; 7% of asymptomatic individuals with BFP test for syphilis ultimately develop SLE.)*

Cryoglobulins, circulating anticoagulants, etc., are evident.

Tests for rheumatoid factor are positive in 35% of patients.

Laboratory findings reflecting specific organ involvement

Urine findings indicate acute nephritis, nephrotic syndrome, chronic renal impairment, secondary pyelonephritis. Patients with azotemia and marked proteinuria usually die in 1–3 years. Sediment is the same as in chronic active glomerulonephritis. With uremia, nephrotic syndrome, or active nephritis the LE test may become negative. High antibody titer to native DNA associated with decreased serum complement indicates lupus nephritis.

CSF findings are of aseptic meningitis (increased protein and pleocytosis are found in 50% of these patients.) *(Rule out complicating tuberculosis and cryptococcosis.)*

Cardiovascular, pulmonary, etc., findings may be present.

Joint involvement occurs in 90% of patients.

Laboratory findings reflecting frequently associated diseases

Hashimoto's thyroiditis (see p. 384)

Sjögren's syndrome (see p. 280)

Myasthenia gravis (see p. 260)

Tissue biopsy of skin, muscles, kidney, and lymph node may be useful.

Drug-induced lupus syndromes (see pp. 526, 545) are due to prolonged administration of

Procainamide

Hydralazine

Isoniazid
Various anticonvulsants (e.g., Dilantin)
Differ from spontaneous SLE in their lower incidence of renal
findings and of anemia and leukopenia. About two-thirds of
patients receiving these drugs develop serologic abnormalities (see p. 123) even though clinical findings and
other laboratory changes are absent. May also occur as allergic reaction to certain drugs (e.g., sulfonamides, methyldopa, birth control pills).

POLYARTERITIS NODOSA
WBC is increased ($\leq$40,000/cu mm), and polynuclear leukocytes
are increased. A rise in eosinophils takes place in 25% of pa-
tients, sometimes very marked; it usually occurs in patients with
pulmonary manifestations.
ESR is increased.
Mild anemia is frequent; may be hemolytic anemia with positive
Coombs' test.
Urine is frequently abnormal.
Albuminuria (60% of patients)
Hematuria (40% of patients)
"Telescoping" of sediment (variety of cellular and noncellular
casts)
Uremia occurs in 15% of patients.
Tissue biopsy
Random skin and muscle biopsy is confirmatory in 25% of
patients; most useful when taken from area of tenderness; if
no symptoms are present, pectoralis major is the most use-
ful site.
Testicular biopsy is useful when local symptoms are present.
Lymph node and liver biopsies are usually not helpful.
Renal biopsy is not specific; often shows glomerular disease.
Serum globulins are increased.
Abnormal serum proteins occasionally occur. BFP test occurs for
syphilis, circulating anticoagulants, cryoglobulins, macroglobulins, etc.
Laboratory findings due to organ involvement by arteritis may be
present—genitourinary system, nervous system, pulmonary,
etc.

WEGENER'S GRANULOMATOSIS
(variant of polyarteritis nodosa)
Anemia is common.
Increased WBC is common; occasionally 50% of patients show
increase in eosinophils.
Serum globulins are frequently increased.
Laboratory findings reflecting specific organ involvement
Kidney. Urine contains protein, RBCs, and RBC casts. Fre-
quently terminal uremia; most patients develop renal in-
sufficiency. There may be laboratory findings of nephrosis
or chronic nephritis.
Central nervous system

Heart
Lungs

TEMPORAL ARTERITIS
WBC is usually slightly increased with shift to the left.
Usually moderate normocytic normochromic anemia is present.
Serum protein electrophoresis may show increased gamma globulins. Rouleaux may occur.
ESR is increased.
Laboratory findings reflecting specific organ involvement
    Kidney
    Central nervous system
    Heart and great vessels
Biopsy of involved segment of temporal artery is diagnostic.
Intracerebral artery involvement may cause increased CSF protein.

SCLERODERMA
Laboratory findings reflect specific organ involvement.
    Malabsorption syndrome due to small intestine involvement
    Abnormal urinary findings, renal function tests, and uremia
        due to renal involvement
    Myocarditis, pericarditis, secondary bacterial endocarditis
    Pulmonary fibrosis, secondary pneumonitis
    Other
Biopsy of skin, esophagus, intestine, synovia may establish diagnosis.
ESR is normal in one-third of patients, mildly increased in one-third of patients, markedly increased in one-third of patients.
Mild hypochromic microcytic anemia may be present in 10% of patients.
Serum gamma globulins are increased in 25% of patients (usually slight increase).
Abnormal serum proteins occasionally occur, as revealed by BFP test for syphilis (5% of patients), positive LE test, positive RA test (35% of patients), cold agglutinins, cryoglobulins, etc.
Antinuclear antibodies in titer of $\geqq 1:16$ are found in 60% of patients.

SCLEREDEMA
WBC, ESR, and other laboratory tests are usually normal.

WEBER-CHRISTIAN DISEASE (RELAPSING FEBRILE NODULAR NONSUPPURATIVE PANNICULITIS)
Biopsy is taken of involved area of subcutaneous fat.
WBC may be increased or decreased.
Mild anemia may occur.

DISCOID LUPUS
Some patients may show
    Decreased WBC
    Decreased platelet count
    Increased ESR

Increased serum gamma globulins
Positive LE cell test (<10% of patients)

SARCOIDOSIS

Kveim reaction (skin biopsy 4–6 weeks after injection of human sarcoid tissue shows histologic picture of sarcoid at that site) is positive in 80% of patients with sarcoidosis; many false negatives are seen in patients who are later proved to have sarcoidosis; a positive reaction is less frequent if there is no lymph node involvement, if the disease is of long standing and inactive, and during steroid therapy; false positive reactions occur in 2–5% of patients.

Tissue biopsy may be taken at several sites.

> Needle biopsy of liver shows granulomas in 75% of patients even if there is no impairment of liver function.
>
> Lymph node biopsy is likely to be positive if lymph node is enlarged.
>
> Muscle biopsy is likely to be positive if arthralgia or muscle pain is present.
>
> Skin lesions occur in 35% of cases.
>
> Other sites of biopsy are synovium, eye, lung, etc.

Serum globulins are increased in 75% of patients, producing reduced A/G ratio and increased total protein (in 30% of patients).

Serum protein electrophoresis shows decreased albumin and increased globulin (especially gamma) with characteristic "sarcoid-step" pattern.

There is positive thymol turbidity, and other tests are affected by increased globulin.

WBC is decreased in 30% of patients. Eosinophilia occurs in 15% of patients.

Mild normocytic, normochromic anemia occurs.

ESR is increased.

Increased urine calcium occurs twice as often as hypercalcemia and may be found even with normal serum calcium. Increased frequency of renal calculi is found, and of nephrocalcinosis in some series of patients.

Serum calcium is increased in >16% of patients.

Serum and urine calcium abnormalities are frequently corrected by cortisone.

Increased sensitivity to vitamin D is often present.

Serum phosphorus is normal.

Increased serum uric acid may occur even with normal renal function in ≦50% of patients.

Mumps complement-fixation test, which is positive in presence of negative mumps skin test (due to dissociation between normal circulating antibodies and defective cellular antibody response), supports the diagnosis but is not specific.

Laboratory findings reflect specific organ involvement.

> Liver. Serum alkaline phosphatase is increased (see p. 222).
>
> Spleen. Hypersplenism may occur (anemia, leukopenia, thrombocytopenia).
>
> Central nervous system. CSF may be normal or may show

moderate to marked increase in protein and pleocytosis (chiefly lymphocytes). Sugar is sometimes decreased.

Pituitary. Diabetes insipidus is evident.

Kidney. Renal function is decreased (because of hypercalcemia or increased uric acid with resultant nephrocalcinosis or renal calculi).

Lung. pO_2 and pCO_2 are decreased.

Other.

AMYLOIDOSIS

Biopsy of tissue may be done at several sites.

Gingival biopsy is positive in one-half to two-thirds of patients.

Rectal biopsy is positive in one-half to two-thirds of patients.

Needle biopsy of kidney is useful when gingival and rectal biopsies are not helpful and there is a differential diagnosis of nephrosis.

Needle biopsy of liver is often positive, but beware of intractable bleeding or rupture.

Skin biopsy is taken from sites of plaque formation.

Other areas of involvement include GI tract, spleen, respiratory tract.

One should use Congo red stain of tissue under polarized light (apple-green birefringence) as well as transmitted light.

Congo red test is positive in one-third of patients with primary amyloidosis and approximately two-thirds of patients with secondary amyloidosis.

Evans blue dye is retained in serum.

Laboratory findings due to primary or associated diseases may occur.

Leprosy (35% of patients)

Rheumatoid arthritis (25% of patients)

Chronic infections (e.g., chronic osteomyelitis, paraplegia with infections of GU tract)

Tuberculosis

Multiple myeloma (10–20% of patients)

Neoplasms (e.g., renal carcinoma, lymphoma)

Familial types of amyloidosis

Familial Mediterranean fever

Other familial types

Laboratory findings associated with involvement of specific organs may be present.

Liver (see p. 222)

Thymol turbidity and cephalin flocculation, SGOT, LDH, serum bilirubin are usually normal.

BSP retention is increased in 75% of patients.

Prothrombin time is occasionally decreased.

Kidney (see p. 448)

Nervous system—peripheral neuropathy

Gastrointestinal system. See Chapter 26 for malabsorption, intestinal obstruction, hemorrhage.

Endocrine system (see Addison's disease, pp. 409–410)
Skin—petechiae, purpura

Increased serum globulin and decreased albumin with reversed A/G ratio are frequent. Serum protein electrophoresis shows decreased albumin and beta and gamma globulins. In familial primary amyloidosis there may be an abnormal peak between alpha$_2$ and beta globulins.

ESR is increased.

Moderate normochromic, normocytic anemia is present.

WBC is frequently increased (>12,000/cu mm).

INFANTILE AMAUROTIC IDIOCY (TAY-SACHS DISEASE)
See p. 373.

SYSTEMIC MAST CELL DISEASE (MASTOCYTOSIS)
This is a rare condition of disseminated mast cell tumor with functional secretion or abnormal proliferation of tissue mast cells.

Progressive anemia and thrombocytopenia are present.

WBC may be increased or (rarely) decreased.

Peripheral blood contains ≦10% mast cells.

Eosinophilia and occasionally basophilia may occur.

Histamine is increased in blood, urine, and tissues.

Gastric acid is increased; there is a higher incidence of peptic ulcer. Hypochlorhydria and achlorhydria have been reported.

Urinary 5-HIAA (hydroxyindole acetic acid) is normal.

Many mast cells appear in bone marrow smears and in metastatic sites.

BASAL CELL NEVUS SYNDROME
Rare disease that shows

Multiple basal cell tumors of skin

Odontogenic cysts of jaw

Bone anomalies (especially of ribs, vertebrae, and metacarpals) and defective dentition

Neurologic abnormalities (calcification of dura, etc.)

Ophthalmologic abnormalities (abnormal width between the eyes, lateral displacement of inner canthi, etc.)

Sexual abnormalities (frequent ovarian fibromas; male hypogonadism, etc.)

Normal karyotyping by chromosomal analysis

Hyporesponsiveness to parathormone (Ellsworth-Howard test)

Rule out presence or development of occult neoplasms (e.g., ovarian fibroma, medulloblastoma).

MALIGNANT NEOPLASMS
Hemorrhage
Anemia
Malnutrition
Hypoproteinemia

Development of autoantibodies, hemolytic anemia, increased ESR, etc.

Tumor cells in bone marrow, liver biopsy, etc.

Metastatic tumor masses (e.g., liver, brain)

Obstruction (e.g., ureters, bile ducts, intestine)

Functional changes due to metastases that interfere with endocrine secretion (e.g., adrenal, pituitary)

Secretion of active hormonal substances by nonendocrine tumors (e.g., bronchogenic carcinoma)

Diseases that occur with particular frequency in association with neoplasms (e.g., polymyositis)

Laboratory findings associated with specific tumors (e.g., carcinoid, thymoma, functioning endocrine tumors, leukemia, melanoma)

OCCULT NEOPLASIA
(e.g., Pheochromocytoma, Hypernephroma, Breast Carcinoma, and Various Benign Tumors)

Rule out presence or development of occult neoplasia in
> Neurofibromatosis
> Sturge-Weber syndrome
> Lindau-von Hippel disease
> Tuberous sclerosis
> Basal cell nevus syndrome
> Polymyositis
> Acanthosis nigricans

BREAST CANCER

Indications for administration of adrenal hormones
> Hypercalcemia
> Metastases
>> To brain or liver
>> Diffuse pulmonary

CONDITIONS DUE TO PHYSICAL AND CHEMICAL AGENTS

NARCOTICS ADDICTION
(usually heroin)

Persistent absolute and relative lymphocytosis occurs, with lymphocytes, often bizarre and atypical, that may resemble Downey cells.

Eosinophilia is seen in 25% of patients.

Liver function tests commonly show increased serum SGOT and SGPT (increased in 75% of patients) and/or increased cephalin flocculation and thymol turbidity tests. Higher frequency of positive tests is evident on routine periodic repeat of these tests. (This probably represents a mild, chronic, intermittently active, usually anicteric serum hepatitis.) Serum protein electrophoresis is usually normal.

Liver biopsy shows abnormal morphology in 25% of patients and foreign particles are particularly suggestive.

HB_sAg is found in 10% of patients.

Laboratory findings due to preexisting glucose-6-phosphate dehydrogenase deficiency may be precipitated (by quinine, which is often used to adulterate the heroin).

Laboratory findings due to malaria transmitted by common syringes may occur. *(Malaria is not frequent; may be suppressed by quinine used for adulteration of heroin.)*

Laboratory findings due to active duodenal ulcer may occur.

Laboratory findings due to tuberculosis, which develops with increased frequency in narcotics addicts, may be present.

Laboratory findings due to staphylococcal pneumonia or septic pulmonary emboli secondary to skin infections or bacterial endocarditis (conditions that are more frequent in narcotics addicts) may be present.

Laboratory findings due to endocarditis
> Right-sided—usually *Staphylococcus aureus* affecting previously normal tricuspid valve
> Left-sided—may be due to *Candida* superimposed on previously normal valve

Oral and IV glucose tolerance curves are often flat (explanation for this finding is not known).

Urinalysis is usually normal unless renal failure due to endocarditis occurs.

Laboratory findings due to syphilis, which occurs with increased frequency in narcotics addicts, may occur. BFP tests for syphilis also occur with increased frequency.

Laboratory findings due to tetanus (which occurs with increased frequency in narcotics addicts because of "skin-popping") may occur. *(Tetanus causes 5–10% of addicts' deaths in New York City.)*

Laboratory findings due to concomitant use of sedative, especially alcohol, barbiturates, and glutethimide (Doriden), may occur.

ALCOHOLISM*
Laboratory findings due to major alcohol-associated illnesses (see
appropriate separate sections)
> Fatty liver, alcoholic hepatitis, cirrhosis, esophageal varices,
> peptic ulcer, chronic gastritis, pancreatitis, malabsorption,
> vitamin deficiencies
>
> Head trauma, Korsakoff's syndrome, delirium tremens,
> peripheral neuropathy, myopathy
>
> Cardiac myopathy
>
> Various pneumonias, lung abscess, tuberculosis
>
> Associated addictions
>
> Other

Laboratory tests due to alcohol ingestion
> Direct
>> Blood alcohol level at any time of >300 mg/100 ml or
>> level of > 100 mg/100 ml in routine examination. *(Blood
>> alcohol level >150 mg/100 ml without gross evidence of
>> intoxication suggests alcoholic patient's increased tol-
>> erance.)*
>
> Indirect
>> Serum osmolality (reflects blood alcohol levels). Every
>> 22.4 increment >200 mOsm/L reflects 50 mg/100 ml al-
>> cohol.
>>
>> Results of alcohol ingestion
>>> Hypoglycemia
>>> Hypochloremic alkalosis
>>> Low magnesium level
>>> Increased lactic acid
>>> Transient increase of serum uric acid
>>> Potassium depletion
>>
>> Thrombocytopenia
>>
>> Anemia—most often due to folic acid deficiency; less fre-
>> quently due to iron deficiency, hemorrhage, secondary
>> to inflammation, etc.

SALICYLATE INTOXICATION
**(due to aspirin, sodium salicylate, oil of wintergreen, methyl
salicylate)**
Increased serum salicylate
> >10 mg/100 ml when symptoms are present
> >40 mg/100 ml when hyperventilation is present
> At ≅50 mg/100 ml, severe toxicity with acid-base imbalance
> and ketosis
> At 45–70 mg/100 ml, death

> *In older children and adults, serum salicylate level corre-
> sponds well with severity; in younger children, correlation is
> more variable.*
> *Gastric lavage may increase salicylate level ≦10 mg/100 ml.*

*Criteria Committee, National Council on Alcoholism, Criteria for the
diagnosis of alcoholism. *Ann. Intern. Med.* 77: 249, 1972.

Early, serum electrolytes and CO_2 are normal.

Later, progressive decrease in serum sodium and pCO_2 occurs. There is combined respiratory alkalosis and metabolic acidosis; change in blood pH reflects the net result. *(Infants may show immediate metabolic acidosis with the usual initial respiratory alkalosis. In older children and adults the typical picture is respiratory alkalosis.)*

Hypokalemia accompanies the respiratory alkalosis. Dehydration occurs.

Urine shows paradoxic acid pH despite the increased serum bicarbonate.

> Ferric chloride test is positive on boiled as well as unboiled urine (thus differentiating salicylate from ketone bodies); it may have a false positive result because of phenacetin.

> Tests for glucose (e.g., Clinistix), reducing substances (e.g., Clinitest), or ketone bodies (e.g., Ketostix) are positive.

> RBCs may be present.

> Number of renal tubular cells is increased because of renal irritation.

Hypoglycemia occurs, especially in infants on restricted diet and in diabetics.

Serum SGOT and SGPT may be increased.

Hypoprothrombinemia after some days of intensive salicylate therapy is temporary and occasional; rarely causes hemorrhage.

BMR is markedly increased.

Hydroxyproline is decreased in serum and urine.

DIFFERENTIATION OF ACIDOSIS IN SALICYLATE INTOXICATION AND DIABETES MELLITUS

Measurement	Salicylate Intoxication	Diabetes Mellitus
Ferric chloride test on urine	Remains positive after boiling	Becomes negative after boiling (volatile acetoacetic acid is removed)
Nitroprusside test for acetoacetic acid in urine	Negative	Positive
Urinary reducing substances	May be due to glucose or other reducing substances (e.g., salicylglucuronide	Due to glucose
Serum ketone level	Usually <20 mg/100 ml.	Often >50 mg/100 ml.
Prothrombin time	Increased	Normal
Serum salicylate level	>40 mg/100 ml.	Negative or increased to nontoxic level

PHENACETIN—CHRONIC EXCESSIVE INGESTION
Laboratory findings due to increased incidence of peptic ulceration, especially of stomach, often with bleeding, may be present.
Laboratory findings associated with increased incidence of papillary necrosis and interstitial nephritis may be present.
Proteinuria is slight or absent.
Hematuria is often present in active papillary necrosis.
WBC is increased in urine in absence of infection.
Papillae are passed in urine.
Creatinine clearance is decreased.
Renal failure may occur.
Anemia is common and frequently precedes azotemia.

BROMISM

Bromism should always be ruled out in the presence of mental symptoms or psychosis.

Serum and urine bromide levels are increased.
CSF protein is increased in acute bromide psychosis.
Serum "chloride" is increased, as indicated by AutoAnalyzer.

If result of chloride determination with AutoAnalyzer is increased out of proportion to result with Cotlove coulimetric titrator, bromism should be ruled out.

SOME POSSIBLE SIDE-EFFECTS OF STEROID THERAPY THAT CAUSE LABORATORY CHANGES
Endocrine effects (e.g., adrenal insufficiency after prolonged use, suppression of pituitary or thyroid function, development of diabetes mellitus)
Increased susceptibility to infections
Gastrointestinal effects (e.g., peptic ulcer, perforation of bowel, infarction of bowel, pancreatitis)
Musculoskeletal effects (e.g., osteoporosis, pathologic fractures, arthropathy, myopathy)
Decreased serum potassium, increased WBC, glycosuria, ecchymoses, etc.

PROCAINAMIDE THERAPY
Procainamide therapy may induce the findings of systemic lupus erythematosus (SLE).
Positive serologic tests for SLE are very frequent, especially in dosage of $\geqq 1.25$ gm/day, and may precede clinical manifestations.
LE cell tests become positive in 50% of patients.
Anti-DNP (anti-deoxyribonucleoprotein) tests become positive in 65% of patients.
Anti-DNA tests become positive in 35% of patients.
One of these tests becomes positive in 75% of patients.

Perform serologic tests for lupus on all patients receiving procainamide.

APRESOLINE REACTION
(in hypertension therapy)
Anemia and pancytopenia occur infrequently.

Prolonged use causes a syndrome resembling lupus erythematosus (microscopic hematuria, leukopenia, increased ESR, presence of LE cells, altered serum proteins with increased gamma globulin). After cessation of drug, remission is aided by administration of ACTH.

ENTERIC-COATED THIAZIDE POTASSIUM CHLORIDE
Laboratory findings due to small-intestine ulceration, obstruction, or perforation.

COMPLICATIONS OF PHENYTOIN SODIUM (DILANTIN) THERAPY
Megaloblastic anemia may occur. It is completely responsive to folic acid (even when Dilantin therapy is continued) but not always to vitamin B_{12}. This is the most common hematologic complication.

Rarely there may occur pancytopenia, thrombocytopenia alone, or leukopenia, including agranulocytosis.

Laboratory findings of hepatitis may be present.

Laboratory findings resembling those of malignant lymphomas may be present.

Laboratory findings resembling those of infectious mononucleosis may occur, but heterophil agglutination is not increased.

PBI is decreased, with increased T-3 uptake, but ^{131}I uptake, PB ^{131}I, BMR, serum cholesterol, etc., are normal (because of competition for binding sites of thyroxin-binding globulin).

Dilantin therapy may induce a lupuslike syndrome.

LABORATORY CHANGES AND SIDE-EFFECTS FROM LIPID-LOWERING DRUGS
Nicotinic acid may cause
  Dramatic lowering (often) of blood triglyceride in hyperlipidemia, Types II and IV and probably also in Types III and V
  Increased blood sugar
  Increased blood uric acid
  Abnormal liver function tests
  Jaundice (rarely)
Cholestyramine in the form of a chloride salt may cause
  Lowering of cholesterol in familial Type II hyperlipidemia
  Mild hyperchloremic acidosis

HYPERVITAMINOSIS A
Increased serum vitamin A level ($\leqq 2000$ μg/100 ml)
May also show
  Increased ESR
  Increased serum alkaline phosphatase
  Decreased serum albumin
  Increased serum bilirubin
  Decreased hemoglobin
  Slight proteinuria

Slightly increased serum carotene
Increased prothrombin time
Bromsulphalein (BSP) retention

CHRONIC ARSENIC POISONING
(from insecticides, rat poisons, or therapeutic arsenic, e.g., Fowler's solution)

Increased arsenic appears in urine (usually >0.1 mg/L; in acute cases may be >1.0 mg/L).
Increased arsenic appears in hair (>0.1 mg/100 mg of hair).
Increased arsenic appears in nails.
Moderate anemia is present.
Moderate leukopenia occurs (2000–5000/cu mm), with mild eosinophilia.
Liver function tests show mild abnormalities.
Urine shows slight proteinuria.
Cerebrospinal fluid is normal.

Arsine gas (hydrogen arsenide) causes hemolysis with hemoglobinuria; may cause oliguric renal failure.

LEAD POISONING

Delta-aminolevulinic acid is increased in urine. Since it is increased in 75% of asymptomatic lead workers who have normal coproporphyrin in urine, it can be used to detect early excess lead absorption.
Increased coproporphyrin in urine is a reliable sign of intoxication and is often demonstrable before basophilic stippling (but one should rule out a false positive reaction due to drugs such as barbiturates and salicylates). This is the most useful rapid screening test.
Confirm diagnosis with determination of blood lead (<20 μg/100 ml is considered normal; 25–40 μg/100 ml is evidence of increased lead exposure; >50 μg/100 ml is a treatable level; 80 μg/100 ml in children is an indication for emergency treatment) and urine lead (normal for children is <80 μg/1000 ml and for adults is <150 μg/1000 ml).
Anemia (slightly hypochromic and microcytic) in chronic exposure may be of moderate degree or may be absent.
Stippled RBCs occur later. Their number is variable; in bone marrow 65% of erythroid cells show stippling.
Urine urobilinogen and uroporphyrin are increased.
Renal tubular damage occurs, with Fanconi syndrome (hypophosphatemia, aminoaciduria, and glycosuria), usually in very severe or very chronic cases. Albuminuria may occur.
CSF protein is increased, with normal cell count in encephalopathy.

MERCURY POISONING

Levels of mercury in serum, urine, and CSF are increased.
95% of asymptomatic normal people (not exposed to mercury) have a urine value <20 μg/L and blood level <3 μg/L. Urine and blood levels are nondiagnostic, in that they vary among patients

with symptoms, and daily urine levels vary in the same patient. Thus in one epidemic, urine levels $\leqq 1000$ μg/L occurred in asymptomatic patients whereas other patients had symptoms at levels of 200 μg/L.

Renal changes may occur (e.g., acute renal failure, nephrotic syndrome, specific tubular defects)

ACUTE IRON POISONING
(occurs in children who have ingested medicinal iron preparations)
Increased serum iron and TIBC. With severe intoxication, serum iron is >500 μg/100 ml within 6 hours of ingestion.

Poor prognostic sign when serum iron greatly exceeds TIBC. Blood for these should be drawn within the first few hours.

Acidosis

ORGANIC PHOSPHATE (INSECTICIDES—PARATHION, MALATHION, ETC.) POISONING
Decreased RBC and plasma cholinesterase by $\geqq 50\%$ (due to inhibition of cholinesterase by organic phosphate pesticides)

In industrial exposure, worker should not return to work until these values rise to 75% of normal. RBC cholinesterase regenerates at rate of 1%/day. Plasma cholinesterase regenerates at rate of 25% in 7–10 days.

MOTHBALLS (CAMPHOR, PARADICHLOROBENZENE, NAPHTHALENE) POISONING
Paradichlorobenzene inhalation may cause liver damage.

Naphthalene ingestion may cause hemolytic anemia in patients with RBCs deficient in G-6-PD (see p. 304).

YELLOW PHOSPHORUS POISONING
(rat poison ingestion)
Acute yellow atrophy of liver occurs.

Vomitus may glow in the dark.

PHENOL AND LYSOL POISONING
Severe acidosis often occurs.

Acute tubular necrosis may develop.

OXALATE POISONING
(due to ingestion of stain remover or ink eradicator containing oxalic acid)
Hypocalcemic tetany (due to formation of insoluble calcium oxalate)

METHYL ALCOHOL POISONING
Onset is 12–24 hours after ingestion.

Severe acidosis

Frequent concomitant acute pancreatitis

MILK SICKNESS ("TREMBLES")
(poisoning from goldenrod, snakeroot, richweed, etc., or from eating poisoned animals)
Acidosis
Hypoglycemia
Increased nonprotein nitrogen (particularly guanidine)
Acetonuria

HEAT STROKE
Uniformly increased SGOT (mean is 20 times normal), SGPT (mean is 10 times normal), and LDH (mean is 5 times normal) reach peak on third day and return to normal by 2 weeks. Very high levels are often associated with lethal outcome.
Cerebrospinal fluid GOT, GPT, and LDH are normal.

Serum potassium varies from decreased levels associated with hyperventilation and respiratory alkalosis to increased levels associated with lactic acidosis or skeletal muscle damage.
Evidence of kidney damage may vary from mild proteinuria and slight abnormalities of urine sediment to acute oliguric renal insufficiency.
Disseminated intravascular coagulation is common in severe cases.

DROWNING AND NEAR-DROWNING
Hypoxemia (decreased pO_2)
Metabolic acidosis (decreased blood pH)
In severe freshwater aspiration
    Decreased serum sodium and chloride
    Increased serum potassium
    Increased plasma hemoglobin
In severe seawater aspiration
    Hypovolemia
    Increased serum sodium and chloride
    Normal plasma hemoglobin

Above-mentioned changes follow aspiration of very large amounts of water. Electrolytes return toward normal within 1 hour following survival, even without therapy.

In near-drowning in fresh water, often
    Normal serum sodium and chloride
    Variable serum potassium
    Increased free plasma hemoglobin; hemoglobinuria may occur
    Oliguria with transient azotemia and proteinuria may develop.
    Fall in RBC, hemoglobin, and hematocrit in 24 hours.
In near-drowning in seawater, often
    Moderate increase in serum sodium and chloride
    Normal or decreased serum potassium
    Normal hemoglobin, hematocrit, and plasma hemoglobin

Blood count may appear normal even when considerable hemolysis is present because usual methodology does not distinguish be-

tween hemoglobin within RBC and free hemoglobin in serum.
Fall in hemoglobin and hematocrit may be delayed 1–2 days.

ACUTE CARBON MONOXIDE POISONING
Arterial pO_2 is normal although O_2 is significantly decreased.
Arterial pCO_2 may be normal or slightly decreased.
Blood pH is markedly decreased (metabolic acidosis due to tissue hypoxia).
Symptoms are correlated with the percentage of carbon monoxide in hemoglobin:

% COHb	Symptoms
0–2%	Asymptomatic
2–5%	Found in moderate cigarette smokers. Usually asymptomatic but may be slight impairment of intellect
5–10%	Found in heavy cigarette smokers. Slight dyspnea with severe exertion
10–20%	Dyspnea with moderate exertion. Mild headache
20–30%	Marked headache, irritability, disturbed judgment and memory, easy fatiguability
30–40%	Severe headache, dimness of vision, confusion, weakness, nausea
40–50%	Headache, confusion, fainting, ataxia, collapse, hyperventilation
50–60%	Coma, intermittent convulsions
>60%	Respiratory failure and death if exposure is long continued
80%	Rapidly fatal

INJURY DUE TO ELECTRIC CURRENT (INCLUDING LIGHTNING)
Increased WBC with large immature granulocytes
Albuminuria; hemoglobinuria in presence of severe burns
CSF sometimes bloody
Myoglobinuria and increased SGOT, serum CPK, etc., indicate severe tissue damage.

BURNS
Decreased plasma volume and blood volume. This decrease follows (and therefore is not due to) marked drop in cardiac output. Greatest fall in plasma volume occurs in the first 12 hours and continues at a much slower rate for only 6–12 hours more. In a 40% burn, plasma volume falls to 25% below preburn levels.
Infection
  Burn sepsis. Gram-positive organisms predominate until the third day, when gram-negative organisms become dominant. By fifth day, untreated infection is active. *Fatal burn-wound sepsis shows no noteworthy spread of bacteria beyond wound in half the cases. Before antibiotic therapy,*

this caused 75% of deaths due to burns; it now causes 10–15% of deaths.

Laboratory findings due to pneumonia, which now causes most deaths that result from infection. Two-thirds of pneumonia cases are airborne infections. One-third are hematogenous infections and are often due to septic phlebitis at sites of old cutdowns.

Local and systemic infection due to *Candida* and *Phycomycetes*.

Laboratory findings due to renal failure. Reported frequency varies—1.3% of total admissions to 15% of patients with burns involving >15% of body surface.

Laboratory findings due to Curling's ulcer. Occurs in 11% of burn patients. *Gastric ulcer is more frequent in general, but duodenal ulcer occurs twice as often in children as in adults. Gastric lesions are seen throughout the first month with equal frequency in all age groups, but duodenal ulcers are most frequent in adults during the first week and in children during the third and fourth weeks after the burns.*

Blood viscosity rises acutely; remains elevated for 4–5 days although hematocrit has returned to normal.

Fibrin split products are increased for 3–5 days.

Other findings that may occur in all types of trauma

Platelet count rises slowly, lasting for 3 weeks. Platelet adhesiveness is increased.

Fibrinogen falls during first 36 hours, then rises steeply for up to 3 months.

Factors V and VIII may be 4–8 times normal level for up to 3 months.

CONVULSIVE THERAPY
(e.g., electroshock therapy)

Increased cerebrospinal fluid GOT and LDH peak (3 times normal) in 12 hours; return to normal by 48 hours.

SNAKEBITE

Pit vipers (rattlesnake, copperhead, water moccasin)

Increased WBC (20,000–30,000/cu mm)

Platelets decreased to approximately 10,000/cu mm within an hour; return to normal in about 4 hours

Burrs on almost all RBCs

Clotting caused by some venoms; normal coagulation prevented by others, which destroy fibrinogen

Albuminuria

Elapidae (coral snakes, kraits, cobras)

Hemolytic manifestations

SPIDER BITE

Black widow spider *(Latrodectus mactans)*

Moderately increased WBC

Findings of acute nephritis

Brown spider *(Loxosceles reclusa)*
   Hemolytic anemia with hemoglobinuria and hemoglobinemia
   Increased WBC
   Thrombocytopenia
   Proteinuria

INSECT BITE
(due to ticks, lice, fleas, bugs, beetles, ants, flies, bees, wasps, etc.)
No specific laboratory findings unless secondary infection occurs.

SERUM SICKNESS
Decreased WBC due to decreased polynuclear neutrophils; occasionally WBC is increased.
Eosinophils are usually normal.
ESR is normal.
Heterophile agglutination test is often positive, and is decreased by guinea pig kidney absorption (see p. 120).

IV

EFFECTS OF DRUGS
ON LABORATORY TEST VALUES

ALTERATION OF LABORATORY
TEST VALUES BY DRUGS

With the coincident ingestion of a large number of drugs and the performance of many laboratory tests (many of which are unsolicited), test abnormalities may be due to drugs as often as to disease. Correct interpretation of laboratory tests requires that the physician be aware of all drugs that the patient is taking. It is important to remember that patients often do not tell their physician about medications they are taking (prescribed by other doctors or by the patients themselves). In addition, there is environmental exposure to many drugs and chemicals.

The classes of drugs most often involved include the anticoagulants, anticonvulsants, antihypertensives, anti-infectives, oral hypoglycemics, hormones, and psychoactive agents.

The following lists of the more frequently performed laboratory test values that may be altered by commonly used drugs are only a general guide to the direction of increase or decrease, not an all-inclusive collection of such information. The selection and arrangement of data by clinical groups provide the most useful, most rapid, and simplest summary of a very complex subject. Only generic names for drugs are used.

The frequency of such modified laboratory test values is variable. A number of causative mechanisms may operate, sometimes simultaneously. Thus some changes are due to interference with the chemical reaction used in the testing procedure. Other changes reflect damage to a specific organ, such as the liver or kidney. In some cases, specific metabolic alterations are induced, such as accelerated or retarded formation or excretion of a specific chemical, competition for binding sites, stimulation or suppression of degradative enzymes, etc. Often the mechanism of these altered laboratory test values is not known.

This chapter is meant only as an illustration of various possible mechanisms of such alterations and as a list of some of the more common responsible drugs. It is not to be considered a complete or exhaustive list, nor should it be used to rule out drug-caused effect on a laboratory test by virtue of a drug's not appearing on the lists. For the most specific information, the reader should consult more detailed sources about an individual drug, such as the manufacturer's insert sheets and data, computer-file based data, and the most current literature available published since this and other compilations.

DRUGS THAT MAY CAUSE MARKED
ELEVATION OF URINE SPECIFIC GRAVITY
Dextran
Radiopaque contrast media
Sucrose

DRUGS THAT MAY ALTER URINE COLOR
Urine coloration due to drugs may mask other abnormal colors (e.g., due to blood, bile, porphyrins) as well as interfere with

various chemical determinations (fluorometric, colorimetric, photometric)

Drug	*Resulting Color*
Acetophenetidin	Hematuria or pink-red due to metabolite
Aminosalicylic acid (PAS)	Discoloration abnormal but not distinctive
Amitriptyline	Blue-green
Anisindione (indandione)	Orange (alkaline urine), pink-red-brown (acid urine)
Anthraquinones	Pink to brown
Anticoagulants	Pink to red to brown (due to bleeding)
Cascara	Brown (acid urine), yellow-pink (alkaline urine), black on standing
Chloroquine	Brown
Chlorzoxazone (metabolite)	Purple, red, pink, rust
Cinchophen	Red-brown
Dihydroxyanthraquinone	Pink to orange (alkaline urine)
Emodin	Pink to red to red-brown (alkaline urine)
Ethoxazene	Orange, red, pink, rust
Furazolidone	Brown
Indomethacin	Green (due to biliverdin)
Iron sorbitol	Brown
Methocarbamol	Dark brown, black, blue or green on standing
Methyldopa	Red darkens on standing, pink or brown
Methylene blue	Greenish-yellow to blue
Metronidazole (metabolite)	Dark brown
Nitrofurantoin and derivatives	Brown, yellow
Pamaquine	Brown
Phenacetin	Dark brown
Phenazopyridine	Orange to red
Phenindione	Red-orange in alkaline urine
Phenolphthalein	Pink to red to magenta (alkaline urine), orange, rust (acid)
Phenothiazines	Pink, red, purple, orange, rust
Phensuximide	Pink, red, purple, orange, rust
Phenytoin sodium	Pink, red, red-brown
Primaquine	Rust yellow to brown
Quinacrine (mepacrine)	Deep yellow on acidification
Quinine and derivatives	Brown to black
Rhubarb	Yellow-brown (acid), yellow-pink (alkaline). darkens
Riboflavin	Yellow
Rifampin	Red-orange
Salicylates	Pink to red to brown (due to bleeding)
Salicylazosulfapyridine	Pink, red, purple, orange, rust

Drug	*Resulting Color*
Senna	Red (alkaline urine), yellow-brown (acid urine)
Sulfonamides	Rust, yellow, or brown
Thiazolsulfone	Pink, red, purple, orange, rust
Tolonium	Blue, green
Triamterene	Green, blue with blue fluorescence

DRUGS THAT MAY CAUSE FALSE POSITIVE TEST FOR URINE PROTEIN

Drugs with nephrotoxic effect. (e.g., gold, arsenicals, antimony compounds)

Drugs that may interfere with sulfosalicylic acid methods
  Cephaloridine
  Cephalothin
  Sulfamethoxazole
  Tolbutamide
  Other

Drugs that may cause false positive turbidity tests
  Chlorpromazine, promazine
  Penicillin (massive doses)
  Radiopaque contrast media (for up to 3 days)
  Sulfisoxazole
  Thymol
  Other

Drugs that react with Folin-Ciocalteu reagent of Lowry procedure
  Aminosalicylic acid (PAS)
  Dithiazine
  Other

Drugs that cause false positive reaction with Labstix because of high pH
  Sodium bicarbonate
  Acetazolamide
  Other

DRUGS THAT MAY CAUSE POSITIVE TEST FOR URINE GLUCOSE

Drugs that may cause hyperglycemia with secondary glycosuria (e.g., corticosteroids, indomethacin, isoniazid)

Drugs that cause renal damage (e.g., degraded tetracycline)

Vaginal powders that contain glucose, causing artifactual false positive (e.g., furazolidone)

Drugs that cause false positive test by reducing action with Benedict's solution and Clinitest but not with Clinistix or Testape
  Acetylsalicylic acid
  Aminosalicylic acid (PAS)
  Cephaloridine (abnormal dark color)
  Cephalothin (brown-black color)
  Chloral hydrate
  Cinchophen
  Other

DRUGS THAT MAY CAUSE FALSE NEGATIVE TEST FOR URINE GLUCOSE
(glucose oxidase method, e.g., Clinistix, Testape)
Ascorbic acid
Levodopa (with Clinistix but not Testape)
Phenazopyridine

DRUGS THAT MAY CAUSE FALSE POSITIVE URINE ACETONE TEST

Ketostix or Acetest Methods	*Labstix, Bili-Labstix, etc.*
BSP	Levodopa
PSP	BSP
Inositol or methionine	
Metformin, phenformin	

DRUGS THAT MAY CAUSE FALSE POSITIVE URINE DIACETIC ACID TEST
(Gerhardt ferric chloride test; Phenistix)
Aminosalicylic acid (PAS)
Chlorpromazine
Phenothiazines
Levodopa
Salicylates

DRUGS THAT MAY CAUSE POSITIVE TEST FOR URINE AMINO ACIDS
ACTH and cortisone
Tetracyclines (degraded) and other nephrotoxic agents
Gentamicin, neomycin, and kanamycin cause spurious spots on
   thin-layer chromatograms (ninhydrin reaction)

DRUGS THAT MAY ALTER URINE TESTS FOR OCCULT BLOOD

Guaiac	*Benzidine*
False positive	False positive
Bromides	Bromides
Copper	Copper
Iodides	Iodides
Oxidizing agents	Permanganate

False negative
   Ascorbic acid (high doses)

DRUGS THAT MAY CAUSE POSITIVE TESTS FOR HEMATURIA OR HEMOGLOBINURIA
Drugs that cause nephrotoxicity (e.g., amphotericin B, bacitracin)
Drugs that cause actual bleeding (e.g., phenylbutazone, indomethacin, coumarin)
Drugs that cause hemolysis (e.g., acetylsalicylic acid, acetophenetidin, acetanilid)

DRUGS THAT MAY CAUSE POSITIVE TESTS FOR BILE IN URINE

Drugs that cause cholestasis
Drugs that are hepatotoxic
Drugs that interfere with testing methods
    Acriflavine (yellow color when urine is shaken)
    Chlorpromazine (interferes with Bili-Labstix)
    Ethoxazene (atypical red color with Bili-Labstix and Icto-test)
    Mefenamic acid
    Phenazopyridine (false positive with Bili-Labstix and Icto-test)
    Phenothiazines (may interfere with Bili-Labstix)
    Thymol (affects Hay's test for bile acids)

DRUGS THAT MAY CAUSE URINE UROBILINOGEN TO BE

Increased	*Decreased*
Drugs that interfere with testing methods	Drugs that cause cholestasis
Aminosalicylic acid (PAS)	Drugs that reduce the bacterial flora in the gastrointestinal tract (e.g., chloramphenicol)
Antipyrine	
Bromsulfalein (BSP)	
Cascara	
Chlorpromazine	
Phenazopyridine	
Phenothiazines	
Sulfonamides	
5-Hydroxyindoleacetic acid	
Bananas	
Drugs that cause hemolysis	

DRUGS THAT MAY CAUSE POSITIVE TESTS FOR URINE PORPHYRINS (FLUOROMETRIC METHODS)

Drugs that produce fluorescence
    Acriflavine
    Ethoxazene
    Phenazopyridine
    Sulfamethoxazole
    Tetracycline
    Other
Drugs that may precipitate porphyria
    Antipyretics
    Barbiturates
    Phenylhydrazine
    Sulfonamides
    Other

DRUGS THAT MAY CAUSE URINE CREATINE TO BE

Increased	*Decreased*
Caffeine	Androgens and anabolic steroids
Methyltestosterone	
PSP	Thiazides

DRUGS THAT MAY CAUSE URINE CREATININE TO BE

Increased
Ascorbic acid
Corticosteroids
Levodopa
Methyldopa
Nitrofurans
PSP

Decreased
Androgens and anabolic
  steroids
Thiazides

DRUGS THAT MAY CAUSE URINE CALCIUM TO BE

Increased
Androgens and anabolic
  steroids
Cholestyramine
Corticosteroids
Dihydrotachysterol, vitamin D
  parathyroid injections
Viomycin

Decreased
Sodium phytate
Thiazides

DRUGS THAT MAY CAUSE FALSE POSITIVE PSP TEST IN URINE

Kaolin
Magnesium
Methylene blue
Nicotinic acid
Quinacrine (mepacrine)
Quinidine
Quinine

DRUGS THAT MAY CAUSE URINE 17-KETOSTEROIDS TO BE

Increased
Chloramphenicol
Chlorpromazine
Cloxacillin
Dexamethasone
Erythromycin
Ethinamate
Meprobamate
Nalidixic acid
Oleandomycin
Penicillin
Phenaglycodol
Phenazopyridine
Phenothiazines
Quinidine
Secobarbital
Spironolactone

Decreased
Chlordiazepoxide
Estrogens
Meprobamate
Metyrapone
Probenecid
Promazine
Reserpine

DRUGS THAT MAY CAUSE URINE 17-HYDROXYCORTICOSTEROIDS TO BE

Increased
Acetazolamide
Chloral hydrate

Decreased
Estrogens and oral
  contraceptives

Increased	*Decreased*
Chlordiazepoxide	Phenothiazines
Chlorpromazine	Reserpine
Colchicine	
Erythromycin	
Etryptamine	
Meprobamate	
Oleandomycin	
Paraldehyde	
Quinine and quinidine	
Spironolactone	

DRUGS THAT MAY INTERFERE WITH DETERMINATION OF URINE CATECHOLAMINES
(by producing urinary fluorescence)
Ampicillin
Ascorbic acid
Chloral hydrate
Epinephrine
Erythromycin
Hydralazine
Methenamine
Methyldopa
Nicotinic acid (large doses)
Quinine and quinidine
Tetracycline and derivatives
Vitamin B complex

DRUGS THAT MAY CAUSE URINE VMA (VANILLYLMANDELIC ACID) TO BE

Increased	*Decreased*
Aspirin	(Values are usually not de-
Aminosalicylic acid (PAS)	pressed to normal in patients
Bromsulfalein (BSP)	with pheochromocytoma)
Glyceryl guaiacolate	Clofibrate
Mephenesin	Guanethidine analogs
Methocarbamol	Imipramine
Nalidixic acid	Methyldopa
Oxytetracycline	Monoamine oxidase (MAO)
Penicillin	inhibitors
Phenazopyridine	
PSP	
Sulfa drugs	

DRUGS THAT MAY CAUSE URINE 5-HIAA (5-HYDROXYINDOLEACETIC ACID) TO BE

Increased	*Decreased*
Acetanilid	Chlorpromazine, promazine
Acetophenetidin	Imipramine
Glyceryl guaiacolate	Isoniazid
Mephenesin	MAO inhibitors

Increased	*Decreased*
Methocarbamol	Methenamine
Reserpine	Methyldopa
	Phenothiazines
	Promethazine

DRUGS THAT MAY CAUSE URINE DIAGNEX BLUE EXCRETION TO BE

Increased	*Decreased*
Aluminum salts	Caffeine benzoate
Barium salts	
Calcium salts	
Iron salts	
Kaolin	
Magnesium salts	
Methylene blue	
Nicotinic acid	
Quinacrine (mepacrine)	
Quinidine, quinine	
Riboflavin	
Sodium salts	
Vitamin B	

DRUGS THAT MAY CAUSE A FALSE POSITIVE URINE PREGNANCY TEST

Chlorpromazine (frog, rabbit, immunologic)
Phenothiazines (frog, rabbit, immunologic)
Promethazine (Gravindex)

DRUG THAT MAY CAUSE A FALSE NEGATIVE URINE PREGNANCY TEST

Promethazine (DAP test)

DRUGS THAT MAY CAUSE THE ERYTHROCYTE SEDIMENTATION RATE (ESR) TO BE

Increased	*Decreased*
Dextran	Quinine (therapeutic effect)
Methyldopa	Salicylates (therapeutic effect)
Methysergide	Drugs that cause a high blood
Penicillamine	glucose level
Theophylline	
Trifluperidol	
Vitamin A	

DRUGS THAT MAY CAUSE A POSITIVE DIRECT COOMBS' TEST

Acetophenetidin	Ethosuximide
Chlorpromazine	Hydralazine
Chlorpropamide	Isoniazid
Dipyrone	Levodopa

Mefenamic acid
Melphalan
Oxyphenisatin
Phenylbutazone
Phenytoin sodium

Procainamide
Quinidine, quinine
Streptomycin
Sulfonamides
Tetracyclines

Illustrative information. For methyldopa, a positive direct Coombs' test occurs in 10–20% of patients on continued therapy. Occurs rarely in first 6 months of treatment. If not found within 12 months, is unlikely to occur. Is dose-related, with lowest incidence in patients receiving ≤ 1 gm daily. Reversal may take weeks to months after the drug is discontinued.

DRUGS THAT MAY CAUSE POSITIVE TESTS FOR LUPUS ERYTHEMATOSUS CELLS AND/OR ANTINUCLEAR ANTIBODIES

Acetazolamide
Aminosalicylic acid (PAS)
Birth control pills
Chlorprothixene
Chlorothiazide
Griseofulvin
Hydralazine
Isoniazid
Methyldopa

Penicillin
Phenylbutazone
Phenytoin sodium
Procainamide
Streptomycin
Sulfonamides
Tetracyclines
Thiouracil
Trimethadione

DRUGS THAT MAY CAUSE THE BLEEDING TIME TO BE INCREASED

Acetylsalicylic acid
Dextran
Pantothenyl alcohol and derivatives
Streptokinase-streptodornase

DRUGS THAT MAY CAUSE THE COAGULATION TIME TO BE

Increased
Anticoagulants
Tetracyclines

Decreased
Corticosteroids
Epinephrine

DRUGS THAT POTENTIATE COUMARIN ACTION (increase prothrombin time)

Anabolic steroids
Chloral hydrate
Chloramphenicol
Clofibrate
Glucagon
Indomethacin
Mefenamic acid
Neomycin

Oxyphenbutazone
Phenylbutazone
Phenyramidol
Phenytoin sodium
Quinidine
Salicylates
D-Thyroxine

DRUGS THAT MAY POTENTIATE COUMARIN ACTION
(increase prothrombin time)

Acetaminophen
Allopurinol
Diazoxide
Disulfiram
Ethacrynic acid
Heparin
Mercaptopurine
Methyldopa
Methylphenidate

Monoamine oxidase (MAO)
   inhibitors
Nalidixic acid
Northriptyline
Sulfinpyrazone
Sulfonamides (long-acting)
Thyroid drugs
Tolbutamide

DRUGS THAT INHIBIT COUMARIN ACTION
(decrease prothrombin time)
Barbiturates
Ethchlorvynol
Glutethimide
Griseofulvin
Heptabarbital

DRUGS THAT MAY INHIBIT COUMARIN ACTION
(decrease prothrombin time)
Adrenocortical steroids
Birth control pills
Cholestyramine
Colchicine
Meprobamate
Rifampin

Patients on long-term coumarin treatment should not take barbiturates, chloral hydrate, chloramphenicol, ethchlorvynol, glutethimide, phenylbutazone (or its congeners), phenyramidon, quinidine, or salicylates. Patients on long-term coumarin treatment should not take any other drugs without consideration of possible drug interaction.

DRUGS THAT MAY INHIBIT HEPARIN
Antihistamines
Digitalis
Nicotine
Penicillin (intravenous)
Protamine
Tetracycline
Tranquilizers (phenothiazine)

DRUGS THAT MAY CAUSE THROMBOCYTOPENIA BY DEPRESSION OF BONE MARROW
Adriamycin
Alkylating agents
Antipurines
Antipyrimadines
Bleomycin
L-Asparaginase

DRUGS THAT MAY CAUSE IDIOSYNCRATIC THROMBOCYTOPENIA

Antibacterial agents
  Isoniazide (INH)
  Sulfonamides
Antibiotics
  Chloramphenicol
  Streptomycin
Anticonvulsant drugs
  Ethosuximide (Zarontin)
  Methylhydantoin
  Paramethadione
  Phenacemide
  Trimethadione
Antirheumatic drugs
  Colchicine
  Gold salts
  Indomethacin
  Phenylbutazone

Hypoglycemic agents
  Carbutamide
  Chlorpropamide
  Tolbutamide
Tranquilizers
  Chlordiazepoxide
  Chlorpromazine
  Meprobamate
  Promazine
Miscellaneous
  Acetazolamide
  Chlorothiazide
  Hydralazine
  Quinacrine
  Tripelennamine
  Quinidine
  Acetaminophen

DRUGS THAT MAY CAUSE ALLERGIC VASCULAR PURPURA WITH NORMAL PLATELET FUNCTION AND NUMBERS

Acetophenetidin
Aspirin
Carbromal
Camphenazine
Chloral hydrate
Chlorothiazide
Chlorpromazine
Colchicine
Coumarin congeners
Diphenhydramine (Benadryl)
Erythromycin

Griseofulvin
Iodides
Isoniazid
Meprobamate
Oxytetracycline
Phenothiazines
Procaine penicillin
Quinidine
Sulfonamides
Tetracycline
Trifluoperazine

DRUGS THAT MAY CAUSE COLOR CHANGES IN STOOL

Drug	*Resulting Color*
Alkaline antacids and aluminum salts	White discoloration or speckling
Anticoagulants (excess)	Due to bleeding
Anthraquinones	Brown staining
Bismuth salts	Black
Charcoal	Black
Dithiazine	Green to blue
Indomethacin	Green (due to biliverdin)
Iron salts	Black
Mercurous chloride	Green
Phenazopyridine	Orange-red
Phenolphthalein	Red
Phenylbutazone and oxyphenbutazone	Black (due to bleeding)
Pyrvinium pamoate	Red
Rhubarb	Yellow
Salicylates	Due to bleeding

Drug	Resulting Color
Santonin	Yellow
Senna	Yellow to brown
Tetracyclines in syrup (due to glucosamine)	Red

DRUGS THAT MAY CAUSE FALSE NEGATIVE TEST FOR OCCULT BLOOD IN STOOL
Vitamin C (usually >500 mg/day)

DRUGS THAT MAY CAUSE INCREASED SERUM UREA NITROGEN

Due To
Nephrotoxic effect (see Table 79, pp. 550–555)
Methodologic interference
> Nesslerization (chloral hydrate, chloramphenicol, ammonium salts)
> Berthelot (aminophenol, asparagine, ammonium salts)
> Fearon (acetohexamide, sulfonylureas)

DRUGS THAT MAY CAUSE DECREASED SERUM UREA NITROGEN

Due To
Methodologic interference—Berthelot (chloramphenicol, streptomycin)

DRUGS THAT MAY CAUSE INCREASED SERUM URIC ACID

Due To
Cytotoxic effect causing increased turnover rate of nucleic acids (e.g., antimetabolite and chemotherapeutic agents in neoplastic diseases [e.g., methotrexate, busulfan, vincristine, azathioprine, prednisone])
Decreased renal clearance or tubular secretion (e.g., various diuretics [thiazides, furosemide, mercurials])
Nephrotoxic effect (e.g., mitomycin C)
Other effects (e.g., levodopa, phenytoin sodium)
Methodologic interference (e.g., ascorbic acid, levodopa, methyldopa)

DRUGS THAT MAY CAUSE DECREASED SERUM URIC ACID

Due To
Decreased production (allopurinol [xanthine oxidase inhibition])
Uricosuric effect (e.g., probenecid, high doses of salicylates, cinchophen, corticotropin, coumarins, thiazine, diuretics, acetohexamide)
Other effects (e.g., corticosteroids, indomethacin)

DRUGS THAT MAY CAUSE INCREASED SERUM BILIRUBIN

Due To
Hepatotoxic effect
Cholestatic effect

Hemolysis and hemolytic anemia (e.g., antimalarials, streptomycin)

Hemolysis in glucose-6-PD deficiency (e.g., primaquine, sulfa drugs)

Methodologic interference

    Evelyn-Malloy (dextran, novobiocin)

    Diazo reaction (ethoxazene, histidine, indican, phenazopyridine, rifampin, theophylline, tyrosine)

    SMA 12/60 (aminophenol, ascorbic acid, epinephrine, isoproterenol, levodopa, methyldopa, phenelzine)

    Spectrophotometric methods (drugs that cause lipemia)

FACTORS THAT MAY CAUSE DECREASED SERUM BILIRUBIN

Presence of hemoglobin

Exposure to sunlight or fluorescent light

Barbiturates (in newborns)

DRUGS THAT MAY CAUSE INCREASED SERUM CHOLESTEROL

Due To

Hepatotoxic effect (e.g., phenytoin sodium)

Cholestatic effect (e.g., androgens and anabolic steroids, thiazides, sulfonamides, promazines, chlorpropamide, cinchophen)

Hormonal effect (e.g., corticosteroids, birth control pills)

Methodologic interference (Zlatkis-Zak reaction) (e.g., bromides, iodides, chlorpromazine, corticosteroids, viomycin, Vitamin C, Vitamin A)

DRUGS THAT MAY CAUSE DECREASED SERUM CHOLESTEROL

Due To

Hepatotoxic effect (e.g., allopurinol, tetracyclines, erythromycin, isoniazid, MAO inhibitors)

Synthesis inhibition (e.g., androgens, chlorpropamide, clomiphene, phenformin)

Diminished synthesis (probable mechanism) (e.g., clofibrate)

Other mechanisms (e.g., azathioprine, kanamycin, neomycin, estrogens, chlorestyramine)

Methodologic interference (Zlatkis-Zak reaction) (e.g., thiouracil, nitrates, nitrites)

DRUGS THAT MAY CAUSE INCREASED SERUM TRIGLYCERIDES

Estrogens and birth control pills, cholestyramine

Due to methodologic interference (enzyme reaction) (glyceraldehyde)

DRUGS THAT MAY CAUSE DECREASED SERUM TRIGLYCERIDES

Ascorbic acid	Clofibrate	Phenformin
Asparaginase	Metformin	Other

Table 79. Effects of Various Drugs on Laboratory Test Values

	Hepatotoxic and/or cholestatic	Nephrotoxic	Intestinal malabsorption	Serum iron	Serum TIBC	Serum folate (inhibit *L. casei*)	Creatinine	BUN	Uric acid	Calcium	Bilirubin	SGOT/SGPT	Glucose
Antihistamines													
Antimony compounds	+	+											
Arsenicals	+	+											
Caffeine											D		I
Cholinergics											I	I	
Cinchophen	+								D				
Clofibrate	+								D				
Coumarins	+								D				
Cyclophosphamide	+												
Dextran				I				I	I		I		I
Phenytoin sodium	+		+			D							I
Heparin										a			
Levodopa									I				
Methotrexate	+					+			Iª				
Procainamide	+												
Propylthiouracil	+								Iª				
Quinacrine	+												
Quinine, Quinidine													
Radiopaque contrast media		+							D		+		
Theophylline									I		I		
VITAMINS — Ascorbic acid							I		I		I	I	I
VITAMINS — Nicotinic acid (large doses)	+										I		
VITAMINS — Vitamin A											I		
VITAMINS — Vitamin D		a											
VITAMINS — Vitamin K													
HORMONES — ACTH				D	D				D				I
HORMONES — Anabolic steroids and androgens	+												
HORMONES — Corticosteroids									D	Iª			I
HORMONES — Estrogens	+					D							I
HORMONES — Birth control pills (estrogens + progestin)	+			I	I	D							
HORMONES — D-Thyroxine													I

See footnotes on p. 555.

Glucose tolerance	Cholesterol	PBI	T-3 uptake	T-4	131I uptake	Amylase/lipase	Sodium	Potassium	Chloride	Phothrombin time	Comments
										D	
I											
						I					I–BSP. Changes due to spasm, sphincter of Oddi
	D									I	D–triglycerides, total lipids, LDH
										I	
											I–protein
D		D	I	D							D–IgA
			I	D						I	aAlters turbidity tests (e.g., thymol) and lipoprotein electrophoresis pattern. May interfere with BSP and calcium
				I							
											aIn gout
			D	D	D					I	aSMA methodology
											I–Diagnex blue
										I	
											I–BSP and protein. Serum protein electrophoresis pattern cannot be interpreted
					D						I–ESR
											D–LDH
	I										
	I										aWith hypervitaminosis D
										D	
D		D		D	D	I	I	D	D		
D			D	I							
	I						I	D	I		
D	D	I	D	I	I						
										D	
	D	I	I	I						I	

Table 79 (Continued)

		Hepatotoxic and/or cholestatic	Nephrotoxic	Intestinal malabsorption	Serum iron	Serum TIBC	Serum folate (inhibit *L. casei*)	Creatinine	BUN	Uric acid	Calcium	Bilirubin	SGOT/SGPT	Glucose
ANTI-INFLAMMATORY, ANTI-GOUT, ANTI-ARTHRITIS	Allopurinol	+								D				
	Colchicine	+		+										
	Gold	+	+											
	Indomethacin	+												
	Phenylbutazone	+												
	Probenecid	+	+							D				
	Salicylates	+	+							Iᵃ				
PSYCHOACTIVE AGENTS	Chloral hydrate								Iᵃ					
	Chlordiazepoxide	+												
	Imipramine	+												
	Phenobarbital						D							
	Phenothiazines													
	Chlorpromazine	+								D				I
	Chlorprothixene	+								D				
	Fluphenazine													
	Thiothixene	+												
NARCOTICS	Codeine										I	I		
	Meperidine (Demerol)										I	I		
	Morphine (heroin)										I	I		
	Marihuana								I	D				D
ANTI-DIABETIC (ORAL)	Acetohexamide (sulfonylurea)	+							I					
	Chlorpropamide	+												
	Tolbutamide	+											Iᵃ	
ANTI-HYPERTENSIVES	Guanethidine analogs								I				I	D
	Hydralazine									I	I		I	I
	MAO inhibitors	+		+										
	Methyldopa	+						I		I				
	Reserpine													I

See footnotes on p. 555.

Glucose tolerance	Cholesterol	PBI	T-3 uptake	T-4	^{131}I uptake	Amylase/lipase	Sodium	Potassium	Chloride	Phothrombin time	Comments
										D^a	[a]On coumarins
		D^a									[a]With some methods
										I	
			I		D					I	
			I	D							[a]High doses decrease uric acid
										D	[a]React with Neisler's reagent
			D		D						
											D–VMA and 5-HIAA
										D	
D											D–5-HIAA. May cause false positive pregnancy test
					I						
					I						I–LDH and BSP. Laboratory changes due to spasm of sphincter of Oddi
					I						
						I	I	I			
											[a]SMA methodology
I							I		I	I	D–VMA
											D–VMA, 5-HIAA
										I	D–5-HIAA
				D							I–5-HIAA

554   IV. Effects of Drugs on Laboratory Test Values

Table 79 (Continued)

	Hepatotoxic and/or cholestatic	Nephrotoxic	Intestinal malabsorption	Serum iron	Serum TIBC	Serum folate (inhibit L. casei)	Creatinine	BUN	Uric acid	Calcium	Bilirubin	SGOT/SGPT	Glucose
DIURETICS													
Acetazolamide									I				
Chlorthalidone		+											I
Ethacrynic acid	+								I				I
Furosemide								I	I				I
Thiazides	+								I	I			I
ANTIBIOTICS. ETC.													
Aminosalicylic acid (PAS)	+					D							
Amphotericin B	+	+											
Ampicillin		+				D							
Cephaloridine		+											
Cephalothin													
Chloramphenicol	+			I	D	D		I or D[a]					
Colistin		+											
Erythromycin	+					D						I[a]	
Gentamicin	+	+											
Griseofulvin	+	+											
Isoniazid	+	+										I[a]	
Kanamycin	+	+	+										
Lincomycin	+					D							
Methicillin		+											
Nalidixic acid	+	[a]											I[b]
Neomycin		+	+										
Nitrofurantoin	+	+											
Novobiocin	+												
Oleandomycin	+												
Oxacillin	+	+											
Penicillin						D							
Polymyxin B		+											
Rifampin	+	+											
Streptomycin		+							D				
Sulfonamides	+	+						I		D			
Tetracyclines	+	+				D							

Glucose tolerance	Cholesterol	PBI	T–3 uptake	T–4	¹³¹I uptake	Amylase/lipase	Sodium	Potassium	Chloride	Phothrombin time	Comments
D										I	
D							D	D	D	I	
D							D	D	D		
D						I	D	D	D		D–PSP and creatinine tolerance
											ªDepends on method
											ªColorimetric method
						D					ªSMA method. D–5-HIAA
											ªNitrogen retention ᵇCopper reduction method
											With massive dosage D–PSP
						D					I–PAH clearance

+ = presence of laboratory test changes due to drug effect on organ; I = values may be increased, elevated, or falsely positive; D = values may be decreased, lowered, or falsely negative.
ª and ᵇ See last column on right.
Hepatotoxic refers to liver damage that may alter one or more laboratory tests of liver function, including alkaline phosphatase, bilirubin, transaminase, cephalin flocculation, thymol turbidity, BSP retention. When this column is marked with a + sign, the individual columns (e.g., bilirubin, SGOT) are not also marked with a + sign.
Nephrotoxic refers to renal damage that may cause changes in BUN, creatinine, urine protein, casts, or cells. When this column is marked with a + sign, the individual columns (e.g., BUN, creatinine) are not also marked with a + sign.

DRUGS THAT MAY CAUSE INCREASED SERUM SODIUM

Due To

Retention of salt and water (e.g., corticosteroids, guanethidine, phenylbutazone)

Alkalosis (e.g., bicarbonates)

Mineralocorticoid effect (e.g., anabolic steroids, cortisone)

Effect on renal tubules (e.g., clonidine, methoxyflurane, tetracycline)

DRUGS THAT MAY CAUSE DECREASED SERUM SODIUM

Due to diuretic effect (e.g., ethacrynic acid, furosemide, thiazides, triamterene, mannitol, ammonium chloride, spironolactone)

DRUGS THAT MAY CAUSE INCREASED SERUM POTASSIUM

Due To

Effect on renal tubules (e.g., spironolactone)

Renal toxicity (e.g., amphotericin B, methicillin, tetracycline)

DRUGS THAT MAY CAUSE DECREASED SERUM POTASSIUM

Due To

Diuretic effect (e.g., ethacrynic acid, furosemide, thiazides)

Increased renal excretion (e.g., corticosteroids)

Other loss (e.g., chronic laxative abuse, aldosterone, licorice)

Alkalosis (e.g., bicarbonates)

DRUGS THAT MAY CAUSE INCREASED SERUM CHLORIDE

Due To

Hyperchloremic alkalosis during prolonged treatment
    Chlorothiazide
    Hydrochlorothiazide

Retention of salt and water (e.g., corticosteroids, guanethidine, phenylbutazone)

DRUGS THAT MAY CAUSE DECREASED SERUM CHLORIDE

Due To

Alkalosis (e.g., bicarbonates, aldosterone, corticosteroids)

Diuretic effect (e.g., ethacrynic acid, furosemide, thiazides)

Other loss (e.g., chronic laxative abuse)

DRUGS THAT MAY CAUSE INCREASED SERUM CARBON DIOXIDE

Due To

Alkalosis (e.g., bicarbonates, aldosterone, hydrocortisone, thiazides, ethacrynic acid)

Diuretic effect (e.g., metolazone)

DRUGS THAT MAY CAUSE DECREASED SERUM CARBON DIOXIDE

Due To
Nephrotoxic effect (e.g., methicillin, nitrofurantoin, tetracycline, triamterene
Acidosis (e.g., dimercaprol, paraldehyde, phenformin)

DRUGS THAT MAY CAUSE INCREASED SERUM AMYLASE

Due To
Spasm of sphincter of Oddi (e.g., codeine, morphine, meperidine, methacholine, cholinergics)
Liver damage (e.g., birth control pills)
Induced acute pancreatitis (e.g., aminosalicylic acid, azathioprine, corticosteroids, dexamethasone, ethacrynic acid, furosemide, thiazides, mercaptopurine, phenformin, triamcinolone)
Methodologic interference (e.g., pancreozymin [contains amylase], chloride and fluoride salts [enhance amylase activity], lipemic serum [turbidimetric methods])

DRUGS THAT MAY CAUSE DECREASED SERUM AMYLASE

Due To
Methodologic interference (e.g., citrate and oxalate—decrease activity by binding calcium ions)

DRUGS THAT MAY CAUSE INCREASED SERUM LIPASE

Due To
Spasm of sphincter of Oddi (e.g., codeine, morphine, meperidine, methacholine, cholinergics)
Induced acute pancreatitis (see preceding section on serum amylase)
Cholestatic effect (e.g., indomethacin)
Methodologic interference (e.g., pancreozymin [contains lipase], deoxycholate, glycocholate, taurocholate [prevent inactivation of enzyme], bilirubin [turbidimetric methods])

FACTORS THAT MAY CAUSE DECREASED SERUM LIPASE

Due To
Methodologic interference (e.g., presence of hemoglobin, calcium ions)

REFERENCES

Christian, D. G. Drug interference with laboratory blood chemistry determinations. *Am. J. Clin. Pathol.* **54:** 118, 1970.
Elking, M. P., and Kabat, H. F. Drug induced modifications of laboratory test values. *Am. J. Hosp. Pharm.* **25:** 485, 1968.
Koch-Weser, J., and Sellers, E. M. Drug interactions with coumarin anticoagulants. *N. Engl. J. Med.* **285:** 547, 1971.
Lubran, M. The effects of drugs on laboratory values. *Med. Clin. North Am.* **53(1):** 211, 1969.

Rayfield, E. J., Cain, J. P., Casey, M. P., Williams, G. H., et al. Influence of diet on urinary VMA excretion. *J.A.M.A.* **221:** 704, 1971.

Sunderman, F. W., Jr. Effects of drugs upon hematological tests. *Ann. Clin. Lab. Sci.* **2:** 2, 1972.

Young, D. S., Thomas, D. W., Friedman, R. B., and Pestaner, L. C. Effect of drugs on clinical laboratory tests. *Clin. Chem.* **18:** 1041, 1972.

BIBLIOGRAPHY

Barnett, H. L. *Pediatrics* (15th ed.). New York: Appleton-Century-Crofts, 1972.

Bloodworth, J. M. B., Jr. *Endocrine Pathology*. Baltimore: Williams & Wilkins, 1968.

Children's Hospital Medical Center, Boston. *Manual of Pediatric Therapeutics*, edited by J. W. Graef and T. E. Cone, Jr. Boston: Little, Brown, 1974.

Conn, H. F., and Conn, R. B., Jr. (Eds.). *Current Diagnosis—4*. Philadelphia: Saunders, 1974.

Davidsohn, I., and Henry, J. B. (Eds.). *Todd-Sanford Clinical Diagnosis by Laboratory Methods* (15th ed.). Philadelphia: Saunders, 1974.

Frankel, S., Reitman, S., and Sonnenwirth, A. C. (Eds.). *Gradwohl's Clinical Laboratory Methods and Diagnosis* (7th ed.). St. Louis: Mosby, 1970.

International Committee for Nomenclature and Nosology of Renal Disease. *A Handbook of Kidney Nomenclature and Nosology*. Boston: Little, Brown, 1975.

Miale, J. B. *Laboratory Medicine: Hematology* (4th ed.). St. Louis: Mosby, 1972.

Popper, H., and Schaffner, F. *Liver: Structure and Function*. New York: McGraw-Hill, 1957.

Stanbury, J. B., Wyngaarden, J. B., and Fredrickson, D. S. *The Metabolic Basis of Inherited Disease* (3rd ed.). New York: McGraw-Hill, 1972.

Strauss, M. B., and Welt, L. G. *Diseases of the Kidney* (2nd ed.). Boston: Little, Brown, 1971.

Thorn, G. W., Adams, R. D., Braunwald, E., Isselbacher, K. J., and Petersdorf, R. G. *Harrison's Principles of Internal Medicine* (8th ed.). New York: McGraw-Hill, 1977.

Wintrobe, M. M., Lee, G. R., Boggs, D. R., Bithell, T. C., et al. *Clinical Hematology* (7th ed.). Philadelphia: Lea & Febiger, 1974.

Ziai, M., Janeway, C. A., and Cooke, R. E. *Pediatrics* (2nd ed.). Boston: Little, Brown, 1975.

Azotemia—*Continued*
  in lupus erythematosus, 516
  in multiple myeloma, 448
  in nephrotic syndrome, 437
  prerenal, 433
  in renal failure, acute, 431
  in thrombophlebitis, septic, 181
  urea nitrogen levels in, 40
  in Waterhouse-Friderichsen syndrome, 411

Bacillary dysentery, 464
Bacillus
  cereus, and gastroenteritis, 197
  in ear, 147
  subtilis, in eye, 149
Bacitracin, and positive test for hematuria or
    hemoglobinuria, 540
Bacteremia
  from anaerobic organisms, 470
  antibiotics in, 478–482
  from coliform bacilli, 460
  in endocarditis, staphylococcal, 459
  gonococcal, 460
  in pneumonia, staphylococcal, 458
  from *Proteus*, 461
  in *Pseudomonas* infections, 462
  in salmonella infections, 464
Bacteria
  in blood. *See* Bacteremia
  in cultures from various sites, 147–151
  gram-negative. *See* Gram-negative bacilli
  in urine. *See* Bacteriuria
Bacterial infections, 457–482
  antibiotics in, 476–482
  C-reactive protein in, 107
  gastroenteritis in, 197
  gastrointestinal manifestations of, 193
  jaundice in, 233
  and leukocyte alkaline phosphatase staining
    reaction, 103
  leukopenia in, 99
  meningitis, 250–251
    recurrent, 251
  monocytosis in, 102
  myocardial disease in, 179
  NBT test in, 104
  oral manifestations of, 193
  pericarditis in, 177
  pneumonia in, 184
  splenomegaly in, 320
  transmission by animals, 515
  vulvovaginitis, 453
Bacteriuria, 128–129
  in pyelonephritis, 441
Bacteroides
  and abscess of brain, 256
  in blood, 149
  in cerebrospinal fluid, 150
  in colon, 148
  infections from, 462
    antibiotics in, 481
  in mouth, 148
  in peritoneum, 151
  in uterus, 150
  in wounds, 151
Bagassosis, 187
Balantidiasis, 501, 507
Balantidium coli, 501, 507
Balkan nephropathy, proteinuria in, 430
Bananas
  and 5-HIAA in urine, 137
  and urobilinogen in urine, 541
  and vanillylmandelic acid in urine, 138, 409
Banti's disease, splenomegaly in, 320
Bantu siderosis, iron deposition in, 111
Barbiturates
  and bilirubin in serum, 549
  in blood, 8, 15

and bromsulphalein retention test, 86
  coma from, 238
  and γ-glutamyl transpeptidase levels, 55
  poisoning from, myoglobinuria in, 133
  and positive tests for urine porphyrins, 541
  and prothrombin time decrease, 546
Barium
  salts, and Diagnex Blue excretion in urine,
    544
  sulfate, and protein-bound iodine levels, 74
Barr bodies, 160
  in Klinefelter's syndrome, 417, 418
  in Turner's syndrome, 415
Bartonella bacilliformis, 471
  and hemoglobinuria, 132
Bartter's syndrome, 407
  hypokalemia in, 346
  plasma renin activity in, 80
Basal cell nevus syndrome, 521
  Ellsworth-Howard test in, 92
  occult neoplasia in, 522
Basal metabolism rate. *See* Metabolism, basal
    rate of
Base, blood, 8, 13
Basophilia, in mastocytosis, 521
Basophilic leukocytes, 101–102
  count of, 4–5
  macrocytes, 107
  stippling of, 107
Bassen-Kornzweig syndrome. *See* A-beta-
    lipoproteinemia
Batten's disease, 373
  mental retardation in, 253
Bauxite fume fibrosis, 187
Beer, cobalt in, cardiomyopathy from, 177
Behçet's syndrome
  HL-A antigens in, 127
  and meningitis, recurrent, 252
BEI, 75, 378, 379
Bejel, 473
Bell's palsy, 258
Bence Jones proteins, 63
  in multiple myeloma, 322, 323
Bence Jones proteinuria, 129–130
Benedict reactions, in urine, 130
  drugs causing false positive test with, 539
  in lactosuria, 366, 367
Bentonite flocculation test
  in larva migrans, visceral, 507
  in schistosomiasis, 511
  in tapeworm infestation, 511
  in trichinosis, 509
Benzene, hematologic effects of, 289
Benzidine, and urine tests for occult blood, 540
Benzol compounds
  pancytopenia from, 288
  thrombocytopenic purpura from, 333
Benzothiadiazines, laboratory findings with,
    166
Beriberi, 349
  cerebrospinal fluid in, 239, 243, 257
  glucose levels in, 39
  and hookworm disease, 509
  hypertension in, 165
  myocardial disease in, 180
  polyneuritis in, 257
  transaminase levels in, 58
Berylliosis, 187
  calcium levels in, 51
  hypoxemia in, 45
Bicarbonate, serum levels of, 48, 345
  in hyperparathyroidism, 390
Bicarbonate therapy
  and carbon dioxide in serum, 556
  and chloride in serum, 556
  and false positive test for urine protein, 539
  and potassium in serum, 556
  and sodium in serum, 556

Measles—*Continued*
  leukopenia in, 99
  lymphocytosis in, 100
  oral manifestations of, 193
  plasma cells in, 102
Meckel's diverticulum, 198
  and rectal bleeding in children, 206
Meconium ileus, in cystic fibrosis, 236
Mediastinal neoplasms, 192
  dermoid cyst, 192
Mediterranean fever, familial, 372, 520
Mefenamic acid
  and positive direct Coombs' test, 544
  and positive tests for bile in urine, 541
Megacolon, aganglionic. *See* Hirschsprung's
    disease
Melanogen, and color of urine, 131
Melanogenuria, 133
Melanoma, malignant, melanogenuria in, 133
Melioidosis, 467
Melituria, 130
Melphalan, and positive direct Coombs' test,
    544
Menetrier's disease, 195
Ménière's syndrome, cerebrospinal fluid in, 239
Meningeal reaction, aseptic, cerebrospinal fluid
    in, 240
Meningioma
  hypopituitarism in, 421
  of olfactory groove, cerebrospinal fluid in,
    249
  of sella, bitemporal hemianopsia in, 259
Meningitis
  acute pyogenic, cerebrospinal fluid in, 240
  aseptic, 251, 486
    in herpes simplex infection, 492
    plasma cells in, 102
  bacterial, 250–251
  cerebral thrombosis in, 247
  in eoccidioidomycosis, 495
  cryptococcal, cerebrospinal fluid in, 241
  from *Haemophilus influenzae*, 465
    antibiotics in, 479
  and lactic dehydrogenase in CSF, 245
  leukocytosis in, 100
  lymphocytic. *See* Meningitis, aseptic
  meningococcic, and septic arthritis, 282
  Mollaret's, 252, 253
  in mumps, 489
  Neisseria meningitidis, antibiotics in, 479
  pneumococcal, 457
  protein electrophoresis in, 67
  recurrent, 251–252
  from *Salmonella*, 464
  seizures in, 239
  streptococcal, 458
    antibiotics in, 476
  syphilitic, 472
  tuberculous, 474
    cerebrospinal fluid in, 240
    and inappropriate secretion of antidiuretic
      hormone, 423
    NBT test in, 104
  uremic, 434
  viral. *See* Meningitis, aseptic
Meningococcal infections, 459
Meningococcemia, purpura in, nonthrom-
    bocytopenic, 334
Meningoencephalitis
  amebic
    cerebrospinal fluid in, 242, 252
    primary, 252
  in mumps, 489
  in trichinosis, 510
  in *Vibrio fetus* infections, 465
Meningovascular disease, in syphilis, 472
Menopause, 415
  and pituitary gonadotropins in urine, 140

Menstruation, 456
  and erythrocyte sedimentation rate, 106
  leukocytosis in, 100
  and plasma renin activity, 80
Mental retardation, 253–254
  and familial iminoglycinuria, 362
  and homocystinuria, 361
  in Lesch-Nyhan syndrome, 372
  and methylmalonic aciduria, 363
  in Prader-Willi syndrome, 395
Mepacrine. *See* Quinacrine
Meperidine
  and amylase in serum, 557
  and laboratory test values, 553
  and lipase in serum, 557
Mephenesin
  and 5-HIAA in urine, 137, 543
  and vanillylmandelic acid in urine, 543
Meprobamate
  allergic purpura from, 547
  and 17-hydroxycorticosteroids in urine,
    543
  and 17-ketosteroids in urine, 542
  and prothrombin time decrease, 546
  thrombocytopenia from, 547
Mercaptopurine
  and amylase in serum, 557
  anemia from, aplastic, 289
  and prothrombin increase, 546
  and uric acid levels, 42
Mercurials
  and calcium in urine, 134
  and triiodothyronine uptake, 74
  and uric acid in serum, 548
Mercuric chloride, and stool color changes,
    547
Mercury
  poisoning from, 528–529
    glycosuria in, 130
    leukemoid reaction in, 101
    leukocytosis from, 100
  purpura from, nonthrombocytopenic,
    334
  radioactive, in spleen scanning, 157
Mesenteric lymphatics, obstruction of, malab-
    sorption in, 199
Mesenteric vascular occlusion, 204
Metabolic diseases, 342–377
  antenatal detection of, 351
  carriers of, detection of, 350–351
  classification of, 349–350
  coma in, 238
  ketonuria in, 130
  malabsorption in, 199
  mental retardation in, 253
  of muscle, 263–265
  renal insufficiency in, 435
  skeletal involvement in, 267
  and urine screening in newborns, 359
Metabolism, basal rate of
  in acromegaly, 420
  in anorexia nervosa, 421
  in hyperthyroidism, 378
  in hypothyroidism, 379
  in leukemia, chronic myelogenous, 316
  in lymphomas, 321
  in pheochromocytoma, 409
  in polycythemia vera, 312
  in pregnancy, 383, 455
  in salicylate intoxication, 525
  in stiff-man syndrome, 265
Metanephrine, in urine, 28
Metaphyseal dysostosis, 270
Metastasis
  Bence Jones proteinuria in, 129
  to bone, 271
    calcium metabolism in, 386
    phosphorus metabolism in, 386